£78.99

Practical Hematopoietic Stem Cell Transplantation

Practical Hematopoietic Stem Cell Transplantation

EDITED BY

Professor Andrew J. Cant
Consultant Paediatric Immunologist
Director of Paediatric Bone Marrow Transplant Unit
Newcastle General Hospital
Newcastle upon Tyne

Dr Angela Galloway
Consultant Microbiologist
Royal Victoria Infirmary
Newcastle upon Tyne

Dr Graham Jackson
Consultant Haematologist
Director of Adult Bone Marrow Transplant Unit
Royal Victoria Infirmary
Newcastle upon Tyne

© 2007 by Blackwell Publishing Ltd
Blackwell Publishing, Inc., 350 Main Street, Malden, Massachusetts 02148-5020, USA
Blackwell Publishing Ltd, 9600 Garsington Road, Oxford OX4 2DQ, UK
Blackwell Publishing Asia Pty Ltd, 550 Swanston Street, Carlton, Victoria 3053, Australia

First published 2007

2 2009

Library of Congress Cataloging-in-Publication Data

Practical hematopoietic stem cell transplantation / edited by Andrew Cant, Angela Galloway, Graham Jackson.
    p. ; cm.
  Includes bibliographical references.
  ISBN 978-1-4051-3401-9
 1. Hematopoietic stem cells--Transplantation. 2. Bone marrow--Transplantation. 3. Hematopoietic system--Diseases. I. Cant, Andrew. II. Galloway, Angela. III. Jackson, Graham, FRCP.
  [DNLM: 1. Hematopoietic Stem Cell Transplantation--contraindications.
2. Hematopoietic Stem Cell Transplantation--nursing. 3. Graft vs Host Disease--prevention & control. 4. Intraoperative Complications--prevention & control. 5. Postoperative Complications--prevention & control. WH 380 P895 2007]

  RD123.5.P73 2007
  617.4'410592--dc22

                                                                                        2006016954

ISBN 978-1-4051-3401-9

A catalogue record for this title is available from the British Library

Set in 9.5/12pt Sabon by Sparks Computer Solutions Ltd – www.sparks.co.uk
Printed and bound in Singapore by Markono Print Media Pte Ltd

Commissioning Editor: Maria Khan
Editorial Assistant: Jennifer Seward
Development Editor: Adam Gilbert
Production Controller: Kate Charman

For further information on Blackwell Publishing, visit our website:
http://www.blackwellpublishing.com

Contents

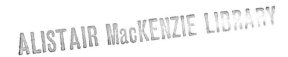

List of contributors

Editors

Prof. Andrew Cant
BSc MB BS MD FRCP FRCPCH
Consultant in Paediatric Immunology and
 Infectious Diseases
Director of Paediatric Bone Marrow
 Transplant Unit
Newcastle General Hospital
Newcastle upon Tyne NE4 6BE

Dr Angela Galloway
BSc MB BS MD FRCPath
Consultant Microbiologist
Royal Victoria Infirmary
Newcastle upon Tyne NE1 4LP

Dr Graham Jackson
MA MB BS MD FRCPath FRCP
Consultant Haematologist
Director of Adult Bone Marrow
 Transplant Unit
Royal Victoria Infirmary
Newcastle upon Tyne NE1 4LP

Contributors

Dr Mario Abinun
MD MSc DSc FRCPCH FRCP (Lond)
Consultant in Paediatric Immunology &
 Infectious Diseases
Newcastle General Hospital
Newcastle upon Tyne NE4 6BE

Maggie Allan
HNC DipSW
Social Worker
Newcastle General Hospital
Newcastle upon Tyne NE4 6BE

Dr Dawn Barge
PhD FIBMS
Consultant Clinical Scientist
Immunology Laboratory
Royal Victoria Infirmary
Newcastle upon Tyne NE1 4LP

Dr Jim Cavet
BA MBBS MRCP MRCPath PhD
Consultant in Haematology/Honorary
 Senior Lecturer
Christies Hospital
Manchester M20 4BX

Carole Charley
SRN/SCM
BMT Nurse Co-ordinator/Quality
 Manager
Chair EBMT (UK) NAP Group
Royal Hallamshire Hospital
Glossop Road
Sheffield S10 2JF

Dr Julia Clark
BMedSci BM BS MRCP DCH FRCPCH
Consultant in Paediatric Immunology &
 Infectious Diseases
Newcastle General Hospital
Newcastle upon Tyne NE4 6BE

Dr Matthew Collin
BM BCh, DPhil
Senior Lecturer in Haematology
University of Newcastle upon Tyne
Framlington Place
Newcastle upon Tyne NE2 4HH

Dr Charles Craddock
MRCP FRCPath DPhil
Professor of Haemato-oncology and
 Honorary Consultant Haematologist
Centre for Clinical Haematology
Queen Elizabeth Hospital
Vincent Drive
Edgbaston
Birmingham B15 2TH

Stephen Fox
RGN
Bone Marrow Transplant Co-ordinator
Royal Victoria Infirmary
Newcastle upon Tyne NE1 4LP

Dr Barbara Fulton
BMedSci (Hons), MBBS, FRCA
Consultant Anaesthetist
Paediatric Intensive Care Unit
Newcastle General Hospital
Newcastle upon Tyne NE4 6BE

Dr Alistair Gascoigne
BSc MBBS FRCP
Consultant in Respiratory Medicine and
 Intensive Care
Royal Victoria Infirmary
Newcastle upon Tyne NE1 4LP

Dr Andy Gennery
MBChB MD MRCP MRCPCH DCH
 DipMedSci
Senior Lecturer/Honorary Consultant in
 Paediatric Immunology
Newcastle General Hospital
Newcastle upon Tyne NE4 6BE

Helen Harvey
RN/DipHE (Child) BSc ENB Higher
 Award
Senior Nurse
Paediatric Bone Marrow Transplant Unit
Newcastle General Hospital
Newcastle upon Tyne NE4 6BE

Dorothy Holder
CQSW
Social Worker
Royal Victoria Infirmary
Newcastle upon Tyne NE1 4LP

Dr Gail Jones
MD MRCP MRCPath
Consultant in Haematology
Royal Victoria Infirmary
Newcastle upon Tyne NE1 4LP

Wendy Larmouth
RGN RSCN
Sister
Paediatric Bone Marrow Transplant Unit
Newcastle General Hospital
Newcastle upon Tyne NE4 6BE

Dr Anne Lennard
MBBS FRCP FRCPath
Consultant Haematologist, Honorary
 Senior Lecturer
Royal Victoria Infirmary
Newcastle upon Tyne NE1 4LP

Angela Reed
BSc (Hons) Nursing Studies (RN)
Senior Infection Control Nurse
Royal Victoria Infirmary
Newcastle upon Tyne NE1 4LP

Dr Rod Skinner
MBChB BSc PhD FRCPCH MRCP DCH
Consultant/Honorary Clinical Senior
 Lecturer in Paediatric Oncology/BMT
Royal Victoria Infirmary
Newcastle upon Tyne NE1 4LP

Dr Mary Slatter
MBChB MRCP (Paeds)
Associate Specialist in Paediatric Bone
 Marrow Transplantation
Newcastle General Hospital
Newcastle upon Tyne NE4 6BE

Dr Gavin Spickett
MA LLM DPhil FRCPath FRCP (Lond)
 FRCP (Edin)
Consultant Immunologist
Royal Victoria Infirmary
Newcastle upon Tyne NE1 4LP

Dr Clive Taylor
BSc PhD FRCPath
Consultant Clinical Scientist in Virology
Health Protection Agency
Newcastle General Hospital
Newcastle upon Tyne NE4 6BE

Dr Andrew Turner
MB ChB Dip Bact FRCPath
Consultant Virologist
Manchester Royal Infirmary
Oxford Road
Manchester M13 9WL

Dr Paul Veys
MBBS FRCP FRCPath FRCPCH
Director Blood and Marrow
 Transplantation
Department of Bone Marrow
 Transplantation
Great Ormond Street Hospital
London WC1N 3JH

Preface

Sixty years ago nuclear weapons were unleashed. In the aftermath of this cataclysmic event, studies were performed to find out how to protect individuals from lethal radiation, and it was discovered that transplanting hematopoietic stem cells could reconstitute the hematological and immunological systems and so prevent death from bone marrow failure. By the 1950s studies in animal models had led to the concept of the pluripotent hematopoietic stem cell and the recognition of the importance of tissue type matching of host and donor to prevent graft-vs.-host disease (GVHD). The first successful hematopoietic stem cell transplants (HSCTs) in humans were carried out in 1968, when children in the USA and Europe were transplanted for severe combined immune deficiency using sibling donors who shared the same tissue type as the parents. In the 1970s HSCT was first carried out for aplastic anemia and then leukemia, but overall the results were poor with only 15% survival due to disease relapse, infection, and GVHD, which remained major threats. By the late 1970s the use of post-transplant immunosuppression to prevent GVHD had been recognized and, in 1981, the first T-cell depleted mismatched HSCTs were performed. Throughout the 1980s and 1990s far more hematopoietic stem cell transplants were performed with increasing success. Donor selection and tissue typing have been greatly refined, so greatly reducing the risk of GVHD. Pre-HSCT conditioning regimens have been modified so as to reduce their toxicity. It is now possible to detect many infections at a much earlier stage and treat them with a greater array of drugs. This has led to greatly increased survival, and with it the increasing use of HSCT for diseases for which it would have previously been deemed too risky. In addition to malignant disease, immunological disorders, metabolic disease, and now auto-immune disease can be cured by HSCT. New sources of stem cells (e.g. umbilical cord blood) have also opened up new possibilities for the treatment of more patients.

Many experienced doctors and nurses still view HSCT as a risky and dangerous procedure to be contemplated only when all else fails. There is a very important message that this is no longer the case, and that the risks from transplant are greatly diminished.

Successful transplantation depends on excellent teamwork and careful attention to detail. There is a huge amount of literature covering the scientific aspects of HSCT, but far less addresses how to plan HSCT and how to care for patients on a day-to-day basis; yet perfecting the art of caring for these patients has a huge impact on outcome. This book sets out to be a practical guide on how to perform HSCT and how to look after patients, set against the background of the history and science of the field. It is aimed at health care workers of all disciplines actively looking after HSCT patients. The authors have found practicing in this field enormously satisfying, as by applying science and good bedside care it is possible to transform the lives of patients with serious disease so that they can be healthy and active members of society. We hope we are able to pass on not only our experience, but also our enthusiasm.

AJC, AG, GJ

Acknowledgments

We would like to thank:
- Deborah Gleadow, for her endless patience, good humor and hard work in helping to prepare the manuscript;
- Penny Taylor, for her thorough, pertinent comments and proof reading;
- our trainees, who helped by telling us what they wanted to read about and how it could best be expressed;
- our families, for their support during hours of reading, writing and editing;
- our patients, who inspired us to find better ways of treating them.

List of abbreviations

aGVHD acute graft-vs.-host disease
ALL acute lymphoblastic leukemia
AML acute myeloid leukemia
APC antigen presenting cells
ARDS acute respiratory distress syndrome
ATG anti-thymocyte globulin
AVN avascular necrosis
BAL bronchoalveolar lavage
BBV blood-borne virus
BCG bacillus Calmette–Guérin
BM bone marrow
BMD bone mineral density
BMT bone marrow transplantation
BO bronchiolitis obliterans
BOOP bronchiolitis obliterans with organizing pneumonia
BuCy busulphan and cyclophosphamide
CGD chronic granulomatous disease
cGVHD chronic graft-vs.-host disease
CML chronic myeloid leukemia
CMV cytomegalovirus
CNS central nervous system
CPAP continuous positive airway pressure
CR complete remission
CRP C-reactive protein
CsA ciclosporin-A
CSF cerebrospinal fluid

CTLpf cytotoxic T-lymphocyte precursor frequency
CVA cerebrovascular accident
CVL central venous line
CVVH continuous veno-venous hemofiltration
CyTBI cyclophosphamide and total body irradiation
DAD diffuse alveolar damage
DAH diffuse alveolar hemorrhage
DAT direct antiglobulin test
DLI donor lymphocyte infusions
EBV Epstein–Barr virus
ECP extracorporeal phototherapy
ELISA enzyme-linked immunosorbent assay
ET endotracheal
FFP fresh frozen plasma
GA general anesthetic
G-CSF granulocyte-colony stimulating factor
GH growth hormone
GRE glycopeptide-resistant enterococci
GVHD graft-vs.-host disease
GVL graft-vs.-leukaemia
GVT graft-vs.-tumor
HC hemorrhagic cystitis
HD Hodgkin's disease
HDSCT high-dependency stem cell transplant
HEPA high-efficiency particulate air

HHV6 human herpes virus type 6
HHV7 human herpes virus type 7
HiB *Haemophilus influenzae* type B
HIV human immunodeficiency virus
HLA human leukocyte antigen
HRCT high-resolution chest tomography
HSCT hematopoietic stem cell transplantation
HSV *Herpes simplex* virus
HTLpf helper T-lymphocyte precursor frequency
HUS hemolytic uremic syndrome
HVG host vs. graft
IA invasive aspergillosis
IBMTR International Bone Marrow Transplant Registry
ICU intensive care unit
IFI invasive fungal infection
IFNγ interferon-gamma
IL interleukin
IPS idiopathic pneumonia syndrome
IVIG intravenous immunoglobulin
JIA juvenille idiopathic arthritis
JMML juvenile myelomonocytic leukemia
LDH lactate dehydrogenase
LOPS late-onset pulmonary syndrome

LRTI lower respiratory tract infection

MDS myelodysplastic syndrome

mHags minor histocompatibility antigens

MHC major histocompatibility complex

MLR mixed lymphocyte reactivity

MMF mycophenylate mofetil

MODS multiple organ dysfunction syndromes

MOF multiple organ failure

MRD matched related donor

MRI magnetic resonance imaging

MRSA meticillin-resistant *Staphylococcus aureus*

MSSA meticillin-sensitive *Staphylococcus aureus*

MTX methotrexate

NBT nitroblue tetrazolium reduction test

NG nasogastric

NHL non-Hodgkin's lymphoma

NIV non-invasive ventilation

NJ nasojejunal

NK natural killer cells

PB peripheral blood

PBSC peripheral blood stem cell collection

PCP *Pneumocystis* pneumonia

PCR polymerase chain reaction

PEEP positive end expiratory pressure

PEG percutaneous endoscopically guided gastrostomy

PFT pulmonary function tests

PH pulmonary hypertension

PHA phytohemagglutinin

PICU pediatric intensive care unit

PID primary immunodeficiency

PIV parainfluenza virus

PML progressive multifocal leukoencephalopathy

PPE personal protective equipment

PTLD post-transplant lymphoproliferative disease

PVOD pulmonary veno-occlusive disease

QoL quality of life

RCT randomized controlled trial

RD related donors

RIC reduced-intensity conditioning

RISCT reduced-intensity stem cell transplantation (RISCT)

RRT regimen-related toxicity

RSV respiratory syncytial virus

RT radiotherapy

SARS severe acute respiratory syndrome

SC systemic candidiasis

SCID severe combined immunodeficiency

SCT stem cell transplantation

SLE systemic lupus erythematosus

TAGVHD transfusion-associated graft-vs.-host disease

TBI total body irradiation

TCD T-cell depleted

TIA transient ischemic attack

TPN total parenteral nutrition

TRALI transfusion-related acute lung injury

TRECS T-cell receptor excision circles

TRM transplant-related mortality

TTP thrombotic thrombocytopenic purpura

UCB umbilical cord blood

URTI upper respiratory tract infection

USCT umbilical cord stem cell transplantation

UTI urinary tract infection

vCJD variant Creutzfeldt–Jakob disease

VISA vancomycin-insensitive *Staphylococcus aureus*

VOD veno-occlusive disease

VRE vancomycin-resistant enterococci

VUD volunteer-unrelated donor

VZV *Varicella zoster* virus

Chapter 1

Why hematopoietic stem cell transplantation and for whom?

A.J. Cant, C. Craddock and R. Skinner

Introduction

Transplantation of allogeneic and autologous hematopoietic stem cells has become an increasingly safe and effective procedure in recent years, and is now established as one of the most important curative strategies in patients with hematological malignancies. It also has an important role to play in the management of acquired marrow failure, hemoglobinopathies, congenital immunodeficiency and metabolic disease.

At first it was thought that HSCT cured patients because increased, myeloablative doses of chemo-/radiotherapy could be given while the risk of permanent marrow aplasia was avoided by giving HSC after the chemo-/radiotherapy. While this remains the sole mechanism of action in autologous transplants it is now clear that in patients transplanted with allogeneic stem cells there can be an additional, immunologically mediated graft-vs.-leukemia (GVL) effect. The growing realization of the potency of the GVL effect has led to:
• the development of reduced-intensity transplants whose curative potential is entirely dependent on the immunotherapeutic potential of the donor immune system;
• an increased interest in the possibility of using allogeneic transplants in the treatment of solid tumors or autoimmune disease

However, since the anti-tumor activity of the GVL effect is mediated by the donor immune system, it is therefore linked with the major complication of allogeneic transplantation: graft-vs.-host disease (GVHD). Thus, although there has been a major expansion in the numbers of patients considered eligible for allogeneic transplantation in the past decade, this procedure still remains associated with major toxicity consequent upon immunosuppression and GVHD.

Historical perspective

Hematopoietic stem cell transplantation has been used to treat humans for nearly 40 years; it was first given in 1968 for an infant with a severe combined immune deficiency who was unable to reject a graft and then a year later in 1969 for a patient with leukemia who had been given lethal total body irradiation. In both cases genetically HLA-identical siblings were used and gave bone marrow. Treatment in these early cases demonstrated that leukemia could be cured, that immune deficiency could be corrected, and that long-term survival was possible. However, problems with infections, graft-vs.-host disease, and graft failure meant that this was considered a very risky technique for many years. In the last 10 years HSCT has become much more successful because of the steady improvements across the field. These have included:
• better tissue type matching of donor and recipient using molecular DNA techniques;
• greater availability of matched unrelated donors;
• refinements in pre-transplant conditioning regimens;
• improved methods for early detection of infection;
• new anti-infective agents, ciclosporin and other immunosuppressive drugs to reduce the risk of graft-vs.-host disease;
• better supportive care, with protective isolation and improved techniques for nutritional support.

No single discovery led to this dramatic improvement in outcome; instead it is the summation of many smaller developments that together have led to very dramatic changes in outcome. For example, in pediatric practice success for transplantation for primary immunodeficiency has risen from 50% to approaching 90% in the last 25 years. This has meant that patients previously considered too ill, too damaged by infection, too old or to have a condition not amenable to transplant are now being considered for HSCT.

Basic principles of hematopoietic stem cell transplantation

Two fundamental principles underpin the development of stem cell transplantation as an effective and relatively safe clinical procedure:
• a combination of drugs and/or radiotherapy are given before the infusion of stem cells, which may include antibodies such as antithymocyte globulin (ATG) that destroy lymphocytes, referred to as the conditioning or preparative regimen; it is essential for disease eradication and the creation of "space" within the marrow cavity to allow engraftment of allogeneic stem cells;
• transplantation of enough stem cell inoculum to ensure lifelong reconstitution of all hematopoietic lineages.

Conditioning regimens

In autologous SCT where there is no genetic difference between the transplanted stem cells and the patient, the only role of the conditioning regimen is tumor eradication. In contrast, in patients transplanted with allogeneic stem cells, whether from a brother/sister or unrelated donor who share the same tissue types (HLA), a potent host-vs.-graft reaction will be generated directed against the transplanted stem cells unless the host immune system is suppressed. Therefore the conditioning regimen serves two purposes in patients undergoing an allogeneic transplant:
• host immunosuppression to prevent graft rejection;

• host myeloablation in order to eradicate malignant hematopoiesis.

Until recently, all patients undergoing an allogeneic transplant received a myeloablative conditioning regimen. In order to achieve the maximum degree of tumor eradication, myeloablative regimens employ high doses of chemo- and/or radiotherapy and are associated with significant side effects (see Fig. 1.1). This means that, even when transplanting young patients with a well-matched donor, 10–20% will die of these side effects (so-called transplant-related mortality). However, the mortality of such intensive regimens rises to unacceptable levels in older patients (greater than 50–55 years old) and so, until recently, allogeneic transplantation has been considered too risky for older patients with leukemia. As hematological malignancies are much more common in older patients, this has profoundly limited the usefulness of allogeneic transplantation. However, the recent demonstration that durable donor engraftment can be reliably achieved using a nonmyeloablative preparative regimen, coupled with increased awareness of the potency of the GVL reaction, has led to the development of a range of reduced-intensity conditioning (RIC) regimens (often referred to as "mini"-transplants, see Fig. 1.2). These regimens are associated with markedly reduced transplant-related mortality (TRM) than would be seen after a myeloablative regimen. As a result, allogeneic transplantation can now be safely performed in many patients in whom it would previously have been contraindicated on the grounds of age or comorbidity. Very rarely for conditions such as severe combined immune deficiency (SCID), it is possible to achieve engraftment of selected cell lineages without the use of conditioning.

Sources of stem cells for clinical transplantation

Sources for hematopoietic stem cells for transplantation include:
• bone marrow;
• peripheral blood stem cells (PBSC) – following mobilization from the bone marrow using granulocyte-colony stimulating factor (G-CSF);
• umbilical cord.

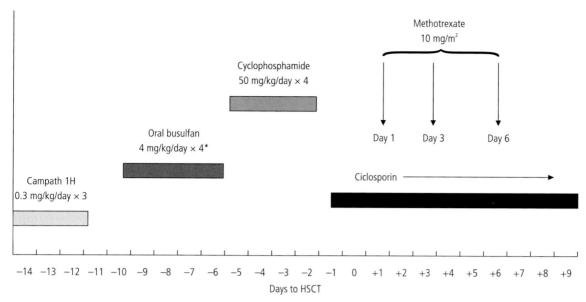

*(or i.v. dose dependent on weight)

Fig. 1.1 Example of standard conditioning regimen (for a child with combined immunodeficiency using whole marrow matched unrelated donor). © Children's Bone Marrow Transplant Unit, Newcastle General Hospital, Newcastle upon Tyne, UK; redrawn with permission.

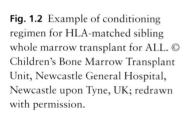

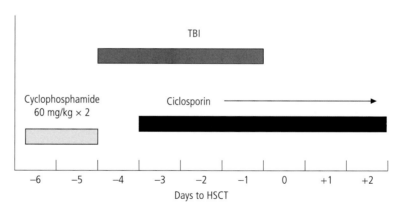

Fig. 1.2 Example of conditioning regimen for HLA-matched sibling whole marrow transplant for ALL. © Children's Bone Marrow Transplant Unit, Newcastle General Hospital, Newcastle upon Tyne, UK; redrawn with permission.

The safe delivery of myeloablative therapy and the genesis of a GVL effect is dependent on the transplantation of long-term reconstituting cells (LTRCs). These cells are defined by their capacity for self-renewal as well as their ability to mature into all hematopoietic lineages; LTRCs differ from more mature hematopoietic progenitors, which have limited ability to self-replicate and are already committed to develop into a specific lineage. LTRCs are rare, however, occurring with a frequency of $1 : 10^4$ or $1 : 10^5$ mononuclear cells in the bone marrow. One of the major determinants of successful stem cell engraftment is the number of stem cells transplanted.

Originally stem cells were obtained from bone marrow by direct puncture and aspiration of bone marrow and the cells obtained were infused intravenously. In recent years stem cells have also been harvested from the peripheral blood and from umbilical cord blood. The term hematopoietic stem cell transplantation (HSCT) is therefore now replacing the term bone marrow transplanta-

3

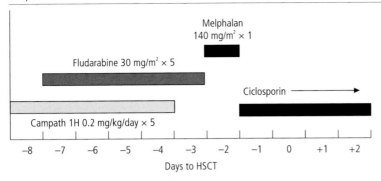

Fig. 1.3 Example of low-intensity conditioning regimen. © Children's Bone Marrow Transplant Unit, Newcastle General Hospital, Newcastle upon Tyne, UK; redrawn with permission.

tion. HSCs are harvested from peripheral blood by giving the donor daily injections of G-CSF for 5 days. The cells are then harvested using a filtration technique called apheresis, which has transformed both autologous and allogeneic SCT (Fig. 1.3 shows a patient undergoing plasmapheresis). The use of G-CSF-mobilized peripheral blood stem cells (PBSCs) makes it possible to transplant significantly higher stem cell doses than is possible if harvested bone marrow is used. Consequently PBSC now play a critical role in optimizing engraftment whether the donor and recipient are HLA tissue type matched or mismatched and where graft enhancing donor T cells have to be removed to prevent GVHD. Incorporating these principles into clinical practice has markedly reduced the risk of graft failure.

Durable engraftment of allogeneic stem cells is also helped by graft-facilitating donor T cells, which usually overcome any residual HVG response generated by host T cells that have survived the conditioning regimen. Thus the major factors determining engraftment are the intensity of host immunosuppression delivered by the conditioning regimen, the numbers of donor T cells in the stem cell inoculum and the degree of genetic disparity between donor and host.

The use of PBSCs is associated with earlier neutrophil and platelet engraftment and in patients with advanced leukemia this may translate into a lower TRM. However, transplantation of PBSC results in an increased incidence of chronic GVHD, reflecting the five- to tenfold greater dose of T cells transplanted if mobilized cells are used in preference to bone marrow-harvested cells. Thus the

use of PBSC has become commonplace in patients being allografted for advanced leukemia where TRM is a major cause of treatment failure, but bone marrow is still preferred in diseases such as aplastic anemia where chronic GVHD is an important cause of treatment failure. The increasing use of PBSC has obvious implications for allogeneic stem cell donors as the G-CSF in the doses used for stem cell mobilization may cause bone pains and splenomegaly.

In the absence of a HVG reaction, graft failure is very rarely observed in autologous transplants providing an adequate stem cell dose is used. Because of their ease of procurement coupled with an increased stem cell dose, PBSCs are now almost universally used in preference to bone marrow harvests in autologous transplants.

Umbilical cord blood (CB) cells, harvested at the time of delivery, have been used as a source of allogeneic stem cells. CB is rich in LTRC and hematopoietic progenitors, and durable engraftment can be reliably obtained in infants and children. Moreover, the incidence of severe GVHD is significantly lower with mismatched CB than would be expected using a comparable unrelated marrow or PBSC donor. It is theoretically possible that the lower numbers of T cells and their naive phenotype contained in CB collections will be associated with a reduced GVL effect, but no increase in relapse risk has yet been reported in CB transplants. Given the difficulties that can be experienced obtaining stem cell collections from unrelated donors, the relative ease of access to CB banks has resulted in this becoming an increasingly important stem cell source in pediatric transplantation. However, in older patients delayed engraftment is commonly observed because of the lower cell doses (per kg body weight) transplanted and this has limited their use in adults. Therefore approaches that improve engraftment, such as *ex vivo* expansion of hematopoietic progenitors, will be needed before CB is widely used in adult transplantation.

Principles of donor choice

Potential donors:
- Autologous (the patient)
- Allogeneic (another person)
  - HLA-identical (matched) sibling
  - Other related donor (RD)
    - HLA-matched
    - HLA-mismatched, including haploidentical (half matched, usually a parent)
  - Unrelated donor (URD)
    - HLA-matched (often termed matched unrelated donor, MUD)
    - HLA-mismatched

Currently accepted indications for hematopoietic stem cell transplantation

Both autologous and allogeneic SCT are now firmly established as important treatments for hematological malignancies. The use of peripheral blood stem cell progenitors, coupled with improvements in supportive care, has reduced the mortality of autografting to below 5% (similar to that of a major surgical procedure) and allowed its extension to patients up to 70 years of age. By contrast, allogeneic SCT remains associated with substantial morbidity and mortality, consequent mainly upon the toxicity of the conditioning regimen and the risk of GVHD, which currently precludes its extension to patients beyond the age of 55. However, this is often outweighed by the increased anti-leukemic effect of an allograft and consequently the decision in any individual patient whether to autograft, allograft or employ chemotherapy alone is often complex and dependent on a range of host and donor factors.

Chronic myeloid leukemia (CML)

Although CML can only be cured by allogeneic SCT, and the long-term disease-free survival rate after HSCT is now in excess of 70% in patients fortunate enough to have an HLA-identical sibling, the encouraging data using the tyrosine kinase inhibitor imatinib has relegated allogeneic transplantation to a second-line option in adults. Nonetheless, a number of patients still wish to proceed immediately to an allograft; a careful analysis of a range of pre-transplant patient and donor details and their influence on HSCT outcome should lead to the best calculated treatment option.

Acute leukemia

The precise role of allogeneic transplantation in patients with AML in first complete remission (1st CR) has been hard to establish. When carrying out studies of the results of HSCT it has proved hard to prevent bias when randomizing patients to HSCT or non-HSCT treatment groups. Furthermore, in many studies the HSCT and non-HSCT groups have not contained the same number of high-risk patients. It is generally accepted that allografting substantially decreases the risk of relapse but whether this benefit outweighs the attendant transplant-related mortality remains controversial. Most groups, however, would consider allogeneic transplantation in all patients in first CR apart from those with good-risk disease (with chromosome markers t : 15 : 17, inv 16 and t : 8 : 21) in whom outcome with conventional chemotherapy is good. There is general agreement that allogeneic SCT is the only curative option in 2nd CR and, in the absence of an HLA-identical sibling, the use of unrelated donor (URD) should be considered.

Allogeneic SCT is also best in patients with myelodysplasia where the outcome after HSCT using a sibling or unrelated donor is better than after conventional chemotherapy. Results are improved if transplantation is performed early in the course of the disease and a number of scoring systems have been used to determine the natural history in order to assist the difficult decision of when to submit an otherwise healthy patient to a life-threatening but potentially curative procedure.

Autologous SCT has been investigated as a method of dose escalation in AML by many groups. Results of the recent MRC study confirmed that autografting using bone marrow cells harvested in remission reduces the risk of relapse in patients with standard risk disease in 1st CR, compared with conventional chemotherapy. However, this effect was blunted by a higher-than-expected transplant-related mortality and current studies are therefore investigating whether the use of peripheral blood stem cells or earlier transplantation will improve outcome.

Most studies indicate that allogeneic HSCT should be considered in all adults with acute lymphoblastic leukemia (ALL) in 1st CR, with the possible exception of those with good-risk disease as defined by white cell count and immunophenotype. In patients with Philadelphia positive ALL and the 4 : 11 chromosome translocation this is effectively the only curative option and unrelated donor transplantation is now indicated in patients in whom an HLA-identical sibling cannot be identified. The role of autologous SCT in the management of patients with ALL remains unclear and is the subject of ongoing randomized studies.

Non-Hodgkin's lymphoma

The superiority of autologous HSCT over salvage chemotherapy in patients with chemosensitive relapses of high-grade non-Hodgkin's disease was confirmed by a recent randomized study. Although it might be expected that dose intensification would benefit patients with poor prognostic features during 1st CR, this has yet to be confirmed by a large randomized study. No randomized studies have examined whether the benefit of autografting extends to patients with follicular NHL, although this is suggested by data from single-center studies. The role of allogeneic transplantation remains controversial. The biology of follicular lymphoma, coupled with the uncertainty surrounding the ability of autologous HSCT to effect a cure, makes allogeneic HSCT using a reduced-intensity conditioning regimen an attractive option and there are encouraging preliminary data in support of this approach.

Hodgkin's disease

Comparison with historic controls suggests that autologous HSCT is superior to conventional chemotherapy in patients with relapsed or refractory Hodgkin's disease. Pilot studies also support the use of autologous HSCT in patients with "high-risk" disease while they remain in 1st CR, and this is the subject of a number of ongoing studies. Allogeneic HSCT using a myeloablative conditioning regimen is usually associated with unacceptably high transplant-related mortality, mostly due to pulmonary complications, and currently has only a limited role although this may change with the advent of reduced-intensity conditioning regimens.

Multiple myeloma

Allogeneic transplantation remains the only curative therapy in multiple myeloma and is capable of producing molecular remissions in up to 30% of patients transplanted. However, the particularly high transplant-related mortality in myeloma and the rarity of the disease in patients under 50 have led to pessimism as to whether it is possible to exploit the undoubted graft-vs.-myeloma experience observed after allogeneic HSCT in more than a small minority of patients with this disease. However, it appears that modifications to the conditioning regimen coupled with improvements in supportive care can substantially reduce the TRM and the age limit in which allografting is considered is currently being extended. By contrast, autologous SCT can be safely performed in patients up to the age of 70 and, although not apparently curative, has been shown to improve both overall and disease-free survival. Best results are obtained in patients with chemosensitive disease, a low presentation betaroglobulin and a normal karyotype. Whether a double autograft is of benefit to patients is currently under investigation, although it appears that such an approach is technically feasible in the majority of patients under 65.

Solid tumors

The role of autologous SCT in the management of advanced breast cancer remains controversial. An early study that suggested benefit in metastatic disease is now discredited and a randomized study of this therapy has failed to show a benefit. The question remains as to whether a subgroup of patients will benefit and the results of a number of ongoing studies are eagerly awaited. There are encouraging data from a number of centers showing that dose intensification with autologous stem cell support improves survival in patients with disseminated germ cell tumors, although this requires confirmation. The possibility of exploiting a graft-vs.-tumor effect in malignancies such as renal cell carcinoma or breast carcinoma is supported by anecdotal reports of responses after allogeneic SCT or donor lymphocyte infusion (DLI) and raises the possibility of extending the benefit of allografting, possibly using a non-myeloablative conditioning regimen, to non-hematological malignancies. Tables 1.1, 1.2, 1.3, 1.4 and 1.5 indicate the types of conditions for which HSCT is used.

Table 1.1 Indications for bone marrow transplantation in children

Malignant conditions	Nonmalignant conditions
Acute leukemia	Bone marrow failure (including inherited monocytopenia)
• Acute lymphoblastic leukemia (ALL)	• Aplastic anemia
• high-risk ALL in 1st CR	• Fanconi anemia
• high- and intermediate-risk relapsed ALL in 2nd CR	• Other constitutional bone marrow failure syndromes
• ALL in ≥3rd CR	• dyskeratosis congenita
• Acute myeloid leukemia (AML)	• congenital amegakaryocytic thrombocytopenia
• poor risk AML in 1st CR	• Schwachman–Diamond syndrome
• AML in 2nd CR†	• Diamond–Blackfan anemia
	• Kostmann syndrome
Chronic myeloid leukemia	Hemoglobinopathy
	• Thalassemia (selected patients)
	• Sickle cell anemia (selected patients)
Myelodysplasia, including juvenile myelomonocytic leukemia	• Primary Immunodeficiency
	• Osteopetrosis
	• Certain metabolic storage diseases
Non-Hodgkin's lymphoma (NHL)	
• relapsed Burkitt's NHL*	
• relapsed diffuse large cell NHL*	
• relapsed anaplastic large-cell lymphoma	
• relapsed T-cell lymphoblastic NHL	
Hodgkin's disease (HD)	
• relapsed/refractory HD (adolescents)*	
• ?multiply relapsed HD	
High-risk solid tumors*	
• stage 4 (or other high risk) neuroblastoma	
• high-risk Ewing's sarcoma	
• high-risk or relapsed medulloblastoma	
• selected patients (in the context of clinical trials) with relapsed or refractory	
• Wilms' tumor	
• germ cell tumor	

Allogeneic HSCT unless indicated otherwise:
* Autologous HSCT
† Autologous HSCT may be indicated in some patients with late relapse (>1 year from initial diagnosis)

Table 1.2 Types of stem cell transplantation

Autologous (autograft)	The patient's own stem cells are harvested and reinfused after the patient has received chemotherapy to kill malignant cells. Used in leukemias, lymphomas and some solid tumors. Also used for immunomodulatory effect in some autoimmune disorders
Allogeneic (allograft)	Stem cells from another individual are infused after the patient's own bone marrow has been destroyed by chemotherapy and/or radiotherapy. Potential allogeneic donors may include: <ul><li>HLA-identical (matched) sibling</li><li>Other related donor (RD)<ul><li>HLA-matched</li><li>HLA-mismatched, including haploidentical (half matched, usually a parent)</li></ul></li><li>Unrelated donor (URD)<ul><li>HLA-matched (often termed matched unrelated donor, MUD)</li><li>HLA-mismatched</li></ul></li></ul>

Table 1.3 Immunodeficiencies suitable for transplantation

SCID
Wiskott–Aldrich syndrome
CD40 ligand deficiency
Other T-cell immune deficiencies
Chronic granulomatous disease
Leukocyte adhesion deficiency
Hemophagocytic syndromes

Table 1.4 Diseases for which allogeneic transplant is used (adapted from Duncombe 1997)

(a) Adults

Sole chance of cure	Improved disease-free survival over conventional treatment
Primary immunodeficiency syndromes	Acute myeloid leukemia (AML) (first or second remission)
Aplastic anemia	Acute lymphoblastic leukemia (ALL) (first or second remission adults only)
Thalassemia	Myelodysplasia
Sickle cell disease	Multiple myeloma
Inborn errors of metabolism	
Chronic myeloid leukemia (CML)	

(b) Children

Sole chance of cure	Anticipation of improved disease-free survival compared to conventional treatment	Prospect of definitive cure in contrast to "disease control"
Chronic myeloid leukemia (CML)	Selected patients with acute lymphoblastic leukemia (ALL)	Selected patients with thalassemia
Myelodysplasia (most patients)	Acute myeloid leukemia (AML)	Sickle cell disease
Juvenile myelomonocytic leukemia (JMML)	Non-Hodgkin's lymphoma	
Fanconi anemia	Hodgkin's disease	
Other constitutional bone marrow failure syndromes		

Table 1.5 Diseases for which autologous transplant is used (adapted from Duncombe 1997)

(a) Adults

Proven benefit in RCT	Probable benefit	Possible benefit
Non-Hodgkin's lymphoma	Relapsed Hodgkin's lymphoma	Chronic myeloid leukemia
Acute myeloid leukemia	Acute lymphoblastic leukemia	Disseminated breast cancer
Multiple myeloma	Relapsed testicular cancer	Disseminated lung cancer
		Other solid tumors
		Severe autoimmune disease

(b) Children

Proven benefit in RCT	Probable benefit	Possible benefit
Stage 4 neuroblastoma	Relapsed/refractory Hodgkin's disease (adolescents)	Relapsed or refractory
	Relapsed Burkitt's NHL	• Wilms' tumor
	Relapsed diffuse large-cell NHL	• Germ cell tumor
	Other high-risk neuroblastoma	
	High-risk Ewing's sarcoma	
	High-risk or relapsed medulloblastoma	

Children

Hematological malignancy
Acute lymphoblastic leukemia (ALL)

Allogeneic HSCT is appropriate in certain groups of children with higher-risk ALL provided that they are in remission at the time of HSCT (high-risk ALL in 1st CR). Some patients with high-risk ALL are transplanted in 1st CR. Ideally an HLA-matched RD or URD should be used, but some centers will accept other closely but not fully matched donors (e.g. one antigen mismatch). High-risk ALL is defined by the following criteria:
• Philadelphia positive (BCR-ABL genetic rearrangement);
• presence of >5% blasts in bone marrow after 4 weeks of induction treatment in children with:
  • near haploid karyotype (≤44 chromosomes in leukemic blasts);
  • MLL gene rearrangement;
• failure to enter remission (i.e. presence of >25% blasts in bone marrow) after 4 weeks of induction treatment.

Allogeneic HSCT is indicated in most children with ALL in 2nd CR, using an HLA-matched or closely matched RD or URD. Three risk groups of relapsed ALL may be defined, based on:

• timing;
• immunophenotype;
• site of relapse.

The risk groups are currently treated according to a risk-stratified approach, as follows.

Standard risk
• *Definition*: late (>6 months after completion of chemotherapy) isolated extramedullary (central nervous system [CNS] or testicular) relapse.
• *Treatment*: chemotherapy and local (testicular or cranial) radiotherapy.

Intermediate risk
• *Definition*:
  • late marrow or combined (i.e. marrow and extramedullary) relapse of non-T-cell ALL; or
  • early (>18 months after initial diagnosis but <6 months after stopping chemotherapy) isolated extramedullary or combined relapse of non-T-cell ALL; or
  • early extramedullary relapse of T-cell ALL.
• *Treatment*: it remains unclear whether chemotherapy (plus local radiotherapy for extramedullary disease) or HSCT is superior in these patients.

High risk
- *Definition*:
  - any very early relapse (<18 months from initial diagnosis of ALL);
  - any marrow or combined relapse of T-cell ALL;
  - early marrow relapse of non-T-cell ALL.
- *Treatment*: HSCT

Although HSCT has often been performed in 1st CR in infants (<12 months of age at diagnosis), in view of the poorer prognosis in comparison to that in older children with ALL, there is no definite evidence that this improves survival. Currently, HSCT in 1st CR is recommended only for high-risk infantile ALL:
- <6 months old at diagnosis;
- MLL gene rearrangement;
- presenting white cell count >300 × 10^9/L.

Autologous HSCT is very rarely performed in children with ALL.

Acute myeloid leukemia (AML)

A meta-analysis of six prospective cohort studies demonstrated statistically significant reductions in relapse risk and improvements in overall and disease-free survival in children with AML in 1st CR undergoing HLA-identical sibling allogeneic HSCT compared to the use of autologous HSCT or chemotherapy alone. However, as the prognosis of children with good- and standard-risk AML treated with intensive chemotherapy protocols has improved greatly, allogeneic HSCT using an HLA-matched donor (RD or URD) is now recommended for AML in 1st CR only in children with poor-risk disease as defined by:
- adverse cytogenetic features (e.g. monosomy 7); or
- resistant disease (>15% blasts in bone marrow) after first course of intensive chemotherapy.

Children with good-risk (favorable cytogenetic abnormalities) or standard-risk AML (not in either good- or poor-risk group) are given intensive chemotherapy only.

Allogeneic HSCT is recommended in most children with AML in 2nd CR who have not had a previous transplant, and the use of mismatched donors may be considered as the prognosis with chemotherapy alone is poor.

Autologous transplants are now performed very rarely in children with AML in the UK, as they probably offer no advantage over intensive chemotherapy.

Chronic myeloid leukemia (CML)

Despite the increasing use of imatinib in the initial treatment of CML in adults, HSCT with an HLA-matched RD or URD is still considered to be the treatment of choice in children in:
- chronic phase (after initial disease control with hydroxyurea);
- advanced phase;
- blast crisis (after initial chemotherapy).

The use of mismatched donors may be appropriate in advanced-phase CML or blast crisis.

Myelodysplasia (MDS)

Although some sub-types of pediatric MDS (e.g. refractory cytopenia) may be relatively indolent, with stable blood counts during prolonged follow-up, others may progress rapidly to AML. Juvenile myelomonocytic leukemia (JMML) is a very rare disease unique to childhood with features of both MDS and myeloproliferative disease. HSCT is generally considered to be the best or even only chance of cure for most children with MDS, especially those with JMML. HLA-matched RDs or URDs may be suitable, and in higher risk MDS (e.g. JMML) the use of mismatched URDs or haploidentical RDs is appropriate.

Non-Hodgkin's lymphoma (NHL)

Autologous HSCT may be appropriate in children with relapsed Burkitt's lymphoma or diffuse large-cell NHL. There are early but promising data about the efficacy of allogeneic HSCT (RD or URD) in relapsed anaplastic large-cell NHL. Children with relapsed T-cell lymphoblastic lymphoma may benefit from allogeneic HSCT, but in practice it is often very difficult to achieve 2nd CR and hence perform a transplant in these patients.

Hodgkin's disease (HD)

Adolescents with relapsed or refractory HD are

usually treated with autologous HSCT, but this is seldom done in younger children as it offers little additional benefit beyond conventional relapse chemotherapy. As in adults, interest is growing in the possible role of reduced-intensity allogeneic HSCT in children and adolescents with multiply relapsed HD.

Non-hematological malignancy

Autologous HSCT, usually with PBSC, is indicated to rescue children from high-dose chemotherapy (occasionally with additional radiotherapy) given for certain relapsed or poor-prognosis solid tumors:
- stage 4 (or other high risk) neuroblastoma;
- high risk Ewing's sarcoma;
- high risk or relapsed medulloblastoma;
- selected patients (in the context of clinical trials) with relapsed or refractory
  - Wilms' tumor;
  - germ cell tumor.

Aplastic anemia, etc.

Allogeneic HSCT is indicated for children with severe or very severe aplastic anemia if an HLA-ID sibling donor is available; if not, intensive immunosuppressive treatment is usually performed initially since URD or mismatched RD HSCT is associated with a relatively high risk of graft rejection or severe GVHD; such transplants are indicated after failure to respond to two courses of immunosuppressive treatment in view of the otherwise very poor prognosis of these patients.

Fanconi anemia (FA)

At present HSCT is the only curative treatment for FA and is indicated when the patient starts to become transfusion dependent, or in the presence of myelodysplastic or leukemic transformation. Until recent years, the results of HLA-identical sibling HSCT were much better than those of URD HSCT due to graft failure and GVHD. However, the introduction of more immunosuppressive conditioning protocols has increased greatly the success rate of alternative-donor HSCTs.

Other constitutional bone marrow failure syndromes

Several inherited bone marrow failure syndromes may be treated by HSCT, including:
- *dyskeratosis congenita* (DKC):
  - HSCT (RD preferred to URD) is the only curative treatment, but is associated with considerable pulmonary and other organ toxicity, necessitating careful choice of conditioning regimen;
- *congenital amegakaryocytic thrombocytopenia* (CAMT):
  - HSCT (RD preferred to URD), usually performed with a standard conditioning regimen, is the only cure;
- *Schwachman–Diamond syndrome* (SDS):
  - HSCT (RD preferred to URD) may cure the hematological but not the other manifestations of SDS, and may be associated with considerable toxicity;
- *Diamond–Blackfan anemia* (DBA):
  - HLA-identical sibling HSCT may cure uncomplicated DBA (i.e. anemia only), but URD HSCT is not recommended;
  - it may be appropriate to consider use of an HLA-matched URD HSCT in DBA complicated by bone marrow failure when no RD is available.

Kostmann's disease (severe congenital neutropenia, SCN)

Although >90% of children with SCN respond satisfactorily to G-CSF, HSCT is the only treatment available for those who fail to respond and who continue to suffer from severe, life-threatening bacterial and fungal infections, and for the minority of patients who develop myelodysplastic or leukemic transformation. Although most HSCTs performed to date have employed HLA-identical sibling donors, there is an increasing number of reports of successful alternative-donor transplants.

Thalassemia

Better transfusion and iron chelation therapy have improved the prognosis for children with thalassemia given optimal treatment from infancy, so an improvement in their quality of life (by avoiding the need for regular blood transfusions and chelation therapy) is the main benefit of HSCT. Therefore the decision as to whether to perform HSCT is complex. Ideally a transplant should be performed in early childhood, when the risk of organ damage due to iron overload from multiple blood transfusions is low. The results of alternative-donor (e.g. URD) HSCT in thalassemia are relatively poor, although this may be considered for carefully selected patients. There is increasing interest in the use of umbilical cord blood as a stem cell source, but a high cell dose is essential.

Sickle cell disease

HLA-identical sibling donor HSCT may benefit patients with high-risk SCD, as suggested by the presence of at least one of the following:
- previous history of:
  - cerebrovascular accident;
  - acute chest syndrome (if hydroxyurea has failed);
- recurrent vaso-occlusive crises (if hydroxyurea has failed).

The following features (unless present in conjunction with the indications above) are no longer considered in the UK to constitute an indication for HSCT in SCD:
- impaired neuropsychological function and abnormal cranial MRI scan;
- sickle nephropathy;
- sickle lung disease;
- bilateral proliferative retinopathy and significant unilateral or bilateral visual impairment;
- osteonecrosis (multiple joints);
- alloimmunization to red cell antigens.

HSCT usually stabilizes and in some cases improves the complications of sickle cell disease, but the high risk of neurological complications (30%) means that this treatment is generally best undertaken in centers with experience in the management of SCID.

Primary immunodeficiencies and metabolic storage disorders

Primary immune deficiency disorders and metabolic storage disorders all arise because of defects in cells derived from the pluripotent hematopoietic stem cell. For this reason they ought to be amenable to cure by HSCT.

Severe combined immune deficiency, the most severe form of primary immune deficiency, from which untreated infants usually die in the first year of life, was one of the first conditions to be successfully treated by HSCT. It was also found that some forms of this condition were amenable to T-cell-depleted mismatched HSCT, even without pre-transplant conditioning. Initially only 50% of HSCTs were successful but particularly in the last 5 years success rates have now risen to approaching 90%. In the light of this success other primary immune deficiencies, which although not immediately lethal in the first months of life still cause serious illness and reduced life expectancy, are now treated by HSCT. The cumulative risk of serious ill health and death during childhood, adolescence and early adult life is now considerably greater than the relatively small risk of HSCT. Indeed, latest data suggest an overall success rate of 80–90% using matched sibling or unrelated donor. Immune deficiencies treated include Wiskott–Aldrich syndrome, chronic granulomatous disease, Chediak Higashi syndrome and hemophagocytic lymphohistiocytosis, as well as less well-defined combined immune deficiencies (Table 1.3).

HSCT has not been as successful with metabolic disorders, although results are improving. In infantile osteopetrosis, HSCT can certainly be very successful but the risk of complications including graft rejection are higher. Subtypes of osteopetrosis with neuroretinal degeneration are not amenable to HSCT, however, as although the bone defect is corrected, neuroretinal degeneration progresses inexorably. HSCT has been attempted for many metabolic storage disorders but patients need to be evaluated very carefully, particularly those with neurological involvement, as although there may be successful engraftment and correction of some features of the disorder, the child may still deteriorate and die from the neurological complications. Of all of the metabolic storage diseases the greatest success has been with Hurler's syndrome (mucopolysaccharidosis type I).

Autoimmune disease

The observation that a patient with severe autoimmune disease improved considerably after HSCT carried out for another reason has led to the development of HSCT for various forms of autoimmune disease. Initially autologous HSCT was performed where the patient's bone marrow was taken, T cells purged (as these are thought to be largely responsible for provoking the manifestations of autoimmune disease) and then the patient's own T-cell-depleted bone marrow returned after conditioning therapy. This has been particularly successful in children with juvenile idiopathic arthritis, most having long periods of disease-free remission, although after some years perhaps up to a third relapse to a greater or lesser extent. More recently, allogeneic transplantation has been attempted and this looks likely to be an important area for future development.

Further reading

Antoine, C. *et al.* (2003) Long term survival in transplantation of haemopoietic stem cells for immunodeficiencies. Report to the European Experience 1968–1999. *Lancet* **361**:553–560.

Ball, S.E. (2000) The modern management of severe aplastic anaemia. *Br J Haematol* **110**: 41–53.

Bleakley, M., Lau, L., Shaw, P.J., Kaufman, A. (2002) Bone marrow transplantation for paediatric AML in first remission: a systematic review and meta-analysis. *Bone Marrow Transplant.* **29**: 843–852.

Brodsky, R.A., Smith, D.A. (1999) *Curr Opin Oncol.*

Chessells, J.M. (2001) The role of bone marrow transplantation in first remission of paediatric ALL. *Front Biosci* **6**: G38–42.

Craddock, C., Chakraverty, R. (2005) Stem cell transplantation. In Hoffbrand, A.V., Catovsky, D., Tuddenham, E. (eds), *Postgraduate Haematology*, 5th edition. Oxford: Blackwell Publishing, pp. 419–435.

Cwynarski, K., Roberts, I.A.G., Iacobelli, S. *et al.* (2003) Stem cell transplantation for chronic myeloid leukaemia in children. *Blood* **102**: 1224–1231.

Gahrton, G. (2005) Progress in hematopoietic stem cell transplantation in multiple myeloma. *Curr Opin Hematol* **12**: 463–470.

Gibson, B.E.S., Wheatley, K., Hann, I.M. *et al.* (2005) Treatment strategy and long-term results in paediatric patients treated in consecutive UK AML trials. *Leukemia* **19**: 2130–2138.

Goldman, J.M., Melo, J.V. (2003) Chronic myeloid leukemia – advances in biology and new approaches to treatment. *N Engl J Med* **349**:1451–1464.

Harrison, G., Richards, S., Lawson, S. *et al.* (2000) Comparison of allogeneic transplant versus chemotherapy for relapsed childhood acute lymphoblastic leukaemia in the MRC UKALL R1 trial. *Ann Oncol* **11**: 999–1006.

Ljungman, P., Urbano-Ispizua, A., Cavazzana-Calvo, M. *et al.* (2006) Allogeneic and autologous transplantation for haematological diseases, solid tumours and immune disorders: definitions and current practice in Europe. *Bone Marrow Transplant* **37**: 439–449.

Locatelli, F., De Stefano, P. (2004) New insights into haematopoietic stem cell transplantation for patients with haemoglobinopathies. *Br J Haematol* **125**: 3–11.

Locatelli, F., Nollke, P., Zecca, M. *et al.* (2005) Hematopoietic stem cell transplantation (HSCT) in children with juvenile myelomonocytic leukemia (JMML): results of the EWOG-MDS/EBMT trial. *Blood* **105**: 410–419.

Peggs, K.S., Hunter, A., Chopra, R. *et al.* (2005) Clinical evidence of a graft-versus-Hodgkin's-lymphoma effect after reduced-intensity allogeneic transplantation. *Lancet* **365**: 1934–1941.

Peggs, K.S., Mackinnon, S., Linch, D.C. (2005) The role of allogeneic transplantation in non-Hodgkin's lymphoma. *Br J Haematol* **128**: 153–168.

Peters, C., Stewart, C.G. (2003) Hematopoietic cell transplantation for inherited metabolic diseases: an overview of outcomes and practice guidelines. *Bone Marrow Transplant* **31**: 229–239.

Pritchard, J., Cotterill, S.J., Germond, S.M., Imeson, J., de Kraker, J., Jones, D.R. *et al.* (2005) High dose melphalan in the treatment of advanced neuroblastoma: Results of a randomized trial (ENSG-1) by the European Neuroblastoma Study Group. *Pediatr Blood Cancer* **44**: 348–357.

Steward, C.G., Jarisch, A. (2005) Haemopoietic stem cell transplantation for genetic disorders. *Arch Dis Child* **90**: 1259–1263.

Yusuf, U., Frangoul, H.A., Gooley, T.A. *et al.* (2004) Allogeneic bone marrow transplantation in children with myelodysplastic syndrome or juvenile myelomonocytic leukemia: the Seattle experience. *Bone Marrow Transplant* **33**: 805–814.

Chapter 2
Pre-transplant assessment

M. Slatter and S. Fox

Introduction

Once a patient's condition is deemed to be best treated by hematopoietic stem cell transplantation (HSCT), the type of transplant to be performed needs to be decided and if it is to be allogeneic, a suitable donor has to be found. The patient's general condition needs to be assessed for both autologous and allogeneic transplants, and for all allogeneic transplants the donor's suitability also needs to be assessed. This chapter details the process of pre-transplant assessment.

Patients may undergo either autologous or allogeneic hematopoietic stem cell transplantation depending upon the condition being treated and the availability of a suitably matched donor. Patient preparation during the immediate pre-transplant phase is similar for both. In the case of autologous transplantation, however, consideration has to be given to the harvesting of stem cells at an appropriate point prior to commencement of conditioning therapy. Donors and patients having autologous transplants may undergo either bone marrow or peripheral blood stem cell harvesting.

Hematopoietic stem cell harvesting is considered a safe procedure. Adverse effects are rare and largely confined to those of anesthesia, which is necessary to harvest bone marrow. A European study of 27,628 donations found two deaths within 30 days of donation (both peripheral blood harvests), giving a death rate of 0.007%, and 18 serious adverse events (rate 0.07%), defined as any unplanned hospitalization within 30 days of donation (Gratwol, 2004). It is essential to perform a pre-harvest examination of the donor looking for anesthetic risk factors (Cleaver *et al.*, 1997). There is no upper age limit for stem cell donation and young infants have successfully been used as donors.

Tissue typing

Tissue typing of the patient should be performed as soon as possible after diagnosing a condition for which allogeneic transplantation is indicated. An accredited laboratory specializing in histocompatibility and immunogenetics should carry out the testing, and a small blood sample will need to be provided. The major histocompatibility complex (MHC) is the term given to genes clustered on the short arm of chromosome six (Fig. 2.1) that form the human leukocyte antigen (HLA) system. This can be thought of as a genetic code that identifies the individual and is therefore significant in the setting of transplantation; when cells carrying the HLA types of two different human beings meet each other there is a risk that an immune response will be provoked. The outcome of such a response may be graft-vs.-host disease (GVHD), in which immunologically active cells from the graft attack body tissues in the transplant recipient (the host), or less commonly graft rejection if the conditioning therapy prior to transplant fails to sufficiently suppress the patient's own immune system.

Modern laboratory techniques allow detailed tissue typing to be performed so that the best matched donor can be chosen. The HLA system comprises both class I and class II antigens. Serological methods can be used to determine low resolution typing of both classes of antigens. Thereafter, DNA techniques using polymerase chain reaction (PCR) allows high-resolution typing to be performed,

Fig. 2.1 Location of the HLA complex on chromosome 6. The complex is divided into three regions: I, II and III. Each region contains numerous genes, only some of which are shown. These are the most significant for allogeneic transplantation. HLA class III are involved in immune function, especially with the serum complement system. © Children's Bone Marrow Transplant Unit, Newcastle General Hospital, Newcastle upon Tyne, UK; redrawn with permission.

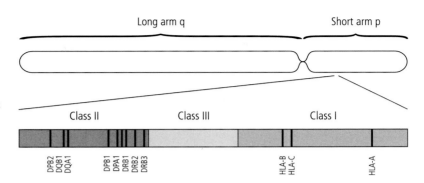

which identifies subtly different tissue types within each broad serological type.

Family donors

When the patient has siblings, they should be tissue typed provided they are of suitable age and fitness to be donors. Due to the way in which HLA types are inherited from parents, there is a 25% chance of any one sibling being a match for the patient (Fig. 2.2). However, the laws of probability mean that no matches are found in families where the patient has many siblings, while in others the patient's only sibling is fully matched. In some families who are closely inter-related it may be possible for a member of the extended family (e.g. first cousin) to act as a donor (Fig. 2.3). Fully matched donors are referred to as being HLA identical, whilst parents are usually haploidentical, meaning half matched. When tissue typing reveals more than one possible donor in the family, other factors such as age, sex, parity, blood group, cytomegalovirus (CMV) status, and general health will be taken into account to help with the final choice. Willingness to donate should not be automatically assumed and all potential donors should have the opportunity to discuss the situation in private with an independent member of the transplant team. Once the final choice has been made and the donor has consented to give stem cells, tissue typing of both donor and recipient should be repeated, sending a fresh blood sample from each to the laboratory. This is known as confirmatory typing and is a safety measure aimed at minimizing the possibility of transplanting from a donor into a recipient who has incorrectly been reported to be matched. Fitness to donate should be assessed by a physician who is independent of the transplant team. Table 2.1 summaries the different donor types.

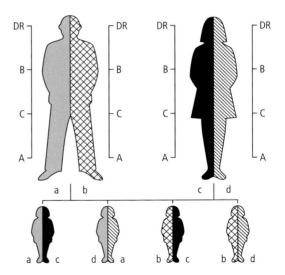

Fig. 2.2 Inheritance of haplotypes. © Children's Bone Marrow Transplant Unit, Newcastle General Hospital, Newcastle upon Tyne, UK; redrawn with permission.

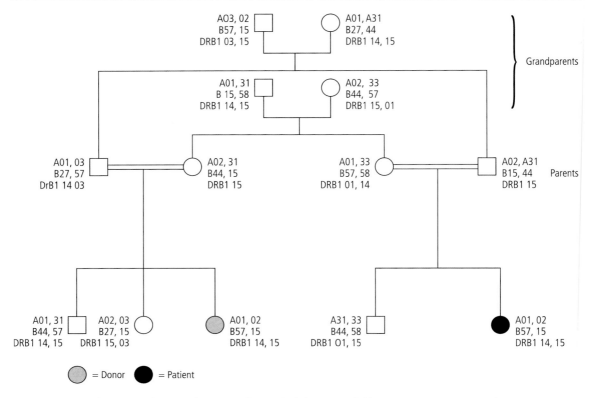

Fig. 2.3 Extended family tree showing phenotypically matched donor. © Children's Bone Marrow Transplant Unit, Newcastle General Hospital, Newcastle upon Tyne, UK; redrawn with permission.

Table 2.1 Donor types

Autologous	Patient's own stem cells
Allogeneic	Family (related donor)
	Unrelated
	Cord (usually unrelated)
	Mismatched related (often haploidentical)

Unrelated donors

When an HLA-matched donor is not available within the family, registers of volunteer unrelated donors may be searched in an attempt to find a match for the patient. In the UK such registers are maintained by the Anthony Nolan Trust (ANT), the British Bone Marrow Registry (BBMR) and the Welsh Bone Marrow Donor Registry (WBMDR). Registries from across the world now exchange tis-

sue type details of potential donors, significantly increasing the chances of finding a well-matched donor.

The first successful marrow transplant from an unrelated donor was performed in 1973 but, at that time, no actual register of such donors existed. The Anthony Nolan Trust register was the world's first register of unrelated bone marrow donors, formed in the early 1970s by the efforts of Shirley Nolan, whose young son Anthony suffered from Wiskott–Aldrich syndrome, an immune deficiency disorder that could have been treated with allogeneic marrow transplantation had a donor been available. As a result of Shirley Nolan raising both awareness and funds, a register was established and grew but, sadly, no donor was ever found for Anthony and he died of his disease in 1979, aged seven. Today, the Anthony Nolan Trust remains an independent charitable organization, operating one of the world's largest HSC donor registers and running the Anthony Nolan Research Institute, an arm of the organization devoted to scientific research into tissue typing and donor selection for HSCT.

The British Bone Marrow Registry operates under the umbrella of the National Blood Service and recruits volunteers from regular blood donors. An advantage of this system is that donors who join the register by this route are already familiar with the principles of donating tissue for the benefit of others and have already shown commitment to doing so by regularly donating blood. In recent years the BBMR has seen steady growth in the number of donors registered so that it too is among the world's largest donor registers.

The Welsh Blood Service operates in a similar way to the NBS and serves most of Wales. Just as the BBMR works as part of the NBS, the Welsh Bone Marrow Donor Registry comes under the auspices of the WBS. The WBMDR maintain a register of volunteer donors and operate associated laboratory services.

All the donor registries either run or have access to tissue typing laboratories so that, as donors are added to the register, their tissue type is recorded. When a transplant center wishes to search for an unrelated donor, it supplies the donor registers with the tissue typing details of the patient and a search of the databases then takes place, looking for any donor recorded who is at least a broad serological match. Increasingly registers record full high-resolution typing of their donors, so reducing the time spent refining the list of potential donors produced in response to the initial search request. Transplant centers may take expert advice from senior staff at their local tissue typing laboratory in deciding which donors to select for confirmatory typing following the initial report from the search. In some areas, the entire process of donor searching may be carried out by the tissue typing laboratory on behalf of the transplant center.

Once a donor has been selected, the donor registries have access to approved centers for medical assessment and harvesting of their donors. The exact arrangements for this vary between the registries. After the harvest has taken place, the reg-

istries arrange for the transport of the harvested product to the transplant center.

All of the unrelated donor registries communicate with each other, so that a UK transplant center only needs to send a search request to one of the registries to receive a report from all three. In the event that a matching donor is not found on any of the UK registers, the search may be extended to registers from other countries. Bone Marrow Donors Worldwide (BMDW) maintains a database of all donor registries and can identify potential overseas donors, enabling the transplant center to contact the registry for more details on the donor. The Anthony Nolan Trust acts as an intermediary in this process, forwarding the patient's details to the registers requested and returning the results to the transplant center for further scrutiny. Table 2.2 summarizes the steps to finding a suitable donor for allogeneic HSCT.

Umbilical cord blood

Umbilical cord blood is a rich source of hematopoietic stem cells (HSC) and in recent years there has been growing interest in using cord blood as an "off-the-shelf" product for transplantation. In response to this, cord blood banks have been developed and expectant mothers are invited to donate the umbilical cord blood to the bank. Additionally, a family who already have a child who suffers from a disease for which HSCT may be appropriate can request that they make a so-called "directed cord blood donation." If this is shown to be a match, the umbilical cord blood may be saved for use in a transplant for the older sibling.

Table 2.2 Steps in finding a suitable donor for allogeneic HSCT

---

1 Establish tissue type of recipient

2 Assess family members for suitability by tissue typing

3 If step 2 is not successful approach a suitable register to look for a match

4 Once donor found, assessment of suitability should be performed (unless umbilical cord blood)

Preparation of the donor for stem cell harvest

Adult donors are increasingly being offered the option of donating peripheral blood stem cells (PBSC) rather than bone marrow. This may be especially useful for donors who may have a medical condition of their own that would increase the risks of general anesthesia. PBSC collection is generally carried out as a day-case procedure and some donors find this prospect less difficult than the short period of hospitalization and general anesthetic needed for bone marrow donation. However, PBSC will require the donor to receive a short course of injections of granulocyte-colony stimulating factor (G-CSF) prior to commencing the first collection. Typically G-CSF at 10 µg/kg is given daily for 5 days before one to two leukapheresis procedures are performed. In the healthy individual, G-CSF will cause rapid proliferation of hematopoietic stem cells. The resulting expansion of the bone marrow can lead to side effects (Table 2.3).

These symptoms generally resolve very quickly once harvesting commences. There have been rare reports of more serious adverse events following administration of G-CSF to healthy donors, including two cases of ruptured spleen, one associated with high-dose G-CSF and the other case due to concurrent Epstein–Barr virus (EBV) infection. Mild side effects from the apheresis procedure itself may occur due to hypovolemia and hypocalcemia. Each PBSC collection will take around 4 h and the donor should be prepared to undergo two or even three collections on successive days. Very rarely, the donor may fail to mobilize sufficient hematopoietic stem cells into the peripheral blood to make a successful collection. By this stage, the transplant recipient will almost certainly have

completed conditioning, therefore making it necessary for the donor to undergo an emergency bone marrow harvest. The donor therefore needs to be appropriately informed and counseled about the risks and benefits of both marrow harvest and PBSC, and PBSC should not be seen as a risk-free option simply because it avoids the need for a general anesthetic. Prior to PBSC, the donor would need to undergo the same medical assessment and laboratory tests as for bone marrow harvest.

Assessment of family donors

A physician or pediatrician who is independent from that of the recipient should perform the pre-transplant assessment of the family donor. A medical history should be taken including:
- vaccinations;
- blood transfusions;
- allergies;
- travel to tropical countries;
- number of pregnancies in women.

A routine physical examination is performed. A chest X-ray and ECG is indicated on all men over 40 and women over 50 years of age (Cleaver *et al.* 1997).

Investigations for donor prior to HSC donation

These are given in Table 2.4.

Thyroid function tests are performed because it is not unusual for patients to have thyroid abnormalities post HSCT and so it is important to exclude donor transfer as a cause. The task to exclude infectious diseases should be completed within 30 days of harvest, but before giving cytoreductive conditioning to the patient. Assessment of venous access is essential for PBSC donors.

vCJD has almost certainly been transferred by blood transfusion in 3 cases. It is not clear whether there will be more cases, nor is it easy to assess the risk. If bone marrow donors have been exposed to vCJD (for example by having received plasma from a blood donor who subsequently developed vCJD) then it is possible they could transmit vCJD and

Table 2.3 Side effects of G-CSF

Common	Dull aching, discomfort especially lower back, hips, upper legs
	Flu-like symptoms
	Mild fever
Rare	Splenic rupture

Table 2.4 Pre-transplant investigations for donor

Hematology	Full blood count
	Coagulation studies
	Blood group, isohemagglutinins
Biochemistry/U&Es	Sodium, potassium, urea, creatinine, calcium, phosphate, glucose
Liver function tests	AST/ALT, alkaline phosphatase, bilirubin, albumin
Thyroid function tests	
Virology	CMV, EBV, HIV 1 and 2, HSV, VZV, measles, hepatitis B surface antigen (HBsAg), hepatitis A (antibody), hepatitis C (antibody), HTLV III (recent recommendation).
Other serology	Syphilis antibodies, toxplasma
Chimerism studies	DNA fingerprinting
Urinalysis	Dipstick
Cardiopulmonary	BP
	Chest X-ray, ECG (Adults)
For recipient with primary immunodeficiency	Immunoglobulins −/+ IgG subclasses

so the possible risk of transmission has to be set against the benefits of using that particular donor.

Bone marrow donation

Written informed consent should be taken from the donor or parent/guardian. The procedure must be explained together with the risks of general anesthesia. Low back pain occurs frequently due to soft tissue and bone trauma, but usually resolves in a few days. Infections, bleeding and thromboembolic events are rare complications of bone marrow harvest. The amount of marrow harvested is strictly controlled but inevitably marrow harvests are associated with significant blood loss. It is no longer routine to take autologous blood for transfusion prior to the harvest. It is very important to avoid allogeneic blood transfusion for the donor and also very important for the team caring for the donor to pay careful attention to correction of fluid losses. It is vital that the donor gets the best possible perioperative care.

Unrelated donors

The examination of the donor will be performed by the donor assessment center. However, the transplant center will need to request blood for confirmatory tissue typing, DNA analysis for post-transplant chimerism studies, and the opportunity is usually taken to check the donor virology and serology status. The donor's fitness to donate must be ascertained before conditioning of the patient begins. The donor center is responsible for the consent of the donor. The donor needs to be fully informed about the procedure for collecting the stem cells, the blood tests that will be performed including HIV status, the possibility of a second donation for the same patient and the emphasis on anonymity for the donor and patient. Anonymity may be relaxed in time and regulations may vary in different countries. The policy for the Anthony Nolan Trust is that two years have to elapse before there can be a donor/recipient meeting and this time period returns to zero if the donor gives lymphocytes or a second donation. Donors are informed that, after two years, if the recipient has progressed well and has exchanged correspondence with the donor, it may be possible to arrange direct contact, but only on the initial instigation of the recipient.

Cord blood donation

At the time of cord collection tests for the following are performed on the mother:
- hepatitis B and C;
- HIV 1 and 2;
- CMV;
- syphilis.

Confirmatory tests 3–6 months after delivery are also performed. The health of the baby is also assessed. Cord blood banks will supply the transplant center with the required viral status of the mother and sometimes the cord blood itself. The cell doses contained within the cord donation and cell viability are also recorded. They will also perform extra tests for confirmatory tissue typing and virology and serology on small aliquots of the cord. Some centers may wish to perform their own confirmatory typing. A small sample is usually taken at the time of thawing for DNA analysis for post-transplant chimerism studies.

Preparation of the patient for stem cell transplantation

The clinical condition of patients undergoing stem cell transplantation varies enormously depending on diagnosis, age, previous treatment including chemotherapy, and organ damage. Once the decision to transplant has been made and a donor selected, each organ system should be assessed so that any organ damage is known about prior to transplant; therefore potential harmful effects of chemotherapy, radiotherapy, risks for GVHD, and recurrence of infections can be anticipated. A full medical history should be taken and a physical examination performed. It is useful to perform the assessment at least 6 weeks before the transplant date in order that any necessary investigations can be arranged. A checklist is essential. Skin and nails should also be assessed for evidence of infection and treated appropriately pre-transplant. It is also useful to perform microbiology screening for resistant bacteria, e.g. meticillin-resistant *Staphylococcus aureus* (MRSA) and glycopeptide resistant enterococci (GRE/VRE). This will depend on unit policy.

Nearly all patients undergoing transplant who receive conditioning will need blood and platelet transfusions and so it is essential to know their transfusion history, blood group, Coombs test and the blood group of the donor and make a transfusion protocol. It is essential to know the viral status of the patient and it is usual to do serological tests for CMV, EBV, hepatitis A, B and C, HIV 1 and 2, VZV, HSV, syphilis, toxoplasma and HTLV III.

A number of infectious agents, particularly viruses, can now be detected by very sensitive molecular techniques such as polymerase chain reaction (PCR) at a much earlier stage of the infectious process. This in turn means that pre-emptive therapy can be given before organ damage, such as life-threatening pneumonitis or hepatitis, occurs.

Such early detection, together with new treatments such as cidofovir for adenovirus, has led to a dramatic improvement in outcome following viral infection. Chapter 7 gives further details on virology infections. Stool and urine samples should be sent for virology and microbiology, and throat and surface swabs should be performed so that colonizing organisms are identified. Blood for DNA genetic markers should be taken for post-transplant chimerism studies. Other blood tests are tailored to the patient's diagnosis. Patients with malignancy may need to have further specific blood tests performed. Examples could include assessment of markers of activity of malignant disease, such as lactate dehydrogenase (LDH) in the case of lymphoma and paraprotein for patients with multiple myeloma. Patients with leukemia should undergo bone marrow biopsy to demonstrate remission status, whilst lymphoma patients should have a CT scan performed. A suggested checklist is provided in Table 2.5. Most patients will have a chest X-ray prior to transplant and lung function tests should be considered. An ultrasound of the abdomen should also be considered. Many centers perform routine ECG and echocardiogram prior to transplant. All patients should have a recent dental check as caries can be an important source of infection. Audiological assessment pre-transplant is useful as a baseline in case damage is caused by drugs used in the transplant process. Ophthalmic assessment pre-transplant may also prove useful as many patients will encounter visual disturbance following transplant, the causes of which may include cataracts in those patients whose conditioning regimen has included total body irradiation, and retinitis in those patients who suffer cytomegalovirus (CMV) infection post transplant. Checklists are given in Tables 2.6, 2.7 and 2.8.

Table 2.5 Disease status checklist

Remission status: CR1/CR2/other(specify)
Assessment: BM/CT/other(specify)
Date and findings:

LDH: Paraprotein:

Table 2.6 Autologous transplant checklist

Test	Date done	Signed	Result	Specify if abnormal
FBC				
Hb				
WCC				
Plts				
Blood group (CMV negative and irradiated)				
U&Es/LFTs				
LDH				
Magnesium				
Serology				
CMV				
HIV				
HEP A				
HEP B				
HEP C				
SYPHILIS				
Chest X-ray				
ECG				
Respiratory function				
EDTA renal clearance				
BP				
Dipstick urinalysis				

Table 2.7 Pre-transplant infection screen for all recipients

	Bacteriology	Result	Virology	Result
Perineal swab				
Stool				
Nose swab/NPA				
Throat swab				
MRSA screen				
GRE/VRE screen				
MSU				

It is essential to address family and psychosocial issues, and so each patient should be referred to a social worker and psychologist. Chapter 15 gives further details of the types of support that can be provided. Each unit will have their own system for information giving, including written information about the transplant procedure, a visit to the unit, and a home visit. It may be appropriate for patients to meet the dietician and physiotherapist prior to transplant. Fertility issues need to be discussed. In particular, sperm banking should be arranged if appropriate. It is vital that written consent is taken once the patient is fully aware of all the aspects of the transplant.

Summary

Thorough assessment of the patient prior to HSCT is essential to ensure that the patient is as well as possible prior to the procedure. Accurate tissue typing of donors for allogeneic transplants

Table 2.8 Allogeneic transplant recipient

	Investigations	
Hematology	Full blood count	
	Coagulation studies	
	Blood group, isohemagglutinins, DCT	
Biochemistry/U&Es	Sodium, potassium, urea, creatinine, LDH, paraprotein, glucose	
Liver function tests	AST/ALT, alkaline phosphatase, gamma GT, bilirubin, albumin	
Thyroid function tests		
Serology	CMV, EBV, HIV 1 and 2, HSV, VZV, measles, HBsAg, hep A, hep C, toxoplasma	
Other serology	Syphilis	
Engraftment studies		
Cardiopulmonary	Chest X-ray and bone age (children)	
	Lung function test	
	ECG	
	Echocardiogram	
Dental check		
Audiology		
GFR	Height:	Weight:

Consider: nutritional studies – zinc, copper, selenium, manganese, vitamin A, vitamin E.
Viral PCRs – CMV, EBV, adenovirus, HHV6.
Abdominal ultrasound scan.
Ophthalmological assessment.

is essential in order to achieve the best possible match. Attention to detail is paramount to ensure the best possible result for the patient.

Further reading

Anthony Nolan Trust. www.anthonynolan.org.uk

Becker, P.S., Wagle, M., Matous, S. *et al*. (1997) Spontaneous splenic rupture following administration of G-CSF: occurrence in an allogeneic donor of peripheral blood stem cells. *Biol Blood Marrow Transplant* **3**: 45–49.

Bone Marrow Donors Worldwide. www.bmdw.org

Cleaver, S.A., Warren, P., Kern, M. *et al*. (1997) Donor work-up and transport of bone marrow – recommendations and requirements for a standardized practice throughout the world from the Donor Registries and Quality Assurance Working Groups of the World Marrow Donor Association. *Bone Marrow Transplant* **20**: 621–629.

Falzetti, F., Aversa, F., Minelli, O., Tabilio, A. (1999) Spontaneous rupture of spleen during peripheral blood stem cell mobilisation in a healthy donor (letter). *Lancet* **353**: 555.

Gratwohl, A. (2004) Severe donor events after stem cell donation. *Bone Marrow Transplant.* 33: Suppl 1, S67.

Platzbecker, U., Prange-Krex, G., Bornhauser, M. *et al.* (2001) Spleen enlargement in healthy donors during G-CSF mobilisation of PBPCs. *Transfusion* **41**: 184–189.

Slatter, M.A., Gennery, A.R., Cheetham, T.D. *et al.* (2004) Hypothyroidism post bone marrow transplantation for primary immunodeficiency syndromes without the use of total body irradiation in conditioning. *Bone Marrow Transplant* 33: 949–953.

Welsh Bone Marrow Donor Registry. www.wtail.org.uk/WBMOR.htm

Chapter 3
The transplant

R. Skinner, A. Lennard and P. Veys

The decision to perform a hematopoietic stem cell transplant (HSCT)

HSCT may offer a realistic hope of curing malignant disease, or it may permanently correct many serious congenital or acquired hematological diseases, a wide variety of immunological deficiencies, and certain inborn errors of metabolism. In so doing, it offers the prospect of improving (and possibly normalizing) life expectancy. In most cases the achievement of cure without the need for further ongoing treatment will improve the patient's quality of life.

In many cases the decision to perform a HSCT is relatively straightforward, typically when the patient has a severe illness at a sufficiently advanced stage to merit transplantation, is medically fit in other respects, and has a readily available well-matched donor to provide allogeneic hematopoietic stem cells (HSCs). However, the situation is frequently much more complicated than this, and a substantial proportion of referrals require very careful evaluation of all the available options. In such cases it is important to be clear what the aim of performing a HSCT is (see Table 3.1), and in particular what benefits might be achieved over and above those offered by alternative non-transplant treatment options.

However, the route to achieving these long-term benefits is associated with many increased risks, predominantly but not exclusively early post-transplant (see Chapters 6, 7 and 9 [early toxicity] and 16 [late effects of treatment]). Transplants may fail, leading to severe morbidity and even mortality, or result in a variety of complications due to:
- conditioning toxicity;

Table 3.1 Potential aims of HSCT

HSCT may:

- Allow rescue from high dose chemoradiotherapy given for cytotoxic effect in malignant disease, with additional benefit from graft-vs.-leukemia (GVL) effect or other graft-vs.-malignancy effect
- Provide normal cells to replace diseased:
  - hematopoietic system (to correct serious non-malignant hematological illness)
  - immune system (to correct immunodeficiency)
  - metabolic/enzymatic capacity (to correct, partially or completely, inborn errors of metabolism
- Permit re-education of autologous stem/T cells (for treatment of autoimmune disease)

- serious infections;
- graft rejection or failure;
- graft-vs.-host disease (GVHD).

However, in many scenarios (particularly in pediatric practice) relapse and subsequent progression of the original malignant disease is the commonest cause of transplant failure and ultimately death.

In its simplest form, the dilemma of whether to perform a transplant may be viewed as being a choice between accepting, or rejecting, a prolonged period of intensive treatment and monitoring with an increased risk of severe illness or death early post-HSCT, in the hope (but not certainty) of achieving a better prospect of long-term survival and, hopefully, cure. In most cases, the alternative scenario of continuing non-transplant treatment is likely (but not guaranteed) to be associated with a lower risk of early severe toxicity and treatment-related mortality, but also less likely to achieve satisfactory long-term disease-free survival and cure. It is often very difficult for clinicians, and especially for patients and their families, to weigh up these conflicting potential benefits and risks to the patient's immediate and future survival prospects.

These already difficult decisions may be made even harder by a variety of factors, including the patient's medical condition, which may preclude some treatment options, especially more intensive transplant treatments. Likewise, although such a scenario is increasingly rare given the wider use of alternative donors and stem cell sources, the inability to identify a suitable allogeneic donor quickly enough may occasionally become a limiting issue in a patient whose condition is very poor or unstable. Other factors influencing the decision of whether to perform a HSCT include the availability (or not) of established alternative treatments and the depth of local expertise in either transplant-based or alternative treatments, as well as wider issues involving national healthcare economics and resource allocation. Perhaps the most difficult issue is the fact that the situation is constantly changing in that improvements in results of HSCT may well be balanced by improvements in the success of alternative treatments, thereby inevitably introducing a degree of uncertainty about the relevance of the most recent results of treatment.

In summary, the decision to perform a HSCT is frequently extremely complex and difficult for all concerned. It is important that such a decision is taken in consultation with the multidisciplinary transplant team (including experienced nursing and social work staff), and particularly with the active involvement of the patient and family.

The hematopoietic stem cell transplant

Overview

The process of performing a HSCT involves several steps (Table 3.2).

Types and choice of donor

HSCT may be:
• *autologous*, where the patient's own HSCs are harvested and then cryopreserved by freezing in liquid nitrogen, with subsequent thawing and

Table 3.2 The stages of performing a HSCT

• Decision to perform HSCT
• Patient and donor selection/evaluation
• Hematopoietic stem cell harvest
• Conditioning
  • chemotherapy
  • radiotherapy
  • immunosuppression
• HSC transplant
• Early post-HSCT care
• Long-term post-HSCT follow-up

reinfusion after the patient has received intensive myeloablative treatment;
• *allogeneic*, where HSCs from another individual (donor) are harvested and infused into the recipient on completion of their conditioning therapy.

Historically, the commonest allogeneic donor has been an HLA-identical sibling, but the last two decades has witnessed a huge increase in the number of transplants performed using alternative donors, including:
• HLA-matched volunteer unrelated donors (URDs);
• HLA-mismatched URDs;
• mismatched related donors (RDs), including haploidentical parental donors for pediatric patients.

Syngeneic (identical twin) donors are rarely available. Although their use is associated with a much lower risk of GVHD, this may have theoretical disadvantages in situations where the graft-vs.-leukemia (GVL) effect may be important, or in genetic disease where the identical twin will suffer from the same disease.

Sources, choice and harvesting of stem cells

The potential sources of HSCs include bone marrow (BM) and peripheral blood (PB) for both autologous and allogeneic transplants, and additionally umbilical cord blood (UCB) for allogeneic procedures. The use of PB and UCB has increased considerably in recent years, especially in adults and children, respectively (Fig. 3.1).

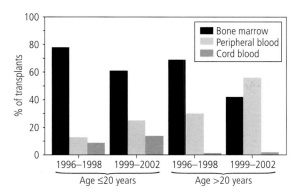

Fig. 3.1 Trends in the proportion of allogeneic HSCTs performed using bone marrow, peripheral blood and umbilical cord blood. Taken from IBMTR Summary Slides 2003, reproduced with permission of International Bone Marrow Transplant Registry (IBMTR).

In autologous transplantation, HSC harvest is performed before commencement of the conditioning regimen, while in allogeneic transplantation, the donor undergoes HSC harvest towards the end of the recipient's conditioning treatment so that the stem cells can be infused into the patient as soon as possible (and no more than 48 hours) after harvest.

Until the late 1980s, BM was the only source of HSCs for either autologous or allogeneic HSCT. Marrow is harvested under general anesthesia by performing multiple aspirates from several bone puncture sites (usually accessed by one skin puncture site) on each posterior iliac crest. Subsequently, the introduction and expanding use of UCB transplants has provided an alternative source of allogeneic stem cells. UCB is harvested from the placenta at the time of birth, and then cryopreserved for future use. A major potential benefit of UCB as a stem cell source is its ready availability, as it is usually much quicker to procure cryopreserved UCB from a cord blood bank than to obtain stem cells from a donor. Furthermore, looking from the perspective of very young potential donors (especially infants), it is clearly more acceptable in medical terms if the stem cells are already available without the donor needing to undergo a harvesting procedure. A further advantage of UCB is the apparent ability to use HLA-mismatched UCB donations with less risk of GVHD when compared to the use of other stem cell sources. However, the number of banked cord blood units remains much smaller than that of potentially available BM or PB URDs accessible via the volunteer donor panels, and the annual number of UCB transplants is still significantly less than that performed using BM or PB (see Fig. 3.1). In part this is due to the relative unfamiliarity of many units with UCB procedures, but the difficulty in achieving an adequate stem cell dose is a limiting factor to UCB transplantation in larger recipients, especially adults. Investigators are exploring possible ways of overcoming this latter issue by *in vitro* "expansion" of individual units or by simply combining two UCB units.

Peripheral blood stem cells (PBSC) were first used as a source of HSCs in the late 1980s and have become the commonest source used in autologous transplants in both adults and children. PBSC are increasingly used in allogeneic transplants, especially when the donor is an adult. PB is harvested using leukopheresis techniques, usually after stem cell mobilization with chemotherapy (autologous) or G-CSF (allogeneic harvest). The use of G-CSF to stimulate the appearance of HSCs in allogeneic PB harvests allows collection of large stem cell (CD34-positive) doses, which maximizes the likelihood of engraftment. This is particularly important in situations where graft failure is more likely:

- HLA-mismatched HSCTs;
- HSCT in conditions known to be associated with an increased risk of rejection, e.g. aplastic anemia.

As acute GVHD is mediated by T lymphocytes, large numbers of which are mobilized during a PBSC harvest, it is necessary to reduce the number of T cells in the harvest (T-cell depletion), or alternatively to positively select CD34-positive cells (i.e. stem cells). Although these techniques have countered the theoretical increased risk of acute GVHD, longer follow-up has shown that chronic GVHD is more common in recipients of PBSC transplants compared with BM transplants.

This trend to increasing use of PBSC and UCB as HSC sources has increased the available donor pool greatly, particularly for children, and it is now relatively unusual not to be able to identify a suitable donor. However, difficulty can arise if the recipient is of mixed racial origin, producing rare combinations of HLA alleles.

The relative advantages and disadvantages of different stem cell sources are summarized in Table 3.3 and a suggested hierarchy for choosing the most appropriate HSC donor and stem cell source is shown in Table 3.4, although this will differ from center to center depending on the level of local experience and expertise available.

Type and intensity of conditioning regimen

Most conditioning regimens may be described as being either myeloablative or nonmyeloablative in nature, whilst the degree of immunosuppression is also of crucial importance. Rarely, no conditioning treatment is used, for example:
• in some forms of severe combined immunodeficiency receiving an HLA-identical sibling HSCT;
• the patient is too ill to tolerate conditioning.

Myeloablative conditioning

This approach depends on a steep dose–response relationship to achieve high cytotoxicity against malignant cells, but at the cost of considerable hematopoietic and systemic toxicity. It has also been employed in many nonmalignant conditions, especially those associated with increased risk of rejection. Regimens incorporating either total body irradiation (TBI) or busulfan (Bu) (both are most frequently given alongside cyclophospha-mide [Cy], as CyTBI or BuCy, respectively) remain the most commonly used, although other high-dose cytotoxic drugs (most commonly alkylating agents, especially melphalan) are sometimes used for myeloablative effect.

Non-myeloablative conditioning

These regimens were developed following observation of the sometimes powerful graft-vs.-leukemia (GVL) effect following donor lymphocyte infusions (DLI) even in the absence of conventional cytotoxic therapy. GVL following DLI is mediated at least in part by allogeneic T cells, although the precise mechanism remains unclear. Nevertheless, it is believed that GVL can occur even in the absence of overt GVHD. Therefore, the underlying principle of nonmyeloablative HSCT is that less intensive conditioning may reduce regimen-related toxicity (RRT) by reducing direct toxicity and limiting inflammatory cytokine release. Therefore the likely severity of GVHD (see Chapter 10) is reduced while sufficient immunosuppressive action is retained to prevent graft rejection and to allow stable engraftment capable of exerting a graft-vs.-malignancy effect. Numerous nonmyeloablative regimens have been described, and most typically incorporate fludarabine in combination with low-dose TBI or chemotherapy (e.g. melphalan or cyclophosphamide). They have been variably divided into "reduced-intensity" and "minimal-intensity" regimens (see Fig. 3.2).

Table 3.3 Potential advantages and disadvantages of different types of hematopoietic stem cell donor

Donor	Availability	Speed of access (feasibility of re-access)	Cost	Rejection risk	Speed of engraftment	GVHD risk	GVL mediated by	Speed of immune reconstitution
Unrelated bone marrow or peripheral blood	10/10 match = 50% ≤9/10 match = 80% ethnic minority = 20%	Slow (possible)	High	Low	Moderate	Moderate	T cells	Moderate
Unrelated cord blood	≥5/6 match = 45% ≥4/6 match = 90%	Fast (no)	Moderate	High	Slow	Low	T cells	Slow
Haploidentical family	>90%	Immediate (yes)	Low	Moderate	Fast	Low	NK cells	Very slow

Table 3.4 A proposed HLA hierarchy and preferred stem cell source to guide choice of the best HSCT donor. RD, related donor; URD, unrelated donor; UCB, umbilical cord blood; BM, bone marrow; PB, peripheral blood.

1 HLA-identical sibling = phenotypically HLA-matched[†] RD = HLA-identical RD UCB*
2 10/10 molecularly HLA-matched[‡] URD = 6/6 HLA-matched URD UCB*
3 9/10 HLA-matched URD = 5/6 HLA-matched RD = ≥4/6 URD UCB*
4 8/10 matched URD = haploidentical RD[§]

*With nucleated cell (NC) dose >3.7 × 10^7/kg recipient weight.
[†]An HLA-matched donor where one haplotype is genotypically identical but the other is not.
[‡]HLA alleles matched using molecular typing techniques.
[§]Most haploidentical family donors for children are parents, as the use of G-CSF in young sibling donors is not encouraged. Choice of parent depends on factors given below and KIR mismatch in myeloid diseases. Options 3 and 4 should only be considered in poor risk patients for whom alternative treatment is unavailable, or has failed.
Option 4 usually requires *in-vitro* T-cell depletion.
Mismatched RDs may be preferred over URDs for certain disorders, e.g. SCID.

Stem cell source

1 HLA-identical sibling[¶] – BM preferred to PB
2 HLA-matched URD[¶] – no preference between BM and PB
3 HLA-mismatched URD/RD – PB preferred to BM

[¶]Adult RDs and URDs should be allowed a choice between donating BM or PB after nondirective counseling by a physician independent of the HSCT program.

CMV status		Gender	
Patient	*Donor*	*Patient*	*Donor*
Positive	Positive preferred to negative	Male	Male preferred to female
Negative	Negative preferred to positive	Female	Male preferred to female

Age	Younger (≤40 years) URDs preferred to older
ABO Blood Groups	Aim for a match in heavily pre-transfused patients

Immunosuppression

Intense immunosuppression is a vital component of conditioning for many alternative donor HSCTs that would otherwise carry an unacceptably high risk of graft rejection (e.g. mismatched unrelated or haploidentical related donor HSCT). Fludarabine

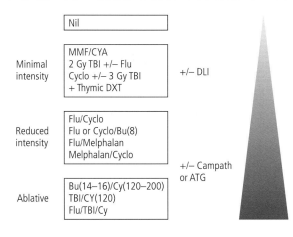

Fig. 3.2 A hierarchy of conditioning regimen intensity.

Table 3.5 Factors affecting the type and intensity of HSCT conditioning regimen

- Underlying disease (malignant or nonmalignant)
- Specific diseases
- Age (especially extremes of life)
- Previous treatment
- General medical condition
- Type of HSCT
- Degree of HLA-matching

and pre-transplant serotherapy (see below) are important elements of enhanced immunosuppression.

The type and intensity of conditioning regimen chosen for any given patient depends on several factors (Table 3.5) including:

- underlying disease;
- patient age;
- nature and timing of prior treatment (especially a previous HSCT);
- pre-transplant medical status.

Underlying disease

Important considerations include:

- non-radiotherapy-containing regimens are preferred in non-malignant disease because of concerns about the perceived greater risk of serious late adverse effects of radiotherapy, especially the risk of secondary malignancy;

- specific diagnoses – examples include the following.
  - Some conditions are associated with an increased risk of graft rejection which may be reduced by more immunosuppressive conditioning; for example, the addition of ATG serotherapy (see below) to conditioning for aplastic anemia (previously usually cyclophosphamide alone) has reduced the previously appreciable graft failure rate.
  - Chemotherapy-only conditioning (e.g. with busulfan, cyclophosphamide and melphalan [BuCyMel]) has led to better event-free survival than CyTBI in children with myelodysplasia and juvenile myelomonocytic leukemia (JMML).
  - Fanconi anemia (FA) patients (who have defective DNA repair) show greatly exaggerated sensitivity to chemotherapy and radiotherapy and should be conditioned with low-dose regimens to reduce the risk of life-threatening regimen-related toxicity (RRT). Recent conditioning protocols for FA have omitted radiotherapy completely in an attempt to reduce the high long-term risk of secondary malignancy.

Patient age

- Infants (<2 years old at transplant) – chemotherapy-only conditioning is usually preferred since TBI is associated with very serious long-term toxicity in this age group, including a high risk of neurocognitive damage and severe growth impairment.
- Older recipients – reduced-intensity conditioning regimens are associated with a lower (but not absent) risk of transplant-related mortality (TRM) in older patients who are more likely to have associated co-morbidities that preclude myeloablative procedures.

Nature and timing of prior treatment (especially a previous HSCT)

Each patient and scenario is considered on an individual basis, but important points include:
- previous use of TBI may preclude use of further radiotherapy;

- previous cranial radiotherapy may increase the risk of neurological toxicity secondary to subsequent TBI, especially in younger children;
- recent myeloablative conditioning treatment (especially within 12 months) increases greatly the RRT and TRM of a second HSCT – nonmyeloablative conditioning is usually preferred in this scenario.

Pre-transplant medical status

Patients with poor pre-transplant medical status, most often due either to complications of the underlying disease or to toxicity of previous treatment, may benefit from reduced or minimal intensity conditioning.

In younger patients, especially children, this approach is most appropriate in conditions where either an effective GVL (or other graft-vs.-malignancy) effect is anticipated, or a degree of mixed chimerism (i.e. partial donor engraftment) is likely to confer an acceptable result of HSCT, e.g. genetic diseases.

Type of HSCT

In general, more intensive conditioning (especially in terms of immunosuppression) is preferred for transplants associated with an increased risk of delayed engraftment or graft failure, e.g. mismatched umbilical cord transplants, when the cell dose may be relatively low.

Degree of HLA matching

Likewise, more immunosuppressive conditioning is preferred for greater degrees of mismatch, with haploidentical donor HSCT as the most extreme example.

The conditioning regimen

The conditioning regimen has two principal goals:
- eradication of diseased cells (especially but not exclusively in the context of malignancy) – usually considered to require myeloablative treatment;
- recipient immunosuppression to allow engraftment of donor stem cells.

Traditionally, it has also been considered that conditioning treatment "creates space" for the incoming donor cells, but the success of nonmyeloablative conditioning regimens (see above) has highlighted the oversimplicity of this belief. The relative ways in which myeloablative and nonmyeloablative regimens achieve these goals is summarized in Table 3.6.

Historically, most conditioning regimens included both chemotherapy and radiotherapy, but there has been a substantial increase in the use of chemotherapy-only regimens in the last two decades. An increasing number of conditioning regimens include elements specifically intended to cause host or donor cell immunosuppression (or both) to reduce the risk of, respectively, graft rejection or graft-vs.-host disease (or both), particularly in alternative donor transplants. In practice there is a spectrum of effects, as many individual elements of the conditioning regimen (e.g. TBI) fulfil both myeloablative and immunosuppressive roles, although some may exert more immunosuppressive than myeloablative effect (e.g. fludarabine), while others have a converse effect (e.g. busulfan).

Chemotherapy

A wide variety of chemotherapy drugs has been utilized to achieve myeloablation in HSCT (see Tables 3.7 and 3.8).

The most important attributes of a cytotoxic drug that permit its use in myeloablative HSCT conditioning are a steep dose–response curve and manageable nonhematopoietic toxicity. The characteristics of a drug's dose–response curve are important in determining its ability to achieve maximum malignant cell kill. Numerous alkylating agents have been employed in this context, but high doses of other cytotoxics (such as etoposide or carboplatin) have also been used, particularly in autologous transplantation.

Certain chemotherapeutic agents are also used to achieve intensive immunosuppression. Traditionally, cyclophosphamide has been regarded as providing the major immunosuppressive component of most conditioning regimens, but in recent years the increasing use of fludarabine has allowed the delivery of profound immunosuppression with acceptable toxicity.

Table 3.6 Principles underlying the mechanisms of action of HSCT

Objective	Mechanism of action	
	Conventional HSCT	Reduced-intensity conditioning HSCT
Prevent rejection	Supralethal chemo/radiotherapy	Pre +/− post-HSCT immunosuppression to achieve tolerance
Create marrow space for donor cells	Supralethal chemo/radiotherapy	Graft-vs.-marrow reaction (may require DLI)
Eradicate malignancy	Supralethal chemo/radiotherapy	Graft-vs.-leukemia (may require DLI)
Cure genetic diseases	Full donor chimerism	Stable mixed chimerism

DLI, donor lymphocyte infusion.

Table 3.7 Cytotoxic agents used in HSCT conditioning regimens

Alkylating agents– interfere with DNA replication by formation of covalent intercalating cross-links between DNA strands:
- busulfan*
- carmustine (BCNU)*
- cyclophosphamide[†]
- ifosfamide[†]
- melphalan*
- thiotepa*
- treosulfan*[†]

Anti-metabolites– inhibit biochemical mechanisms involved in cell division
- Fludarabine[†]

Epipodophyllotoxins – inhibit topoisomerase II during DNA replication and transcription
- Etoposide (VP-16)[†]

Platinum agents – bind with DNA, interfering with replication
- Carboplatin
- Cisplatin

Radiotherapy – direct cytotoxicity
- TBI 12–14.4 Gy*
- TBI 2–3 Gy[†]

Taxanes – inhibits dissolution of microtubules, blocking mitosis
- Paclitaxel

NB: Although most cytotoxic agents are both myelosuppressive and immunosuppressive, some are used primarily for myeloablative effect* and others predominantly for immunosuppressive effect[†].

Table 3.8 Transplant conditioning regimens and their early toxicities

Disease	Donor	Age (years)	Protocol	Agents	Doses	Toxicity
ALL >2 years CML (ap)	MSD, URD MSD	>2 >2	Cy/TBI*	}Cyclophosphamide }	60 mg/kg x 2	Hemorrhagic cystitis, inappropriate ADH, cardiac failure
CML (cp), AML	MUD	>2		}TBI	12 Gy in 6 # 14.4 Gy in 8 #	Parotitis, erythema, mucositis, somnolence, pneumocystis
ALL >2 years	MSD, URD	>2	VP16/TBI	}VP16 }TBI	60 mg/kg	Mucositis, veno-occlusive disease, hemorrhagic cystitis
				}TBI	12 Gy in 6 # 13.2 Gy in 11 #	As above
ALL AML MDS	MMURD, haplo-identical	>2 >2	Flu/Cy/TBI *	}Fludarabine }Cyclophosphamide }	120 mg/m^2 60 mg/kg x 2	Occasional neurotoxicity Hemorrhagic cystitis, inappropriate ADH, cardiac failure
				}TBI	14.4 Gy in 8 #	As above
ALL <2 years CML (cp)	MSD, URD MSD	Any	Bu/Cy	}Busulfan	16–20 mg/kg	Veno-occlusive disease, seizures, pulmonary fibrosis, skin changes
AML	MSD			}Cyclophosphamide	50 mg/kg x 4	As above
AML, ALL JMML/MDS	Haplo-identical	<2	Flu/Bu/Cy	}Fludarabine }Busulfan }Cyclophosphamide	125 mg/m^2 14 mg/kg 50 mg/kg x 4	As above As above As above
AML (cardiac dysfunction)	MSD	<2	Bu/Melph	}Busulfan }Melphalan	16–20 mg/kg 140 mg/kg	As above Mucositis, renal impairment
JMML/MDS AML	MFD/URD	Any	Bu/Cy/Melph	}Busulfan }Cyclophosphamide }Melphalan	16 mg/kg 120 mg/kg 140 mg/kg	As above As above As above
Poor organ function 2nd HSCT	MFD/URD		Flu/Melph	}Fludarabine }Melphalan	150 mg/m^2 140 mg/m^2	As above As above

MSD = HLA-matched sibling donor; URD = HLA-matched unrelated donor; MMURD = HLA-mismatched unrelated donor; MFD = other HLA-matched related donor; # = fractions; ap = accelerated phase; cp = chronic phase.
*Order reversed to TBI/Cy in some centers.

Radiotherapy

Total body irradiation (TBI) is primarily regarded as a myeloablative component of conditioning regimens, although lower-dose TBI schedules are used in some nonmyeloablative regimens (see below). In addition, TBI also offers substantial immunosuppressive effect.

The maximum tolerated dose of TBI is limited by both acute and chronic toxicity, but the use of fractionated dose schedules (i.e. dividing the total dose into a number of daily or twice daily doses for 3–4 days) is believed to permit the use of higher doses with a reduced risk of toxicity, especially late adverse effects. This is particularly important for younger children, who are especially vulnerable to chronic toxicity adversely affecting neurocognitive function and growth potential.

Immunosuppression

As indicated above, chemotherapy and radiotherapy both provide important immunosuppressive effects to reduce the risk of graft rejection and GVHD. The increasing use of alternative donor HSCTs has necessitated the development of conditioning regimens with additional immunosuppressive effect. Initially, this was principally provided by *in vivo* serotherapy (monoclonal or polyclonal antibodies directed against T lymphocytes) or *in vitro* T-cell depletion techniques, or a combination of both (see below). More recently, the increasing use of fludarabine has provided extra immunosuppression with relatively little extra acute or chronic toxicity. Initially fludarabine was used predominantly in nonmyeloablative conditioning regimens, but increasingly it is now a component of conventional myeloablative regimens.

Prevention of GVHD

GVHD is a major cause of morbidity and mortality in allogeneic HSCT recipients. Various strategies have evolved to prevent, reduce and treat this significant complication. Acute GVHD occurs by definition in the first 100 days post transplant and chronic GVHD after this period. In practice, however, these cut-offs are not absolute and patients can present with symptoms typical of chronic GVHD in the early weeks after transplant and with symptoms typical of acute GVHD at times beyond day 100.

The best means of reducing the risk or severity of GVHD is to use a well-matched donor, ideally an HLA-identical sibling donor. However, this approach severely limits the number of patients in whom a transplant can be performed, as only about 25–30% of individuals in the UK have a fully HLA-matched sibling donor. The use of alternative donors, especially mismatched RDs and matched or mismatched URDs, has greatly increased the pool of available donors, and it is now possible to identify a potential donor for most patients (especially children in whom greater degrees of mismatch are likely to be tolerated) in urgent need of a transplant. However, the increasing use of such alternative donors has necessitated the development of increasingly sophisticated techniques to prevent GVHD in order to reduce the incidence of severe acute or disabling chronic GVHD. It has become very important to seek the optimal balance of GVHD and GVL in the context of HSCT for malignancy, where some degree of a GVL or other graft-vs.-malignancy effect is important.

The three main methods used to achieve GVHD prophylaxis are:

Pre- and peri-HSCT serotherapy

Acute GVHD is mediated by donor T lymphocytes reacting against antigenically distinct host tissues (see Chapter 10). Serotherapy involves the use of antibodies directed against these lymphocytes to achieve T-cell depletion. The antibodies used most commonly are:
- ATG (anti-thymocyte globulin) – a polyclonal antibody made by inoculating either rabbits or horses with human T lymphocytes;
- Campath (alemtuzumab) – a family of monoclonal antibodies directed against the CDw52 antigen, which is expressed on a wide range of B and T lymphocytes and monocytes.

In vivo ATG or Campath serotherapy is given as daily intravenous infusions, usually for 4 or 5 consecutive doses before HSCT (starting early, e.g. day −14, or late, e.g. day −6, in the conditioning regimen), but occasionally "across the graft" (typically days −2 to +2). Both antibodies have half-lives of 2–3 weeks and therefore act on both host (thereby reducing the risk of graft rejection) and donor (reducing GVHD) lymphocytes. There is no definite evidence that either ATG or Campath is superior or inferior in terms of efficacy or toxicity, although there are theoretical grounds for expecting that the use of ATG might lead to a greater risk of post-transplant B-cell lymphoproliferative disease (since Campath depletes both B and T cells, whereas ATG depletes only T cells). Both ATG and Campath can cause significant early reactions or later side effects (Table 3.9).

Table 3.9 Adverse effects of ATG or Campath serotherapy

Early reactions (commonest after first dose)
- fever
- rash
- cardiovascular
- respiratory
- gastrointestinal disturbances, most often occurring after the first dose

Late adverse effects (weeks to months after treatment)
- serum sickness
- prolonged severe lymphopenia (associated with a significant risk of potentially serious viral infections, e.g. disseminated adenovirus infection)

Table 3.10 Side effects of ciclosporin A and tacrolimus

- Nephrotoxicity – glomerular impairment, hypomagnesemia
- Hypertension
- Neurotoxicity* – variable manifestations, ranging from severe headache and visual disturbance to convulsions and encephalopathy
- Hypertrichosis*
- Gum hypertrophy*
- Impaired glucose homeostasis
- Marked immunosuppression

* especially ciclosporin A.

In vitro *T-cell depletion*

BM and PBSC harvests may be depleted of T lymphocytes *in vitro* by a variety of physical and immunological techniques. Historically, physical methods to remove T cells have included:
- sheep red blood cell rosetting;
- counterflow centrifugal elutriation (a separation process based on the cells' physical properties);
- fractionation on a density gradient.

Immunological techniques to achieve T-cell depletion have included:
- antibody-mediated purging (e.g. using Campath 1M, activated via complement);
- immunomagnetic positive selection (e.g. of CD34-positive cells) to give a stem cell population;
- immunomagnetic negative selection (e.g. of CD3-positive cells) to remove T cells.

Post-HSCT immunosuppression

This may include the use of:
- ciclosporin A;
- methotrexate;
- tacrolimus (FK 506);
- corticosteroids;
- mycophenolate mofetil (MMF).

The commonest immunosuppressive drug used post-HSCT has been ciclosporin A, sometimes with the addition of a short course of intravenous boluses of methotrexate (3 or 4 doses, over the first 6–18 days post-HSCT). Ciclosporin is given intravenously initially, with the dosage adjusted by measuring trough blood levels, and converted to oral administration once tolerated (usually once mucositis has resolved). The duration of ciclosporin varies from 1 to 12 months (occasionally longer), and depends on:
- type of HSCT, and hence the risk of GVHD (continued longer when risk of GVHD is higher);
- indication for HSCT (usually withdrawn earlier in high-risk malignancies);
- the occurrence (or not) of acute GVHD (continued for longer).

Occasionally, ciclosporin may need to be continued for longer in patients with chronic GVHD. Tacrolimus is increasingly used as an alternative to ciclosporin. Both of these drugs have many side effects, some of which may be severe (Table 3.10).

Corticosteroids, especially methylprednisolone, are used in many protocols, particularly those for UCB transplants. Mycophenolate mofetil (MMF) is sometimes used for GVHD prophylaxis usually in combination with ciclosporin.

Peri-transplant care

Chemotherapy administration

Patients undergoing HSCT require central venous access (see Chapter 2). There are many types of central venous catheter (CVC) available and the exact choice depends on the preference of the operator performing the insertions, the proposed duration of use and patient acceptability. The most suitable devices will have double or triple lumens to allow simultaneous infusion of medications, electrolyte solutions, blood products, and parenteral nutrition if required.

The exact schedule for chemotherapy administration will depend on the regimen chosen for conditioning the patient. Regimens using chemotherapy alone will be administered entirely within the transplant center but regimens including TBI may require patients to be transferred between centers. It is essential that where this happens there is good communication between the centers to ensure timely administration of other constituents of the conditioning regimen, peri-transplant immunosuppression and prophylactic medications.

Transplant centers should have written protocols for each regimen specifying:
• date and timing of drug administration;
• exact doses of drugs;
• volume and nature of diluent;
• recommended infusion schedule.

These can be adapted for each individual to take account of pre-transplant laboratory findings, and the individualized patient transplant plan circulated to all members of staff involved in the care of the patient during their admission. Due to the potentially severe toxicity of the agents used, attention to detail is essential.

Regimen related toxicity

As HSCT conditioning regimens frequently include high doses of chemotherapeutic drugs and/or total body irradiation (TBI), side effects are common and frequently severe. The toxicities occurring after HSCT may be classified as:
• early – occurring within the first few days and weeks after conditioning;
• late – occurring months to years after transplantation.

An exhaustive list of possible toxicities caused by HSCT conditioning regimens is beyond the scope of this text, but some of the more common manifestations of early toxicity are described below and summarized in Table 3.11. Others are described in more detail in Chapter 9. Delayed toxicities are described in detail in Chapter 16.

Table 3.11 Side effects of conditioning regimens

• Nausea and vomiting
• Alopecia
• Gastrointestinal
    • Oral mucositis
    • Esophagitis
    • Diarrhea
    • Typhlitis
• Hepatic veno-occlusive disease
• Pulmonary
    • Idiopathic pneumonitis
    • Infection
• Renal
• Cardiac
• Allergic or idiosyncratic reactions
• Hemorrhagic cystitis

Side effects common to most conditioning regimens

Nausea and vomiting

These are most troublesome during administration of chemotherapy/TBI and the following few days. Conditioning treatment should be accompanied by antiemetic prophylaxis according to unit protocols, usually incorporating 5-HT$_3$ antagonists, and breakthrough nausea and vomiting usually responds to alternative or additional antiemetic agents. Occasionally nausea and vomiting may be severe and prolonged, especially if patients have experienced profound symptoms during prior courses of chemotherapy.

Alopecia

This is virtually universal after myeloablative regimens and common but not inevitable after reduced-intensity conditioning.

Gastrointestinal

These are caused by both high-dose chemotherapy and TBI.

Mucositis

Mucositis usually starts to develop about 48–72

hours post-chemotherapy/TBI, and may persist until neutrophil recovery. It may affect both the oral mucosa and the esophagus, as well as contributing to diarrhea as a result of enteritis. The period of mucositis may be prolonged by the post-transplant inclusion of methotrexate as GVHD prophylaxis. The severity of mucositis varies from patient to patient and is difficult to predict, but it may be severe enough to restrict or prevent oral intake of food, drink and medication. It may be necessary to provide sufficient calories by the parenteral route and to give all medications intravenously. Mucositis is the cause of much morbidity in transplant patients and is often the side effect that most declare to be the worst part of the whole transplant experience. In severe cases patients are unable to swallow their own saliva and severe pain may require high doses of opiate analgesia for several days.

There are no universally effective strategies to prevent mucositis. Some conditioning protocols recommend that patients should suck on ice cubes or ice lollipops during infusion of the chemotherapy drug to lower the temperature in the mouth, causing vasoconstriction and reduced blood flow. The dose of chemotherapy delivered to the oral mucous membranes is thus reduced and the potential for severe oral mucositis limited. This approach is only of practical use in conditioning regimens where chemotherapy is administered over a short period of time, e.g. melphalan, and does not significantly reduce esophagitis.

Superadded infection can occur, the two most likely organisms being *Candida* and *Herpes simplex*. Antifungal and antiviral prophylaxis are therefore routinely used.

Diarrhea

This is common in the early post-transplant period and is most often secondary to direct toxic effects of chemotherapy and/or radiotherapy causing enteritis, which may occur alongside mucositis and esophagitis. Enteritis is commonly aggravated by superadded infection and/or GVHD.

Typhlitis (neutropenic enterocolitis)

This can occur during the neutropenic phase post-transplant, usually as a result of bacterial or rarely fungal infection penetrating intestinal mucosa damaged by chemo-radiotherapy. Patients have profuse diarrhea accompanied by abdominal pain and fever. Abdominal X-ray or CT scan shows dilated large bowel. Colonoscopy may be necessary in some patients, revealing mucosal hemorrhage and ulceration. The differential diagnosis includes acute gastrointestinal GVHD and pseudomembranous colitis due to *Clostridium difficile*. Stool and blood should be cultured for bacteria, fungi and viruses, and broad spectrum antibiotics and antifungal agents should be introduced as indicated, together with other supportive measures and intravenous fluids. Conservative management is usually preferred as surgery is extremely risky in these patients, although typhlitis is itself associated with significant risk of mortality from bowel perforation or hemorrhage.

Hepatic veno-occlusive disease (VOD)

This potentially fatal early complication of HSCT is more common in the allogeneic than the autologous setting. Risk factors for development of VOD include pre-existing liver disease and intensive conditioning regimens, especially those that include busulfan or other alkylating agents. Classically, VOD presents with:
- jaundice;
- hepatomegaly;
- weight gain and/or ascites.

Monitoring of daily weight in the early post-transplant period can alert the physician to any rapid gains and the possibility of VOD. The investigation and treatment of this complication are outlined in more detail in Chapter 11.

Pulmonary complications

These are common in the post-transplant period. Many are related to infection but the conditioning regimen may also cause direct toxicity. Fractionated TBI, which has fewer pulmonary complications than unfractionated treatment, and the use of lung compensators to standardize the dose received by pulmonary tissue, is now standard practice to reduce the pulmonary toxicity of TBI. Nevertheless, idiopathic pneumonitis can still occur, presenting with:

- shortness of breath;
- dry or productive cough;
- interstitial shadowing on chest X-ray.

Patients presenting with such symptoms may need to undergo high-resolution CT scan of the lungs and/or bronchoalveolar lavage (BAL). The diagnosis of idiopathic pneumonitis is made by excluding infective or cardiac causes and by the absence of pulmonary hemorrhage on BAL. Patients with a previous history of pulmonary problems, or with previous exposure to known pulmonary toxins such as bleomycin, are at particular risk of interstitial pneumonitis.

Renal

Cytotoxic agents used in transplant conditioning regimens may cause significant alterations in renal function. However, other drugs used in the early post-transplant phase, such as aminoglycoside antibiotics, antifungal agents and ciclosporin, can also affect renal function and it can be impossible to determine which agent is primarily responsible. Careful screening of renal function pre-transplant can help to identify those patients at highest risk, and dosages of renally excreted or potentially nephrotoxic drugs can be adjusted accordingly.

Cardiac

Similarly, cardiac toxicity can be multi-factorial. However, regimens utilizing high-dose cyclophosphamide have occasionally been reported to cause acute cardiac failure. Pericarditis is uncommon but should be considered in the differential diagnosis of retrosternal symptoms.

Allergic or idiosyncratic reactions

These are varied, sometimes severe (e.g. anaphylactic reaction to ciclosporin, which may follow the first dose) and, by their very nature, difficult to predict.

Other common regimen-specific toxicities

Hemorrhagic cystitis

This can be caused by a number of cytotoxic agents but is most commonly seen after cyclophosphamide or ifosfamide, which are metabolized to acrolein, a toxic product that causes ulceration of the urothelial mucosal membrane, leading to:

- hematuria;
- pain;
- urinary frequency.

High-dose cyclophosphamide (as used in HSCT conditioning regimens) or ifosfamide should never be given without simultaneous intravenous hyperhydration and infusion of mesna (2-mercaptoethanesulphonate), which binds to acrolein, rendering it inactive. Regular dipstick surveillance for hematuria should be performed during conditioning with cyclophosphamide. Despite prophylactic hyperhydration and mesna, breakthrough problems can occur during the first few weeks after cyclophosphamide administration. Although the polyoma BK virus is often detected by PCR in the urine of patients suffering from hemorrhagic cystitis, its involvement in the pathogenesis of the condition remains unproven.

The treatment of established hemorrhagic cystitis includes adequate analgesia, aggressive blood and platelet transfusion support (to maintain a platelet count $>50 \times 10^9/L$), and the maintenance of a high urinary flow rate to reduce the formation of vesical blood clots that may cause urethral obstruction and painful clot retention. It is important to seek early involvement of an urologist to advise on the need for bladder irrigation or in extreme cases nephrostomy. Estrogens may be useful in some cases.

Peri-HSCT nutrition

As described above, intensive conditioning regimens frequently cause severe nausea, mucositis, esophagitis, and diarrhea leading to poor oral intake of fluids and food, and poor absorption of those that are ingested due to disruption of the intestinal membrane transport mechanism. The development of acute GVHD as engraftment occurs can further exacerbate gastrointestinal symptoms, and post-transplant medication such as steroids, ciclosporin or tacrolimus can interfere with glucose metabolism.

Patients undergoing HSCT have increased calorie needs, because intensive conditioning induces a catabolic state. Development of infection or acute GVHD will further increase nutritional requirements. The need for nutritional support in HSCT patients depends on:

- severity of the gastrointestinal symptoms;
- type of transplant (greater need after allogeneic than after autologous HSCT);
- pre-transplant nutritional status;
- likely duration of the post-transplant neutropenia.

The choice of how best to deliver nutritional support to transplant recipients is usually a simple one. Those most in need of support are those who typically have the most severe gastrointestinal side effects in whom it is inappropriate to deliver or rely on enteral nutrition. Total parenteral nutrition (TPN) can be given through the multiple-lumen CVC. However, there are no published guidelines on when or in whom to use nutritional support, and few randomized controlled trials on its effectiveness.

Reports in the 1980s claimed that bone marrow transplant recipients given TPN had a superior outcome to those not given TPN. It has been postulated that certain lipid constituents of TPN can reduce acute GVHD, and that oral or intravenous supplementation with glutamine can reduce mucositis, but these reports have not been confirmed.

Some transplant units initiate TPN in all allograft recipients from day one post-transplant whereas others have no standard procedure and decide on a case by case basis depending on the severity of gastrointestinal symptoms. In most centers TPN is not routinely prescribed for autograft recipients.

The transplant unit should have access to a trained dietician who can assess patients' calorie, nitrogen balance and other nutritional needs and who can supervise the ordering of TPN. Daily monitoring is essential as fluid and nutritional requirements can change quickly.

Patients receiving TPN are not usually prevented from taking small amounts of nutrition orally if they are capable. Indeed, continued enteral intake is actively encouraged in view of recent evidence that it facilitates gastrointestinal recovery from the acute effects of mucositis. Delivery of enteral feed via a nasogastric tube, or occasionally a gas-

trostomy, is now considered a standard part of the feeding strategy in children undergoing HSCT.

TPN is discontinued when there is evidence of mucosal recovery and the patient is taking at least a proportion of the required calories orally. Prolonged administration of TPN can depress appetite, and problems can occur with fluid overload, infected central venous catheters, glucose intolerance requiring simultaneous administration of insulin, and disturbances of liver function.

Blood product support

Most if not all patients undergoing transplantation will at some stage require red cell and platelet transfusion support. Requirements will vary from patient to patient and will generally be greater in high-intensity allogeneic recipients than reduced-intensity allogeneic and autograft recipients

CMV infection

Cytomegalovirus infection as a consequence of immunocompromise post-HSCT is a significant risk to patients, as it can cause potentially fatal organ damage, although PCR testing and preemptive antiviral therapy has greatly reduced this. Consequently, potential HSCT candidates who are CMV negative (or whose CMV status is as yet unknown) should be given CMV-seronegative blood products to minimize seroconversion. Use of such CMV-negative blood components in CMV-negative recipients is associated with a low risk of reactivation (1–3%); such breakthrough infection may be due to low antibody levels in previously exposed donors or recent blood donor infection (or very occasionally primary infection post-HSCT via oropharyngeal contact). Leukocyte depletion (as practiced throughout the UK to reduce risk of variant CJD) also reduces CMV transmission by blood products, although there is some uncertainty about whether it is completely effective, and so most HSCT units still give CMV-negative blood components to CMV-negative recipients of autologous grafts or CMV-negative allogeneic grafts.

Transfusion-associated GVHD (TAGVHD)

Persistence and proliferation of blood donor-derived lymphocytes in immunocompromised recipients can lead to TAGVHD, with fever, skin rash, jaundice, and diarrhea leading to very high mortality. The lymphocyte dose required to cause TAGVHD may be below that generated by leukodepletion, hence gamma-irradiation to 25 Gray is necessary for cellular products (but not for FFP). Individuals whose blood components require gamma-irradiation include:

- autologous recipients: from 7 days prior to harvest until 3 months post-HSCT (6 months if TBI conditioning);
- allogeneic recipients: from conditioning until off immunosuppression and free from GVHD or lymphopenia (1×10^9/L);
- donors of marrow for allogeneic recipients: at time of harvest;
- all HLA-matched platelet transfusions (or donations from first/second-degree relatives).

ABO incompatibility

Around 20–25% of HLA-identical related donor–recipient pairs differ at ABO blood group, with a higher proportion amongst unrelated donor transplants. ABO incompatibility in HSCT brings particular problems, related to both acute and delayed hemolysis (potential delay of engraftment occurs, but appears largely confined to reduced-intensity HSCT). Major mismatch consists of recipient possession of isohemagglutinins reactive against new antigen(s) from the donor (e.g. A, B or AB donor into O recipient, and AB donor into A or B recipient); minor mismatch involves new isohemagglutinin from the donor reactive against recipient red cell antigen(s) (e.g. O donor into A, B or AB recipient, and A or B donor into AB recipient). Major and minor mismatch can coexist when there is bidirectional isohemagglutinin present (e.g. A donor into B recipient, or vice versa).

In major ABO incompatibility, acute intravascular hemolysis can be reduced by ensuring that the graft is depleted of potentially reactive red cells. Red cell depletion of bone marrow graft can be performed by density gradient centrifugation, gravity sedimentation or automated cell separation (the latter gives more reproducible separation and has the advantage of a closed system). Associated loss of stem cells occurs, but stem cell/mononuclear count recovery should be at least 75%. Red cell depletion is not necessary for most apheresis PBHSC harvests, as erythroid contamination is low level (hematocrit <10%; <20 mL red cells). Reduction of recipient isohemagglutinin titer can be performed by recipient plasma exchange (or immunoadsorption) prior to marrow reinfusion; unfortunately, rebound production of isohemagglutinin can occur early post-transplant. Blood product support after ABO-mismatched HSCT is summarized in Table 3.12.

In minor ABO-incompatibility donor isohemagglutinin reactive with recipient red cells can be removed by plasma depletion of the marrow graft (apheresis of PBHSC reduces plasma burden to acceptable levels). Delayed hemolysis is not uncommon, and not always predicted by pre-transplant isohemagglutinin titers. Delayed hemolysis may be due to synthesis of antibody by lymphocytes and plasma cells in the graft (hence greater risk with PBHSC rather than BM, due to higher lymphoid cell burden), or subsequent production from the engrafted lymphoid compartment. Agents suppressing lymphoid proliferation, including the antimetabolites methotrexate and mycophenolate mofetil used for GVHD prophylaxis, reduce this risk of delayed hemolysis. Use of Campath (alemtuzumab) also reduces anamnestic antibody production via B-cell depletion. Reduced-intensity HSCT may have increased rates of hemolysis compared to full-intensity HSCT, with reports of slower decline in anti-donor isohemagglutinins and delayed erythroid engraftment. ABO mismatch in reduced-intensity HSCT may be linked to higher mortality.

Non-ABO incompatibility

Rhesus-D (RhD) incompatibility can also cause difficulties with blood product administration in HSCT. RhD-negative components should be administered to RhD-positive recipients with RhD-negative HSCT donors, as there is a 10–15% incidence of hemolysis following minor Rhesus-mismatched HSCT. However, RhD mismatch does not appear to

	1	2		3	4	

Table 3.12 Blood components in ABO-mismatched HSCT

ABO incompatibility

Major

Red cells RRRRRRRRRRRRRRRRRRRRRRDDDDDDDDDDDDDD

Platelets/plasma RRRRDDDDDDDDDDDDDDDDDDDDDDDDDDDDDD

Minor

Red cells RRRRDDDDDDDDDDDDDDDDDDDDDDDDDDDDDD

Platelets/plasma RRRRRRRRRRRRRRRRRRRRRRRRRRRRRDDDDD

Major and minor

Red cells RRRROOOOOOOOOOOOOOOOOODDDDDDDDDD

Platelets/plasma RRRRABABABABABABABABABABABABABABDDD

Groups: R=Recipient; D=Donor; O=Group O; AB=Group AB

Time points

1 Commencement of conditioning

2 Infusion of graft

3 Anti-donor RBC antibodies undetectable; direct Coombs negative

4 Recipient RBC no longer detectable

affect engraftment, GVHD or overall survival. Alloantibodies have also been described post-HSCT against Kidd and MNS antigens; anti-Jk^a antibody in particular can cause an unpredictable and severe delayed hemolysis. Auto- and alloantibody production can occur in conjunction with GVHD, and may flare in association with tapering of immunosuppression. Vigilance and close immunohematological monitoring of LDH, direct antiglobulin test, liver function, blood count, and film are vital in the care of HSCT patients (reticulocytosis is not a good guide to hemolysis in the early post-HSCT).

Platelet transfusions

Platelet transfusions are likely to be needed in all allogeneic recipients and the vast majority of autograft patients.

In most transplant units platelets are transfused prophylactically in accordance with published guidelines (BCSH), below a threshold of 10,000/μL. The threshold may be adjusted upwards in the presence of sepsis or hemorrhage. Strict ABO matching is not as essential as for red cell transfusions. Advice on which group to transfuse should be sought from the hospital blood bank but options may be limited by reduced availability. Random donor platelet pools are usually adequate, except where HLA antibodies are present when HLA matched platelet pools must be obtained.

Infection prophylaxis and treatment of infection in the transplant patient

Patients undergoing all types of HSCT are at risk of bacterial, viral and fungal infections. The risk is related to the degree of immunosuppression and the duration of cytopenia post-transplant. Thus patients undergoing allogeneic procedures are at greater risk than those receiving autografts.

As well as physical isolation and hand washing by healthcare workers and visitors, prophylactic medications are used to decrease the risk of infection. Regimens vary from unit to unit, but patients undergoing allogeneic transplants will usually receive prophylaxis against *Herpes simplex* (aciclovir) and fungal (azoles) infections. Gut decontamination (e.g. with ciprofloxacin and colistin) is widely but not universally employed.

Patients who are cytomegalovirus (CMV) antibody negative with CMV-negative donors are protected by the transfusion of CMV-negative blood products. A CMV surveillance program is instigated early in the post-transplant period for those patients at risk of CMV reactivation or those with

CMV-positive donors. Pneumocystis prophylaxis is started on admission for HSCT or introduced at the time of engraftment, and then continued until immunosuppression is stopped and/or there is evidence of immune reconstitution.

Infection prevention, prophylaxis and treatment of bacterial, viral and fungal infections are covered in greater detail in Chapters 5, 6, 7, and 8.

Monitoring and surveillance

General monitoring

It is good clinical practice to medically assess HSCT recipients twice daily while they remain as in-patients, and at other times when asked to do so by nursing staff. Symptom assessment, clinical examination and review of charts can help to identify potential problems at the earliest possible stage and lead to prompt institution of correct therapy or timely organization of further investigations.

Blood counts, liver and renal function, and CRP should be monitored daily, and serum magnesium, bone chemistry, and clotting checked on alternate days or more often when clinically indicated. Some units perform routine surveillance blood, respiratory secretion, urine, and other cultures on a regular basis according to written protocols, while others only take samples when clinically indicated.

Transplant specific surveillance

Allograft recipients require:
• CMV surveillance (usually by blood PCR) if reactivation or primary infection is a possibility;
• blood PCR for adenovirus and EBV;
• monitoring of immunosuppressive drug treatment, for example, ciclosporin levels;
• monitoring of galactomannan antigenemia and/or aspergillus PCR to enable early detection of invasive fungal infections is becoming more widely available, and should be undertaken according to local protocols.

The frequency of monitoring varies from unit to unit, according to local availability of tests, and between adult and pediatric practice. Exact recommendations should be part of the transplant unit's written protocol.

Engraftment

Engraftment is defined as the attainment of:
• sustained neutrophil count of $>0.5 \times 10^9$/L;
• transfusion independent platelet count of $>20,000 \times 10^9$/L.

The time to achieve engraftment will vary from patient to patient, depending on:
• type of transplant (allogeneic usually longer than autologous HSCT);
• cell dose of graft (quicker with higher cell dose);
• product infused (BM usually longer than PB);
• type of post-transplant GVHD prophylaxis (methotrexate delays engraftment);
• post-transplant use of growth factors (e.g. G-CSF) (speeds engraftment);
• presence or absence of other features such as infection in the recipient.

According to the above criteria most patients will achieve engraftment 2–4 weeks post-transplant. Failure to engraft is now uncommon. Reconstitution of the immune system post-transplant takes much longer. Patients remain at risk of severe infection for many months and may require long-term or even lifelong prophylactic antibiotics (see Chapter 14).

Summary

Conditioning regimens involve the use of potentially extremely toxic chemotherapy and radiotherapy, and need to be tailored to the needs of individual patients. The HSCT team need to be aware of specific issues relating to each patient in order to minimize the risk of severe toxicity and to maximize the likelihood of achieving the transplant's aims. Supportive care, especially during the period of pancytopenia, is essential to optimize the chances of a good outcome of HSCT.

Further reading

Ascioglu, S., Rex, J.H., de Pauw, B. *et al.* (2002) on behalf of the Invasive Fungal Infections Cooperative Group of the European Organization for Research and Treatment of Cancer and Mycoses Study Group of the National

Institute of Allergy and Infectious Diseases. Defining opportunistic invasive fungal infections in immunocompromised patients with cancer and haematopoietic stem cell transplants: an international consensus. *Clin Infect Dis* **34**: 7–14.

Benito, A.I., Diaz, M.A., Gonzalez-Vicent, M., Sevilla, J., Madero, L. (2004) Hematopoietic item cell transplantation using umbilical cord blood progenitors: review of current clinical results. *Bone Marrow Transplant* **33**: 675–690.

Bensinger, W.I. (2004) High-dose chemotherapy and chemoradiotherapy preparative regimens. In: Atkinson, A., Champlin, R., Ritz, J., Fibbe, W.E., Ljungman, P., Brenner, M.K. (eds), *Clinical Bone Marrow and Blood Stem Cell Transplantation*, 3rd edn. Cambridge, Cambridge University Press, pp. 337–356.

British Committee for Standards in Haematology, Blood Transfusion Task Force (Chairman P. Kelsey) (2003) Guidelines for the use of platelet transfusions. *Br J Haematol* **122**: 10–23.

Casper, J., Camitta, B., Truitt, R. *et al.* (1995) Unrelated bone marrow donor transplants for children with leukaemia or myelodysplasia. *Blood* **85**: 2354–2363.

Dreger, P., Schmitz, N. (1999) Allogeneic transplantation of peripheral blood stem cells. In: *Baillière's Clinical Haematology* **12**(1–2): 261–278.

Eapen, M., Horowitz, M.M., Klein, J.P. *et al.* (2004) Higher mortality after allogeneic peripheral-blood transplantation compared with bone marrow in children and adolescents: The Histocompatibility and Alternate Stem Cell Source Working Committee of the Interantional Bone Marrow Transplant Registry. *J Clin Oncol* **22**: 4872–4880.

Giralt, S., Khouri, I., Champlin, R. (2004) Non-myeloablative conditioning: induction of graft-vs.-host disease effect as a therapeutic modality. In: Atkinson, A., Champlin, R., Ritz, J., Fibbe, W.E., Ljungman, P., Brenner, M.K. (eds), *Clinical Bone Marrow and Blood Stem Cell Transplantation*, 3rd edn. Cambridge, Cambridge University Press, pp. 357–368.

Heslop, H.E. (1999) Haemopoietic stem cell transplantation from unrelated donors. *Br J Haematol* **105**: 2–6.

Korbling, M., Anderlini, P. (2001) Peripheral blood stem cell versus bone marrow allotransplantation: does the source of hematopoietic stem cells matter? *Blood* **98**: 2900–2908.

Laughlin, M.J. (2001) Mini-review: Umbilical cord blood for allogeneic transplantation in children and adults. *Bone Marrow Transplant* **27**: 1–6.

Muscaritoli, M., Conversano, L., Torelli, G.F. *et al.* (1998) Clinical and metabolic effects of different parenteral nutrition regimens in patients undergoing allogeneic bone marrow transplantation. *Transplantation* **66**:610–616.

Pinkel, D. (1993) Bone marrow transplantation in children. *J Pediatr* **122**: 331–41.

Schloerb, P.R., Skikne, B.S. (1999) Oral and parenteral glutamine in bone marrow transplantation: a randomised, double-blind study. *J Parenteral Enteral Nutr* **23**: 117–122.

Skubitz, K.M., Anderson, P.M. (1996) Oral glutamine to prevent chemotherapy induced stomatitis; a pilot study. *J Lab Clin Med* **127**: 223–228.

Soiffer, R.J. (2004) T-cell depletion to prevent graft-vs.-host disease. In: Blume, K.G., Forman, S.J., Appelbaum, F.R. (eds), *Thomas' Hematopoietic Cell Transplantation*, 3rd edn. Oxford: Blackwell Publishing, pp. 221–233.

Veys, P., Amrolia, P., Rao, K. (2003) The role of haploidentical stem cell transplantation in the management of children with haematological disorders. *Br J Haematol* **123**: 193–206.

Veys, P., Rao, K. (2004) Allogeneic stem cell transplantation. In: Pinkerton, R., Plowman, P.N., Pieters, R. (eds), *Paediatric Oncology*. London, Arnold, pp. 513–537.

Warkentin, P.I. (1983) Transfusion of patients undergoing bone marrow transplantation. *Hum Pathol* **14**: 261–266.

Weisdorf, S.A., Lysne, J., Wind, D. *et al.* (1987) Positive effect of prophylactic total parenteral nutrition on long-term outcome of bone marrow transplantation. *Transplantation* **43**: 833–838.

Worel, N., Kahls, P., Keil, F. *et al.* (2003) ABO mismatch increases transplant-related morbidity and mortality in patients given nonmyeloablative allogeneic HPC transplantation. *Transfusion* **43**: 1153–1161.

Chapter 4
Care of the transplant patient

C. Charley and W. Larmouth

Introduction

During the past three decades caring for patients undergoing hematopoietic stem cell transplant (HSCT) has undergone numerous changes in an effort to meet the needs of an increasingly diverse and complex patient group. HSCT is now a potentially curative treatment for many more previously lethal conditions including hematological malignancies, solid tumors and non-malignant conditions such as aplastic anemia, autoimmune disorders, congenital immunodeficiency syndromes, and disorders of metabolism. Chapter 1 highlights the range of conditions for which HSCT is now being used. HSCT patients now come from a broader age range, more diverse backgrounds and are suffering from a wider range of conditions, the aetiology of which are now more fully understood.

Medical advances in supportive treatments and the growing diversity of patients' conditions continue to challenge nurses in the specialty. There is a need to be innovative and questioning in the approach to patient management and to the interventions we offer, in order to provide best standards of practice for this patient group. Care of HSCT should be carried out by a team of specialist nurses who are trained specifically in the management of HSCT patients. It is no longer enough for patients to survive HSCT – the quality of that survival needs to be constantly assessed by healthcare professionals and by the patients themselves.

The innovations in the field of HSCT have led to reduced length of hospital stay, and the environment in which the patients are nursed is now more varied. This may vary from strict isolation bubbles/rooms or single rooms to patients being nursed in their own home environment immediately after autologous HSCT. For this reason "protective care" is used in preference to isolation. Whatever form of protective care is provided for patients, the care given needs to have an emphasis on psychological support as well as administering treatment and monitoring the patients for very early signs of complications.

This chapter describes the care concerns and interventions commonly used, for both adult and pediatric patients during their hospital stay for HSCT.

Care of the central venous line (CVL)

Prior to HSCT all patients undergo insertion of a skin tunneled central venous line. This is an essential tool used for assessment, monitoring, support, and treatment of the patient. The use of the CVL is not without well-documented risk to the patient. The main complications following CVL insertion are:
- infection;
- thrombus formation.

The number of lumens and the frequency with which they are accessed influences the risk of infection. It is therefore of critical importance that everyone accessing CVLs employs meticulous standards of care; this must include:
- scrupulous sterile precautions when accessing the CVL;
- care in securing CVL;
- care in cleaning and dressing the CVL;
- microbiological surveillance of the CVL and exit sites as per unit policy;
- when blood cultures are taken these should be from each lumen.

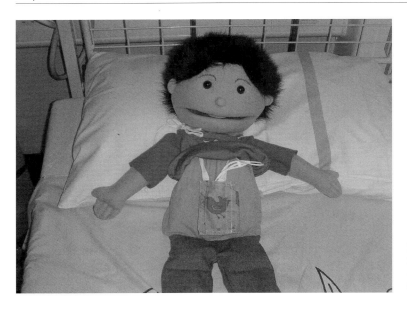

Fig. 4.1 Small pouches made of cotton to keep the ends of the Hickman line out of sight can be especially useful for children.

Young children may be inclined to play with their line or chew it. To avoid this it is often helpful to keep the ends of the line out of sight by using a pouch made from cotton (easily washable), which can be worn round the neck (Fig. 4.1).

Education of healthcare staff in the importance of CVL care is essential. Rates of infection greatly decline with the introduction of standardized aseptic care. Each unit policy should have a method of CVL care and training and on-going assessment of the competence of staff. Units should monitor their own infection rates to ensure compliance with their policies.

Control of body temperature and management of pyrexia

Body temperature is one of the most critical indications of wellbeing in the HSCT patient and should be recorded not less than 4-hourly using the same site (oral, axilla or ear). Recording ear temperatures may be inaccurate in infants under one year of age. Changes in mouth or skin integrity caused by rash or mucositis may require an alternative site to be used. The site where the temperature is taken should be recorded.

While the normal body temperature applies to HSCT patients, alterations in the usual pattern for the individual patient's temperature may be the first indication of a serious infection; however, absence of fever does not exclude infection. In addition, patients may suffer with flushing or chills during specific treatments, e.g. with Campath. Causes of changes in body temperature are given in Table 4.1.

Table 4.1 Causes of changes in body temperature

Conditioning phase (pre-transplant)	Conditioning drug therapy, e.g. serotherapy lysing cells
	Total body irradiation
	Stem cell infusion
	Infection – bacterial/viral/fungal
Neutropenic phase (usually during transplant)	Infections – bacterial/viral/fungal
	Engraftment syndrome
	Underlying disease
	Blood product support
	Acute GVHD
Non-neutropenic phase (post-transplant)	Infections – bacterial/viral/fungal
	Relapse
	Acute GVHD

Therapies that may mask increase in body temperature include:

- antipyretic agents used for analgesia, which should be used with caution and in line with the transplant unit protocol, as there is significant risk of inadvertently masking pyrexia;
- steroid therapy for the treatment of acute graft-vs.-host disease (GVHD);
- pre-medication prior to blood product support.

Body temperature control may be difficult to maintain due to drafts from positive-pressure ventilation systems, especially when hair loss has occurred; therefore, maintaining an appropriate ambient temperature is very important.

Management of pyrexia

The presence of fever, i.e. temperature >38°C on one occasion or of >37.5°C after two readings taken 2 hours apart, should be taken as a sign of possible infection that requires urgent further investigation and treatment. Each unit needs to have a protocol for the management of febrile episodes in HSCT patients. The nurse may be required to obtain blood samples for culture, serum C-reactive protein (CRP) and other specimens as part of an infection screen, prior to the administration of antimicrobial therapy. This should include broad-spectrum antibiotics as per unit protocol. Patients who become pyrexial may require extra platelet support and increased calorific intake. Chapter 8 outlines management of febrile neutropenia. Nursing observations and prompt actions taken in reporting fevers, obtaining appropriate samples and commencing therapy are of paramount importance in preventing septic shock in the neutropenic phase.

Nutrition

All patients should be encouraged to be in optimal physical condition and weighed prior to admission as there are several factors that may cause loss of weight during transplant care. A dietician can assist in choosing an appropriate diet for the patient.

During transplantation nutritional intake is often poor and enteral feeding may be required.

Table 4.2 Causes of poor nutritional state during transplant

- Mucositis
- Nausea and vomiting caused by chemotherapy/radiotherapy
- Acute or chronic gastrointestinal GVHD
- Poor absorption of food following total body irradiation
- Dental health problems
- Infection of gastrointestinal tract
- Altered taste and dry mouth
- Dislike of food offered and lack of availability of favorite foods
- Anxiety or distress

Mucositis is the commonest cause of poor nutritional intake (Table 4.2).

Conditioning regimens frequently cause severe nausea, mucositis, esophagitis, and diarrhea leading to poor oral intake of fluids and food, and poor absorption of those food and fluids that are ingested because of disruption of the intestinal membrane transport mechanism. Preventative measures such as regular mouth care using soft toothbrushes and sponges, prevention of infection, and adequate pain control are vital. An oral assessment tool may be used to monitor mucosal health and guide treatment.

The development of acute GVHD as engraftment occurs can further exacerbate gastrointestinal (GI) symptoms, and post-transplant medication such as steroids, ciclosporin and tacrolimus can interfere with glucose metabolism.

Patients undergoing HSCT have increased calorific needs, because high-intensity conditioning induces a catabolic state. Development of infection or acute GVHD will further increase nutritional requirements.

The need for nutritional support in transplant patients depends on the severity of the symptoms, the type of transplant (greater need after allogeneic than after autologous HSCT), the pre-transplant nutritional status and the likely duration of the post-transplant neutropenic period.

Enteral feeding

There are no published guidelines on when to use nutritional support or in whom, and few randomized controlled trials on its usefulness. Artificial feeding, such as nasogastric (NG), nasojejunal (NJ) tube or PEG tube, may be unit policy to prevent poor nutritional intake, supplement poor fluid intake and preserve gut integrity in high-risk transplantation, e.g. matched unrelated allogeneic transplants. The frequency of tube changes should be dictated by the manufacturer's recommendation and the patient's platelet count. These procedures should be performed prior to transplant, while the platelet count is above 100×10^9/L or performed with platelets support. It should be explained to patients that continued enteral feeding should reduce the risk of gut GVHD and shorten the length of stay. Intravenous feeding may prove necessary in some patients.

Total parenteral nutrition (TPN)

Some transplant units initiate TPN in all allograft recipients from day one post-transplant, whereas others have no standard procedure and decide on a case by case basis depending on the severity of gastrointestinal symptoms. In most centers TPN is not routinely prescribed for autograft recipients. TPN can be given through the multiple lumen central venous catheter already in place. The following criteria can be used to define the need for TPN:

- severe malnutrition at admission;
- at least 7–10 days of minimal oral intake;
- weight loss of more than 10% during treatment.

The transplant unit should have access to a trained dietician who can assess the patients' calorific, nitrogen balance and other nutritional needs, and who can supervise the ordering of TPN. Electrolytes, minerals, vitamins and trace elements (chromium, zinc, copper, manganese, selenium) are added to the TPN according to the recommended daily amount. Daily monitoring is essential since fluid and nutritional requirements can change quickly. Table 4.3 summarizes the monitoring that is needed for TPN patients.

Patients receiving TPN are not usually prevented from taking small amounts of nutrition orally if they are capable. TPN is discontinued when there is evidence of mucosal recovery and the patient is taking at least a proportion of required calories orally. Prolonged administration of TPN can de-

Table 4.3 Monitoring required for patients receiving TPN

Daily	Once a week	Once a month
Weight	Lipid profile	Serum zinc,
Fluid balance	Calorie and protein	copper, selenium,
Serum electrolytes	intake	manganese, B12,
Serum urea & creatinine		folate, iron, ferritin
Liver function tests		
Serum magnesium		
Serum calcium		
Serum phosphorus		

press appetite, and problems can occur with fluid overload, infected central venous lines, glucose intolerance requiring simultaneous administration of insulin, and disturbances of liver function.

Transaminases often rise 1–2 weeks after the start of TPN. Increases in bilirubin and alkaline phosphatase generally occur 1–2 weeks later. These changes often resolve spontaneously without long-term consequences, especially if the period of administration of TPN is short (< 3 months). However, elevated liver enzymes have multiple causes in HSCT and the differential diagnosis may be difficult. Shortening the period of infusion of TPN from 24 hours to 12–20 hours, decreasing the non-protein calorie intake and commencing treatment with ursodeoxycholic acid may help.

Potential benefits of nutritional support in allogeneic transplant recipients

Reports in the 1980s claimed that HSCT patients given TPN had a superior outcome to those not given TPN. In addition, it has been postulated that certain lipid constituents of TPN can reduce acute GVHD, and that oral supplementation with glutamine can reduce mucositis. Subsequent studies have failed to confirm the beneficial effects of oral or intravenous glutamine and further studies in homogeneous groups of patients are required to fully evaluate its usefulness.

Nursing intervention to improve nutritional intake:

- Provide small frequent meals, offering patient's chosen menu whenever possible.

- Provide patient information on diet. Determine with patients which food to avoid, if unit policy is to provide a low-bacterial diet.
- Determine which other foods to avoid that would cause irritation of the GI tract, e.g. spicy food.
- Administer anti-emetics prophylactically, in combination, and at a frequency that prevents nausea and vomiting.
- Use a mouth care program to provide adequate pain relief for oral health problems.
- Consider artificial saliva.
- Encourage high-calorie drinks.

Patients receiving steroids may gain excessive weight due to abnormal fat deposits and this may require dietary adjustment. For some transplant patients the ability to maintain or gain weight may remain a problem in the post-transplant period, especially if re-admission for post-transplant complications occurs.

Mouth care

Maintaining good oral hygiene is important in preventing and treating mucositis, which may occur as a consequence of chemotherapy. Mucositis can be very painful, therefore early and adequate pain relief is important to help maintain oral fluid intake and nutrition. An oral assessment tool may be used to monitor mucosal health and guide treatment.

- Teeth and oral cavity should be assessed pre-transplant and any dental work carried out and infections treated prior to HSCT.
- Regular mouth care should be performed even when not eating.
- Antibacterial mouth rinses, e.g. chlorhexidine, should be used.
- A soft toothbrush should be used to prevent bleeding gums.
- Lips to be kept moist to prevent cracking.

The patient or the carer should report to the nursing staff:
- dry, cracking lips;
- signs of cold sores (herpes infection);
- ulcers;
- thrush;
- mucositis and changes in mucosal epithelium (may indicate GVHD).

Management of diarrhea

Diarrhea is a common complication during transplant and may be due to a variety of factors, such as the following.
- High-dose chemotherapy or radiotherapy conditioning regimens are common causes of diarrhea in the first week post-transplantation.
- Milk intolerance is a consequence of damaged gut epithelium and cell degeneration in the gut caused by the conditioning regimens, especially if total body irradiation is part of the conditioning regimen.
- Acute GVHD is the most common cause of diarrhea post-engraftment.
- In adults infection due to *Clostridium difficile* is the commonest infection. In children viral infections are more common, e.g. adenovirus, norovirus and parasites such as *Cryptosporidia* may cause persistent diarrhea until engraftment occurs. GI infections are considered in Chapter 8.

Nurse interventions

- Ensure strict fluid balance and record body weight at least daily.
- Modify oral diet to reduce bowel mobility, e.g. minimize caffeine, cooked fruits and vegetable, and some lactose containing products.
- Monitor serum electrolytes and administer electrolyte replacements as prescribed.
- Monitor stool characteristics and appearance for infections, bleeding, and GVHD. Samples should be measured and sent for virology and microbiology testing as appropriate.
- Monitor the perineal area for breakdown of tissue and infection.
- Encourage good personal hygiene, keeping the area dry. A wound specialist team can be involved to give advice on barrier cream treatment as per local policies.
- Anti-diarrheal agents may be indicated once a diagnosis has been made and antibiotics and GVDH treatments as prescribed.
- Observe the patient for abdominal pain in association with vomiting or diarrhea. These must be reported and investigated immediately as they may

indicate bowel obstruction and require immediate treatment.

• The patient may require to be nil by mouth if there is excessive diarrhea with or without abdominal cramping.

• Administer platelet transfusion as prescribed, if the patient is thrombocytopenic or blood is present in stools.

• Ensure that the patient and family carer are informed of the reasons for changes in stool characteristics.

• Ensure that they understand the reasons for good personal hygiene in maintaining intact skin and preventing spread of infection (particularly washing hands during care episodes and when leaving the patient's area).

Post-transplant phase

Depending on the cause of abnormal stool characteristics, it may take many months for normal bowel movements to occur. Therefore poor weight gain in the post-transplant period can persist.

Prevention of respiratory complications

Due to their underlying condition or previous treatment, patients undergoing HSCT are likely to be at risk of respiratory complications. An awareness of actual or potential problems prior to the commencement of conditioning is essential. Pre-transplant assessment of the patient allows baseline readings of respiratory function to be recorded and for patients or carers to highlight concerns regarding respiratory function, e.g. contact with infected individuals.

Prior to admission to the transplant unit, the insertion of the central venous line (CVL) or other surgical interventions may afford an opportunity to perform bronchoalveolar lavage (BAL) to look for opportunistic infection. Samples sent for microbiological culture and virological studies help to identify infective agents such as cytomegalovirus (CMV). This is especially useful for patients with severe immunodeficiency who may be infected or colonized with a range of bacterial, viral or fungal pathogens prior to HSCT.

Table 4.4 Symptoms and signs of respiratory problems

• Respiratory rate
• Breathing pattern
• Chest wall movement, use of ancillary muscles and breath sounds
• Oxygen saturation
• Skin colour – remember that anemic patients are unable to become cyanosed
• Sputum – increase production/change in colour
• Coryzal symptoms – cough, increased nasal secretions

Regular observation of the above will help detect the early signs of respiratory problems (see Table 4.4). These may be due to drug or blood product reactions, fluid overload, interstitial pneumonitis, respiratory infection, compromised cardiac status or anemia. To help prevent respiratory complications the patient should be encouraged to be as mobile as possible in their protective environment by performing the following:

• regular and deep breathing exercises;
• aerobic exercise, e.g. stationary bicycle;
• changes in positioning, e.g. sitting, lying, or turning.

The unit physiotherapist can also organize an exercise program that takes into account the patient's condition and any factors, such as thrombocytopenia, that may make the patient more susceptible to bleeding.

Nursing actions

• Encourage exercises.

• Perform regular observations of breathing pattern and act upon abnormal findings.

• Administer medications via the prescribed routes. Intravenous drugs required may include antibacterial, antifungal and antiviral agents, and drugs to assist with symptom control (to reduce respiratory compromise), e.g. diuretics to decrease pulmonary edema and bronchodilators.

• Ensure that only sterile water is used for inhalation and for rinsing respiratory equipment, as mains tap water may contain *Legionella* bacteria and pose a risk of infection.

• Administer oxygen as prescribed, safely.

- Maintain a strict fluid balance and body weight record. The frequency will be dictated by the patient's symptoms or recorded daily.
- Obtain blood samples for CMV monitoring as per unit protocol.
- Collect samples of respiratory secretions if infection is suspected.

Sputum samples, if available, should be collected from adults or older children for bacterial and fungal culture. Nasopharyngeal secretions should be collected from children and adults with coryzal symptoms. Immunofluorescence staining of respiratory secretions or nasal washing can give a rapid diagnosis for viral pathogens, e.g. influenza A, influenza B, parainfluenza I–III, respiratory syncytial virus (RSV), measles. Further details are given in Chapter 7.

Inhaled medications are given for their direct effect on the respiratory system. All apparatus involved in the administration of inhaled therapies, e.g. nebulizers and masks, will harbor microorganisms between use if they are not decontaminated. Equipment therefore should either be single use and discarded, or decontaminated. A steam sterilizer may be used for this purpose; each patient should be allocated one for themselves on an individual patient basis.

After the administration of steroid-based inhaled medication it is recommended to clean the patient's face, mouth and eyes to remove any drug debris. (Rinsing the mouth will help to prevent a dry mouth and hoarseness of the voice.)

Prevention of renal and urinary tract complications

Renal insufficiency is a frequent complication post-transplant and its etiology is often multifactorial (Table 4.5).

Nurse interventions

These include the following.
- Monitor oral and intravenous intake.
- Weigh daily or more frequently if necessary (e.g. patients with veno-occlusive disease).
- Ensure appropriate renal blood flow by monitoring and controlling blood pressure.

Table 4.5 Causes of renal insufficiency during transplantation

- Nephrotoxic agents, e.g. ciclosporin, amphotericin
- Chemotherapy and total body irradiation conditioning regimens
- Dehydration
- Hemorrhagic cystitis
- Veno-occlusive disease
- Capillary leak syndrome
- Viral infections, e.g. polyoma BK virus (causing hemorrhagic cystitis)
- Bacterial infection
- Infusion of autologous stem cells that have been frozen
- Tumor lysis

- Monitor volume, frequency and odor of urine.
- Test urine for pH, ketones and blood daily. If thawed autologous stem cell infusion is given, the patient may experience pain over the kidney area as fragmented red cells are being excreted; hematuria may also occur.
- Send urine samples for bacteriology and virology as appropriate.
- Encourage oral intake of fluids if urinary output is low; if intake is low due to nausea or mucositis, administer fluids via nasogastric or intravenous routes as appropriate.
- Fluid restriction may be required in the case of renal failure.
- In severe cases of hemorrhagic cystitis, bladder irrigation may be required. A suprapubic catheter may need to be inserted surgically to facilitate this in some patients.

If intravenous cyclophosphamide or ifosfamide is prescribed as part of the conditioning regimen, extra precautions are required. These include:
- high hydration before, during and post cyclophosphamide/ifosfamide infusion to prevent bladder irritation;
- administration of mesna to prevent urothelial toxicity caused by intravenous cyclophosphamide and ifosfamide;
- monitoring every urine sample for pH and blood and reporting abnormal findings immediately, so that changes to intravenous input rate and mesna administration can be prescribed (urinalysis should show alkaline urine and "false ketones" from mesna therapy);

• more frequent weighing of patient during conditioning if there is a positive fluid balance;
• administration of i.v. diuretics if there is fluid overload;
• extra monitoring of electrolytes and i.v. replacement if required;
• bladder irrigation and administration of platelets if hematuria persists.

Skin care

Pre-transplant assessment of skin for infections should be carried out and any skin condition treated to reduce the infection rate during the transplant phase. Abnormal areas of skin, e.g. eczema, are likely to be heavily colonized by bacteria; swabbing patients pre-transplant may be helpful in deciding if skin decontamination is required pre-transplant. Each unit should have a protocol for management of patients colonized by resistant bacteria, e.g. MRSA. This needs to be considered at the pre-transplant assessment (see Chapter 2). Good skin care is essential during transplantation. This should include:

• care of central venous line site and surrounding skin (as above);
• strict hand washing after the use of the toilet;
• daily showers;
• keeping the perineal and perianal area dry;
• use of non-scented soaps if total body irradiation is used as part of the conditioning regimen;
• use of moisturizing non-scented body creams is recommended;
• keep fingernails short;
• dry shave only;
• as alopecia will occur, head protection such as a hat or scarf may be worn to keep the head warm, as the ventilation systems can cause a draught;
• if the patient has not previously had chemotherapy, a hair sample should be retained if the patient chooses to have a wig;
• the patient and any family carer should be asked to point out any change in skin integrity to staff.

The nurse should also regularly observe the skin for changes. This should include:

• dry and cracking skin;

• rashes, especially early signs of GVHD, e.g. maculopapular rash, dryness, scaling puritis, redness or itchy palms of hands and soles of feet;
• bruising or petechial hemorrhages;
• sore perianal area;
• signs of infection around any *in situ* artificial lines, e.g. CVL, PEG tubes.

Administration of blood products and stem cells

Although blood products are all leukocyte depleted, it is important that everyone is aware of the patient's and donor's cytomegalovirus (CMV) status, so the correct CMV status blood products are given.

In pediatric HSCT all the blood products used are CMV negative and irradiated as well as leukocyte depleted. In adults all blood products are irradiated and CMV-negative products are used for CMV-negative recipients

As detailed in Chapter 1, HSCT can now be performed using a variety of products (peripheral blood stem cells, bone marrow or umbilical stem cells) which are delivered to the unit either ready to infuse or frozen and in need of regeneration by laboratory trained nursing or medical staff, prior to immediate administration. The volume and nature of product containing stem cells can vary from 45 mL of clear fluid containing positively selected CD 34-positive cells to up to 1 L of whole marrow. This presents challenges to staff administering the cells, who must give the product in a safe and controlled way. The time scale for infusion will range from a few minutes for thawed cells to several hours for fresh large volume harvests. Patients are commonly premedicated with an antihistamine such as chlorpheniramine to lessen the risk of a reaction, while some are also given hydrocortisone, particularly to prevent reactions to the agents used to preserve the stem cells. Prehydration is not usual in pediatric patients or adults with good renal function. The administration of the stem cells is often viewed with apprehension by the patient and is generally seen as an anticlimax. The patient and family may wish to record the event with photographs or express a wish for a particular person to be present. This is most likely when a family donor is used. It is advisable to ask the patient before the day of the transplant if they have any specific wishes so that appropriate preparations can be made.

Reactions and side effects of infused stem cells

Patients receiving fresh stem cell infusions should be observed in the same way as they would during any other fresh blood product infusion.

Reactions and side effects for patients receiving thawed stem cells are the same as for fresh stem cells, plus the following:
• flushing of the face often occurs if given too quickly;
• altered taste due to the preservative (DMSO);
• hematuria post-infusion;
• pain around the kidney area as red blood cells are passed through the kidney;
• excretion of the DMSO through the skin and breath for several days. Patient, family and visitors should be warmed of this.

Maintaining a safe environment

All patients undergoing HSCT will undergo some period of protective isolation; this is likely to have an adverse effect on their emotional and psychological wellbeing. Staff are likely to be required to balance risk between the patient's physical and psychological wellbeing. Chapter 5 deals with aspects of prevention of infection, including maintaining a clean environment.

The length of stay in hospital will depend on the indication for transplant, the type of HSCT performed, the condition of the patient, the type of protective care utilized within the department, and the complications encountered during HSCT. Patients should be encouraged to "personalise" their space with personal items (which should be in good order), either to use or to place on the notice boards, etc. This can often cause the facility to become overcrowded and difficult to keep clean; therefore storage should be carefully selected and managed. In an effort to prevent patient and staff

injury, the following should be considered during each nursing shift.
• The patient's room should be kept as tidy as possible to facilitate cleaning and to allow easy access.
• Surfaces, equipment, and floors should be cleaned daily and a record of this kept to ensure compliance and communication between staff.
• Disposable items such as bedpans and urinary bottles should be changed frequently.
• Staff must be able to ensure that they have easy access to emergency equipment within each patient's area.
• Electrical and phone cables from hospital and patient equipment must not obstruct free movement.
• The works department should check any electrical equipment that has been brought into the facility.
• Encourage the patient to move with care when their platelet counts are low.
• Patients should be discouraged from walking barefoot.
• It may be necessary to use cot sides to prevent falls in patients who may become drowsy or confused due to the effects of medication or illness.
• There should be a clear policy regarding visiting by children and casual, non-family visitors, or any visitors with potential infections. Numbers of visitors may need to be restricted to lessen the risk of nosocomial infection (see Chapter 5).

To help provide an environment free from infection, the following remain important:
• good hand washing technique prior to entering the patient's area;
• wearing of protective clothing;
• daily change of bedding, patient clothes, and towels;
• patient dedicated nursing and medical equipment that will be required throughout the transplant period, e.g. monitoring equipment;
• patients may be required to use a particulate filter facemask (SF2) when they are required to leave their protected environment for any reason during the neutropenic phase of transplant or if they are at high risk of fungal infection (e.g. receiving high dose steroids for GVHD) – this is particularly important if there is building work in the vicinity of the transplant unit.

Mobilizing

While the patient is not likely to be restrained in any way during transplantation, full activity is inhibited by:
- pain or discomfort;
- medication;
- attachment to an infusion device;
- limited space in isolation;
- psychological distress: fear or anxiety.

However, mobilization is essential whenever possible in order to maintain:
- muscle strength and bulk;
- balance;
- optimal circulatory and respiratory function;
- good skin integrity.

Mobilization is also essential in the child for:
- developmental progress;
- spatial awareness.

The physiotherapy team should be involved in helping the patient to plan and follow an exercise regime that can be adapted to use in bed, or while sitting or standing. Awareness of the patient's platelet count is important when encouraging mobilization so as not to encourage activities that could cause bleeding.

The introduction of dance mats and exercise bicycles can be helpful, especially if offered in an innovative or interesting way, e.g. planning an imaginary route to a pleasant destination or a reward system for achieving time or distance targets set by the patient. Post-discharge, the patients may find it very beneficial to be part of a rehabilitation program that includes an exercise program.

Daily living

Personal hygiene and dressing

Personal hygiene is very important, especially in the neutropenic phase, as most infections the patients acquire are from their own body flora. Advice should be given pre-transplant and again emphasized while in hospital.

A patient's stay in hospital during the transplant phase will vary from 3 weeks for patients undergoing autologous HSCT up to several months for allogeneic HSCT. It is very important that the patient should have some control of their daily activities and time for privacy. Personal hygiene and dressing is one of these activities.

Prior to admission, it may be helpful to discuss how the patient and family carers will cope with the protective care and length of stay from an inclusive and practical viewpoint. Individualizing their single room with their personal belongings and bringing in "day clothes" to wear during the day may help to give some structure to the day. If washing and drying of day clothes is a problem for relatives then it should be stressed that night-clothes can be worn. All clothes should allow easy access to central venous lines.

Discharge from the transplant unit

The patient must be aware that personal hygiene remains important, as they will still be prone to infections and GVHD if they have received an allogeneic transplant. Further details on prevention of infection post-transplant are given in Chapter 14.

Sleeping

During the process of HSCT nursing interventions are usually required throughout the 24-hour period. Efforts must be taken to minimize disturbance during night hours. Even on busy units staff should ensure that the unit environment changes to reflect day and night time, with reduced lighting and noise levels at night while giving patients the same level of supervision and nursing care.

Patients should be encouraged to change clothing, as if at home, during the 24-hour period. Normal sleep patterns may be disrupted by fears or anxieties, which may be presented to the nurse during the night. Where fluid intake is strictly controlled it is essential to allow for the patient to drink when they awake should this be required. Total body irradiation may cause increased sleepiness, especially about 6 weeks post-transplant, and fatigue is also a common side effect of HSCT, so this should be explained to the patient.

The following may help improve the patient's comfort and ability to sleep.
- Continuation of familiar bedtime rituals can be comforting and promote wellbeing and so sleep.

• It is helpful to inform the patient if it is likely they will be disturbed during the night, e.g. for the administration of a medication, so that they are not alarmed by an unexpected intrusion.

• Appropriate analgesia or strategies should be used to reduce nausea and itching.

• Steroid therapy for GVHD often disturbs sleeping pattern. Administration of steroid during the early part of the day, instead of at night, may improve this side effect of treatment.

Patients may want to bring in their own duvets, pillows and bedding. This will depend on unit policy.

Communicating and psychological support

During transplant, patients and their relatives differ in the amount of information they require and can understand. Some patients and parents appreciate as much written information as possible and use the internet as a resource; other patients and families ask for only limited and purely practical information. While all those in our care should expect honest and open communication, it is inappropriate to offer information in a situation that is not pertinent to the particular patient, which will increase anxiety or distress. Patients and their families and carers should receive both written and verbal information about the transplant prior to admission. The use of recorded tapes or videos may also be appropriate. It is very important to give the patient or family carers the opportunity to discuss on a daily basis up-to-date progress of their transplant, concerns and anxieties, and side effects of any treatment, and to provide appropriate psychological support. Provision of photographs on the transplant unit of all staff on the unit may help carers to get to know all those involved in the transplant team and to understand their roles (Fig. 4.2).

Where a patient or family has a poor grasp of the native language used in the transplant unit, it may be unwise to use a family member as an interpreter as, no matter how well meaning, important details may not be translated in an effort to spare the patient or their family undue anxiety.

The patient's ability to communicate verbally may be adversely affected by oral mucositis. This side effect of some conditioning regimes is likely to be severe enough to require opioid analgesia for several days. The patient can be reassured that this will pass and the use of mouthwashes and gels can be actively encouraged to promote healing, prevent infection and as symptomatic relief.

Confidentiality is essential, as in all healthcare settings, but can be difficult to maintain when

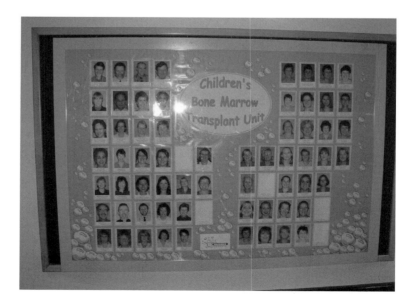

Fig. 4.2 Photographs of all staff on the unit can help patients and their carers understand the roles and responsibilites of the staff.

patients and family members compare and contrast their information and experiences with those of others on the unit; often forgetting that what applies to one patient may not apply to another.

It should be remembered that, during planned admission, patients will have been given information at each visit prior to transplant. This is often excellent but, when added to the information given on admission, can result in information overload, be misunderstood or misinterpreted, or some patients may simply forget some of the details offered previously. It is important to give consistent information and deviations from the expected course must be explained. Written information is very important and is easily accessible from patient support organizations; in addition, the unit should provide more specific written information.

If you are nursing a patient who requires very little information, it is very important that they receive information that they will act on, especially in the post-transplant period. Some patients will discuss their thoughts with everyone; others will find one person with whom they have a good rapport.

During the transplant phase, communication with the outside world is important; facilities within their room should help maintain contact, e.g. telephone, television, internet. Daily newspapers, post, and seeing friends and family are also important to help maintain a good quality of life.

Good communication, both written and verbal, across the multidisciplinary team is paramount in order to achieve seamless care for the patient. A culture of mutual respect between co-workers in all disciplines and parts of the service allows any professional concerns to be resolved to the benefit of the patient and staff.

Working and playing

The healthy individual often defines or describes themselves in terms of their occupation. This part of their life is often the part that is first to be threatened by illness, particularly when this is life threatening or involves complex treatment such as HSCT. The nurse and social worker are often able to assist the patient to develop strategies that en-

able them to work around the illness to a degree, should the patient and his employer agrees to this. Employers will sometimes allow patients to work part-time or flexible hours. Chapter 15 deals with the social aspects of care for the HSCT patient.

During the process of HSCT children and teenagers often wish to continue their school work and meeting the hospital teacher at the time of admission enables them to contact the child's school to plan how best to assist the patient to keep up with peers during their hospitalization. The teacher will usually visit daily during term time and will assess the appropriate amount of school work in the light of the child's condition at that time. The use of the computer and internet can be valuable in keeping in touch with classmates as well as researching lesson topics.

The nursery nurse or hospital play specialists (HPS) have vital and valued roles within the children's HSCT unit. Previous health problems may mean that children coming to HSCT have delayed development compared with healthy peers. By careful assessment of the child's developmental stage and an appropriate but imaginative play plan, the sick child can be assisted in reaching his developmental potential. The role of the HPS can encompass play preparation for procedures or treatment, which can help the child to understand what is to happen and to make their wishes known beyond the scope of their expressive language. The HPS or NN will often become the child's best friend, allowing time for them to be a child and have fun rather than just a patient requiring hospitalization. In the very young child or infant, careful and detailed documentation of the child's achievements during early days, such as first smiles and the ability to sit or stand, can produce a treasured record for a parent who is resident in hospital with the infant and unable to share pride in the child's achievement with the extended family as would normally happen at home.

Toys and games should be provided to stimulate young children. Figure 4.3 shows a cot under laminar flow which contains all the usual toys suitable for a young child. Toys and games can, however, be a source of cross-infection, particularly with gastrointestinal viruses, and so will need to be carefully selected with this in mind. Soft toys can usually be

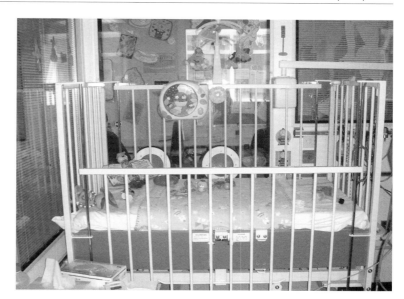

Fig. 4.3 A child's cot (under laminar air flow) can be made more friendly by the addition of the toys and brightly coloured equipment.

machine washed, as can some construction bricks and plastic toys with small parts. Other hard toys can be cleaned with detergent or alcohol wipes. Toys should not be shared among children on the unit.

Adult patients should be encouraged to bring in favorite activities, computer games, sewing machines, play stations or handicraft work. Mothers may use the telephone to maintain the daily activities at home. Older patients may bring in a laptop computer to continue work or use the phone.

Sexuality

Depending on the age of the patient, considering high-dose chemotherapy with stem cell transplant, sexuality issues will vary from what colour blankets or Babygro is to be used for the very young child to fertility issues for those of reproductive age.

Team members should be able to discuss issues regarding sexuality and give accurate information, act as an advocate and make appropriate referrals. It is helpful to have identified members to lead on fertility issues. Team members should not make assumptions, as some patients may not want information, but informed consent for the transplant process must be obtained and patients should be

aware of the side effects of the treatment that are likely to affect fertility. Chapter 16 discusses issues around fertility for the HSCT patient.

There may be other issues that can affect sexuality. These include damaged body image and change in role in the family:
• hair loss, weight loss, weight gain, central venous lines;
• husband not being able to provide for the family;
• mother not being able to fulfill her role as mother and housewife.

Team members should have some knowledge on the effects of treatment and to whom to refer the patients. They should know what is available for males and females and where to go if they do not have the answers. Support can also be given through written information, psychological support and items of clothing such as wigs or special head wear.

Dying

Patients approach treatment from all aspects of humanity and encompass all manner of diversity in their wishes and expectations. Religious belief and attitudes surrounding death may be privately held or publicly declared. It is usually the role of the nurse to ascertain the individual patient's attitude and to broach the subject in an appropriate and sensitive manner.

The prognosis for patients undergoing HSCT has improved dramatically in recent years. The conditions treated with HSCT are still considered to be fatal in nature, causing most patients and their families to consider mortality from a very personal perspective. Some patients may wish to consider HSCT as an opportunity to extend life; others may consider treatment to be another threat.

Death may occur during a period of acute deterioration in health during the transplant period, or more insidiously several months post-transplant. Graft-vs.-host disease or intractable infection are factors that can lead the vulnerable patient into multiple organ failure. In the active phase of treatment this is likely to cause the patient to require some degree of life support, with mechanical ventilation or inotropic support in the intensive care setting, which will offer the opportunities to consider the planned suspension or withdrawal of active treatment. Chapter 9 deals in detail with the management of patients requiring intensive care.

The role of the transplant nurse at this time is one of support for all those involved, especially when the patient is not being treated within the transplant facility.

The high dependency or intensive care units can intensify feelings of isolation to relatives of patients who are "institutionalized" in the transplant unit, so it is important that transplant and intensive care staff meet frequently and work together with the patient and relatives.

This phase of the patient's treatment can also affect the transplant nurse, who would often like to continue caring for the patient and family, and may feel excluded or a lack of conclusion when the patient is no longer in their care. In the ideal situation transplant nurses may be able to continue the physical care and emotional support of the patient and family alongside the intensive care team.

Once a decision has been made to withdraw active treatment the pathway of care for the dying patient should be followed, which may use specific treatments to make the patient comfortable and pain free. Whether death occurs as an acute event or following a drawn-out period of terminal care, the patient should be allowed to die with dignity.

Conclusion

Care of the HSCT patient during transplant involves not only ensuring that they survive the transplant and its complications but also that the quality of life is maintained as far as possible, working within the constraints of a transplant unit.

Further reading

Apperley, J., Carreras, E., Gluckman, E. *et al.* (eds). (2004) Supportive care. In: *Haematopoietic stem cell transplantation: EBMT Handbook*. Paris: European School of Haematology, pp 119–131.

O'Grady, N.P., Alexander, M., Patchen-Dellinger, E. *et al.* (2002) Guidelines for the prevention of intravascular catheter related infections. *Clin Inf Dis* 35: 1281–1307.

Otto, S.E. (2001) *Oncology Nursing*, 4th edn. London: Mosby, Chapter 24.

Roper, N., Logan, W.W. and Tierney, A.J. (2000) *The Roper–Logan–Tierney Model of Nursing: Based on the Activities of Living*. London: Churchill Livingston.

Tschudin, V. (ed.) (1996) *Nursing the Patient with Cancer*, 2nd edn. London: Prentice Hall in association with the Oncology Nursing Society of the RCN.

Twycross, R. (1997) *Symptom Manangement in Advanced Cancer*, 2nd edn. Oxford: Radcliffe Medical Press.

Whedon, M B., Wujcik, D. (1997) *Blood and Marrow Stem Cell Transplantation. Principles, Practice and Nursing Insights*, 2nd edn. Sudbury, MA: Jones & Bartlett.

Chapter 5

Prevention of infection during hematopoietic stem cell transplantation

W. Larmouth and A. Galloway

Introduction

Infection is a major cause of morbidity and mortality in hematopoietic stem cell transplantation (HSCT) patients and some risk may be lifelong. Attention to preventative strategies in the most vulnerable period before engraftment is essential and the highest standards of care are required to ensure a safe environment. Risk factors that make the patient more susceptible to infection during transplantation are shown in Table 5.1. The design of the transplant facility is crucial for ensuring that a unit can be kept as clean as possible. There is a place also for recognizing the needs of the individual patient and the requirement to protect the patient should be balanced against their holistic needs.

Methods to prevent infection

These include the following:
• prevention of exogenous organisms colonizing/infecting the patient (protective isolation, control of the air, inanimate environment, food, water);
• prevention of patient's endogenous organisms causing infection (prophylactic antimicrobials, gut decontamination, personal hygiene);
• reduction in invasive procedures that breach body's defenses (i.v. catheters, enemas, suppositories);
• augmentation of host defenses (colony stimulating factors, e.g. G-CSF, leukocyte infusion, i.v. immunoglobulin).

The following areas will be considered:
• clean environment;
• clean air;
• inanimate environment;

Table 5.1 Risk factors for infection in HSCT patients

Underlying condition and pre-transplant factors

Defects in T- and B-cell immunity
Hematological malignancy
Older age
Extensive antibiotic use
Higher radiation dose
Infection prior to conditioning
Relapsed disease
Prior use of live vaccines (e.g. BCG)

• water;
• food;
• personal hygiene;
• visitors;
• staff health;
• protective clothing;
• surveillance cultures;
• prevention of specific infections;
• prophylaxis for infection;
• spirituality.

Clean environment

The patient should be nursed in a single room. Where the patient is nursed and what protective measures are employed depend on the needs of the individual patient. The age of the patient, the underlying condition, and the wellbeing of the patient are critical factors. The type of hematopoietic stem cell product used and the degree of manipulation will affect the rate of recovery; the more complete the stem cell product the faster the recovery of immunological function. Oncology patients' response to previous chemotherapy regimes may help predict potential complications and problems. In immune-deficient patients the type and site of existing infection will affect the rate of recovery and the risk of graft-vs.-host disease (GVHD) requiring further immunosuppression at the time of engraftment. Isolation facilities should conform to the latest Department of Health standards (HBN4).

The room in which the patient is nursed should be clutter free and have adequate storage for reasonable amounts of the patient's property and equipment in frequent use. Overstocking should be avoided. Equipment, surfaces and floor within the room must be cleaned frequently and this can only be achieved if they are accessible. Drug cupboards and fridges within the patients' room should only contain current stock and should be cleaned on a regular basis. While the responsibility for the hygiene within the patient's room is usually assumed by the nurse, domestic services or the patient's carers are likely to assist in undertaking chores.

Flowers and plants

Flowers and plants shed a large number of fungal spores; also, flower water rapidly becomes colonized by *Pseudomonas* and other environmental Gramnegative organisms, and may be a source of infection. For these reasons it is recommended that flowers and plants are not allowed in the transplant unit.

Clean air

It is essential to protect the patient from airborne infection during HSCT. The most serious risk is from invasive fungal infection, especially *Aspergillus*. Invasive *Aspergillus* (IA) has an overall mortality of >90% in HSCT patients. Prevention of IA includes:
- HEPA filtration
- Anti-fungal prophylaxis (see below)

HEPA filtration

High-efficiency particulate airflow (HEPA) is essential for patients requiring allogeneic HSCT. The requirement of HEPA filtration for autologous transplant patients is not clear but should be considered desirable, especially for those with prolonged neutropenia, as this is a major risk factor for IA. HEPA filtration filters air up to 0.3 μm with an efficiency of >99.9%. It is recommended by CDC that the patient should be nursed in a sealed room with HEPA filtration and air changes >12/h. The system should have controls for temperature and humidity and air is delivered via a duct or grill in the ceiling of the patient's room or lobby and therefore clean air flows across the patient towards a low-level extract. The windows, walls, ceiling and doors provide a physical barrier to the non-patient area. The isolation room should be at positive pressure with reference to the corridor. This can be provided by either the source of HEPA-filtered air being from the lobby or directly to the isolation room. The lobby is required to maintain positive pressure and prevent air from the corridor entering the isolation room. The door from the lobby to the corridor and from the airlock to the cubicle should not be open at the same time to prevent air flow into the isolation room. The staff should be aware of the normal pressures and flow rates, and an alarm should enable staff to detect any loss of pressure, which may occur with a systems failure.

Figure 5.1 shows a typical lobby facility. Visitors to the isolation room would enter the lobby, wash their hands, and put on protective clothing (usually apron and in some instances gloves) before going into the cubicle. Outside visitors (family and friends, etc.) would be expected to remove outdoor clothing before entering the airlock, and also to wash hands and put on protective clothing.

Laminar air flow

This provides a high number of air changes (>200/hour) and is a mechanism for directing HEPA-filtered air either vertically or horizontally. This type of system requires the same specification as above. The aim is for filtered air to move over the patient and be drawn away at low level to ensure protection within the patient's living space. The use of laminar flow may be used as a less confining form of isolation, as the patient can see and communicate directly with staff or named visitors inside the room while remaining protected behind

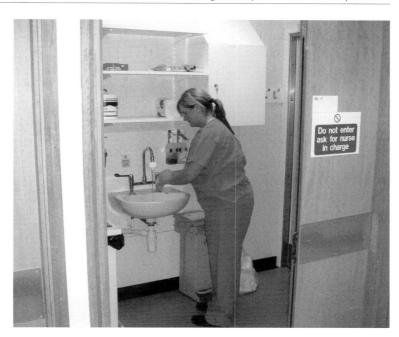

Fig. 5.1 Lobby (air lock) facility for an isolation room on a transplant unit. All staff and visitors should wash their hands before entering the isolation room.

the air curtain. Figure 5.2a shows an isolator that was previously commonly used for transplant patients and Fig. 5.2b shows a room with laminar air flow providing an invisible air curtain around the patient. For most patients receiving HSCT, laminar flow is not generally considered to give significant extra protection to that given by standard HEPA filtration, but has been shown to provide added protection for patients especially when building work is being performed on the hospital site.

Masks

Special face masks, HEPA particulate SF2 filter masks, which afford a high degree of protection to the wearer from the outside air, should be used for patients who need to leave the protected environment provided by HEPA-filtered air. They need to be carefully fitted on the face.

Building work

If building work (construction or demolition) is planned on the transplant unit or nearby then the infection control team should be involved in discussions with ward staff and the estates department to agree on the precautions that will be taken to protect vulnerable patients. There are several reports of outbreaks of *Aspergillus* involving immunosuppressed patients during building work, especially those on transplant units. HEPA filtration alone may not be adequate to prevent hospital-acquired infection, and attention should be paid to environmental cleaning and other aspects of prevention. Policies to control *Aspergillus* should be in place to ensure that vulnerable patients are protected at all times.

The inanimate environment

Walls

These need to be kept in a good state of repair to prevent release of organisms. A form of protective cladding should be used to prevent damage and facilitate easy cleaning. All surfaces should be nonporous and readily cleanable – unlaminated wood should be avoided.

Ceilings

These should not be suspended and need to be cleanable. Light fittings should be flush with the

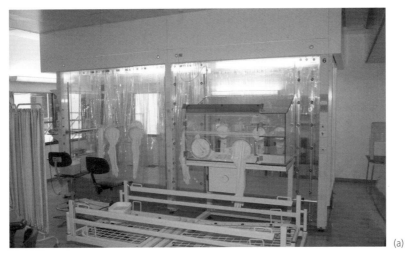

(a)

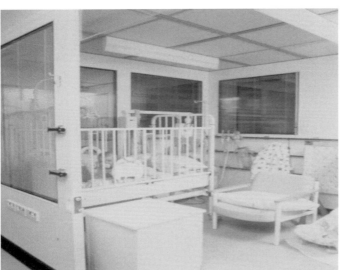

(b)

Fig. 5.2 (a) Isolator previously in common use to provide a protective environment. The patient is effectively in a clean air chamber. (Picture courtesy of Dr L.M. Ball, Leiden.) (b) Baby in protective isolation using laminar air flow provided from vents in the ceiling allows easy access and a more natural environment.

ceiling and easy to access for repair. Access to facilities should be made available.

Ensuite bathroom facilities

The surface should be smooth and readily cleanable (extensive use of tiling should be avoided). If there are concerns regarding *Legionella* in the water supply, the water from the shower or bath taps should be run at least daily when the patient is not in the bathroom. Showerhead filters (Pall®)

are also available that provide safe water (Fig. 5.3a). Plastic rather than wooden shower seats should be provided for ease of cleaning, and bath mats should be of material that is readily machine washable. Shower curtains, if used, should also be changed frequently and readily washable.

Fabrics and furnishings

Blinds, curtains and soft furnishings are not recommended. Blinds, if used, should be enclosed in glass as they are difficult to clean. Patients are often requested to bring personal items to hospital to individualize their space; however, the items brought in should be clean and in a good state of repair. Efforts must be taken not to damage the environment by applying adhesive material to surfaces and patients should be required to remove personal items, artwork and stickers before discharge. Maintenance teams should be readily available to perform repairs and should have an understanding of the HSCT patient's safety needs.

Toys and games

HSCT is often associated with a lengthy inpatient stay. Games and pastimes are essential to the well-being of the patient and smaller children/infants require stimulation to help their normal development. Items should be in good order and not exchanged between patients, particularly as this is an often overlooked source of cross-infection. Soft toys can be laundered should they become soiled or in need of cleaning. Hard plastic games parts can be cleaned by alcohol wipes and small games parts, e.g. plastic construction bricks, can be machine washed in a suitable bag or closed pillowcase. Strict attention should be paid to cleaning control units of televisions, videos, etc., as these can be a source of cross-infection.

Water

Drinking

Sterile drinking water should be provided in the pre-engraftment period. This can be boiled and cooled (cheapest option); filtered (added expense but convenient) or purchased (most expensive option). The decision to offer sterile water during transplant will be based on the patient's degree and duration of cellular reconstitution and is recommended by the Department of Health for all lymphopenic patients.

Figure 5.3a shows a Pall® filter in place on a bathroom basin. Filters need to be changed weekly or more often if used frequently, e.g. if used in a unit kitchen to supply sterile drinking water to several patients.

Cryptosporidia may be present in the mains water supply and will not be killed by chlorination. *Legionella*, *Aspergillus* and *Pseudomonas* may also be present in mains water. Water used for cleaning teeth should be of the same quality as drinking water.

Washing and bathing

Washbowls, baby baths, and toothbrushes should be cleaned and disinfected regularly, and stored dry to prevent infection. Damaged equipment

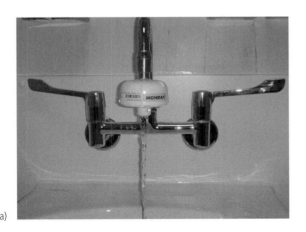
(a)

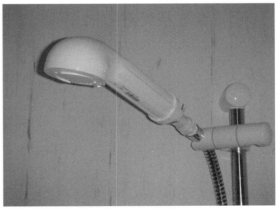
(b)

Fig. 5.3 (a) A Pall® filter on a sink tap in an isolation cubicle provides microbiologically safe water suitable for drinking and brushing teeth. (b) Pall® filters can also be fitted to showers in the form of a shower head, providing microbiologically safe water for showering.

should be replaced. Wash cloths should be single use and disposable. Showers and baths should be kept clean and dried. Care must be taken to decontaminate waste pipes and sink U-bends. Baths or washbasins should not have an overflow outlet. *Legionella* may be present in many hospital water systems and may cause infection. If there are concerns, then filtered shower heads are available that provide clean water (Fig. 5.3b).

Care must be taken not to submerse the end of the Hickman line in bath water. For children it may be useful to make a temporary cover for the Hickman line using a latex glove. This is demonstrated in Fig. 5.4.

Hand hygiene

Hand hygiene is the single most important procedure to prevent spread of infection and should be carried out regularly by healthcare workers, the patient and their visitors. Anyone entering the isolation room should wash their hands before entering and also on leaving the room. As well as being very susceptible to infection, the patient may be exposed to infections, such as norovirus, that may be easily transmitted by door handles, television controls, etc.

An antiseptic hand wash with water, or alcohol rub if hands are non-soiled, should be used to decontaminate hands. Attention to hand care is especially important for healthcare workers who may be washing their hands several times a day.

Food and diet

A low-microbial or sterile diet is recommended during transplantation.

Foods excluded during HSCT include:
- unpasteurized milk;
- uncooked or part-cooked eggs;
- live cheeses;
- fresh fruit and vegetables;
- hand-squeezed juices;
- shellfish;
- buffet foods;
- yoghurts;
- takeaway foods;
- spices, peppers, nuts and seeds that are uncooked;
- soups, snacks, etc., that are made by adding boiled water without further cooking.

Indications for a clean or sterile diet will be made on an individual patient basis depending on the integrity of the patient's gastrointestinal (GI) tract and the degree and duration of the patient's cellu-

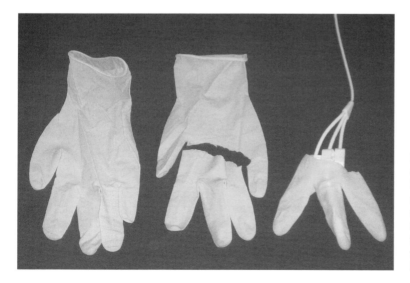

Fig. 5.4 A temporary waterproof dressing can be made for the Hickman line using a latex glove with the three middle fingers cut out. The lumens of the Hickman line are placed in the middle finger of the cut-off glove and the two remaining fingers are tied together to secure the latex covering in place.

lar recovery. In recent years the range of frozen and tinned products that are acceptable to the patient has increased, as has the range of small cooking appliances available, enabling the patient to choose food and have this freshly prepared whenever required. Nasogastric or gastrostomy feeds are commonly used to maintain weight and preserve GI function. Crockery and cutlery can be patient dedicated to reduce potential cross-infection. The use of an appropriate dishwasher can improve the quality of cooking and eating utensils. The use of steam sterilizers for the feeding equipment of infants and small children is essential.

Personal hygiene

As the skin harbors a number of organisms that may be pathogenic in the transplant setting, attention to personal hygiene is essential.
• The patient should have a daily bath/shower with a suitable body wash.
• Topical antibacterial agents e.g. mupirocin ointment (Bactroban®) may be applied to the line site if there is evidence of superficial inflammation (note that nasal preparation must be used, as standard mupirocin contains polyethylene glycol, which attacks plastic). An iodine preparation (e.g. Betadine®) may be used if there are concerns regarding the development of mupirocin resistance.
• Topical antifungal agents should be used if there is evidence of nappy rash or groin infection.

Visitors

All visitors must be free of communicable infection, e.g. respiratory tract infection, and follow good infection control practices at all times. The importance of hand washing must be emphasized for all visitors to the patient (clinical and non-clinical). In addition, visitors who may be incubating a communicable disease, e.g. *Varicella zoster*, should be excluded from contact with the patient. Those receiving oral polio vaccine should be excluded for at least 3 weeks post-vaccination.

Family and carers

The patient and family will be asked to name the individuals who are to support and care for the patient during the transplant. These named individuals need to commit to fulfill their role for the duration of the patient's admission and they should not be changed to include substitutes. The carers will be asked to shower and change clothes daily and should remove outer clothing when entering the transplant cubicle. They are taught methods of assisting the patient to undertake personal tasks and need to comply with unit hygiene standards and hand washing. Carers should also be briefed to report any problems, particularly infections and contact with infections, which may lead to their exclusion until full health has been regained. Young children are likely to carry potentially infectious viruses and should be discouraged from having contact with the HSCT patient.

Healthcare personnel

Healthcare personnel should always have a reason for entering the patient environment to limit contact. However, each nursing intervention should be used as an opportunity to interact with the patient to prevent depression, fear, anxiety, misinformation, and other effects of isolation in the face of illness. A doctor will see the patient at least daily for a detailed examination, and during this time the patient and family carers will have an opportunity to discuss progress and ask questions.

Other visitors

Other visitors should be welcomed to the unit but avoid physical contact with the patient. The patient should be provided with means of contacting the outside world through the use of an intercom, telephone, computer, etc. Visitors should be encouraged to offer support to the patient and family; this can be in offering practical help through shopping or laundry needs, or offering assistance with the care of the family's children. The casual visitor could offer the family carer time out by accompanying them for coffee or a meal. All visitors to the unit should be asked to wash hands on entry to the unit.

The infected patient

In the HSCT setting preventing infection is paramount but the patient may be infected with communicable infections prior to transplant and be a risk to other patients and staff. Patients infected with community respiratory viruses, e.g. influenza B, or respiratory syncytial virus, may continue to excrete the virus for several weeks/months until engraftment occurs. Similarly viral infection, e.g. with parvovirus or adenovirus, may be excreted for a prolonged period; indeed, clearing of infection is often a sign of successful engraftment. Strict infection control procedures need to be followed (especially hand washing and cleaning of the environment) to ensure that infection does not spread from patient to patient and cause an outbreak on the unit that may have disastrous consequences.

Staff health

It is essential that healthcare workers having direct patient contact should observe the following.
• They should be free from obvious infection.
• They should report any potentially infectious illness, or close contact, to the senior nurse as soon as possible so that appropriate treatment and exclusion can occur if necessary. This includes sore throat, herpetic lesions (cold sores and whitlows), diarrhea with or without vomiting, respiratory tract infection or rashes suspected to be a viral infection.
• They should be up to date with current vaccinations as defined by the Department of Health and local policy. Generally healthcare workers should be immune to measles, mumps, rubella, influenza and varicella. In the UK evidence of BCG vaccination is also usually required.
• Vaccine program may vary between countries and some staff may have missed out on what are now routine childhood vaccinations. Occupational health should play an active role in ensuring staff are vaccinated appropriately for their work.

• In UK newly employed staff with direct contact with HSCT patients will usually be screened for carriage of meticillin-resistant *Staphylococcus aureus* (MRSA) prior to employment and eradication therapy will usually be given before contact with patients is allowed.

Protective clothing

Personal protective equipment (PPE) should be used by staff attending a transplant patient, to protect the patient. Also the patient may be a source of infection and PPE will protect staff. If the patient is infected, PPE should be disposed of in the patient's cubicle and not brought out of the protected environment.

Personal protective equipment may include:
• gowns;
• aprons;
• masks;
• head covers;
• gloves;
• shoe covers.

The use of these will vary between units. The most important infection control procedure is hand hygiene, and the use of plastic aprons and gloves is also very important when direct patient contact occurs.

Plastic aprons

Plastic aprons are widely accepted as a requirement to protect the patient. The plastic apron may be worn under a long-sleeved cotton gown when caring for an infant or young child. The gown offers no further protection to the patient but is used for patient comfort. It also holds the plastic apron in place as it is likely to move away from the carer's lap or stick to the child's legs when being held.

Gloves

The use of gloves is usually dictated by hospital policy, but can be summarized by the use of non-sterile gloves when the staff member is to be protected and sterile gloves for any invasive procedure to be undertaken. Gloves should be put on in the patient's room after hand washing, and removed in the room before hand washing on leaving the room. Contaminated gloves should be changed before touching a clean area or accessing the central venous line.

Surveillance specimens

Patient

Taking routine surveillance specimens (for bacterial and fungal culture) is not widely accepted, so the frequency and type of surveillance specimens from patients should be determined by local policies, taking into consideration the underlying condition of the patient, the type of transplant used, and the prevalence of resistant organisms. Specimens may be taken routinely or only in response to a clinical indicator (e.g. appearance of a skin rash, diarrhea or pyrexia). Table 5.2 indicates the type of specimens that may be useful. In many instances, for patients in isolation a colonizing organism rather than a newly acquired organism will be the cause of an infection. Monitoring organisms and their antibiotic sensitivities colonizing patients may help decide which antibiotic to give the patient if they become febrile. HSCT units will each have a policy for treatment of a febrile neutropenic patient, which should be commenced promptly on suspicion of sepsis (see Chapter 8). Units will need to develop a policy for screening for resistant organisms e.g. MRSA and vancomycin-resistant enterococci (VRE). Screening for resistant organisms should be performed prior to admission for transplant

so that, if appropriate, eradication therapy can be started and completed before hospital admission for transplant. If patients remain carriers, repeated screening may be warranted during transplant. MRSA screening may involve taking swabs from the following:

- nose;
- throat;
- perineum;
- line site or any abnormal area of skin;
- urine if catheterized.

A VRE screen will usually involve culture of feces; occasionally throat swabs may also be useful.

Screening for viral infections, e.g. cytomegalovirus (CMV), is important during HSCT, to detect reactivation or primary infection from blood products. Screening for other viruses, e.g. Epstein–Barr virus (EBV), human herpes virus type 6 (HHV6), and adenovirus, is indicated for patients in primary immunodeficiency requiring HSCT. Chapter 7 deals in detail with the investigation of viral infections.

Environmental screening

The environment for each patient should be serviced and cleaned prior to the admission of the new patient. This would involve washing the walls, washbasins, bathroom facilities, and floor. While this can be done effectively with standard detergent-based products, chlorine-based products are recommended if the previous occupant of the room had a proven or suspected viral infection. The equipment to remain within the room should be serviced regularly (including entertainment equipment, e.g. television, video recorder, DVD, etc). Bath and washbasin drains should be disinfected regularly, as Gram-negative bacilli such as *Pseudomonas* survive well in the moist environment. It is possible to install sink traps which can be boiled to heat-disinfect the trap.

Air sampling for Aspergillus in a HEPA-filtered environment

Air sampling and settle plates are useful indicators of the air quality of the environment. Although not

Table 5.2 Surveillance specimens

Specimen	Useful to detect
Sputum or nasopharyngeal secretions (NPS)	Bacteria, respiratory viruses
Throat swabs	Bacteria
Blood cultures	Bacteria
Blood for viral screen	Especially CMV
Feces	Colonization with resistant bacteria; *Candida*

routinely recommended, this can prove particularly useful in monitoring the efficacy of HEPA filtration. In a HEPA-filtered environment no fungal spores should be found. Monitoring can be easily performed using an air sampler that samples a large volume of air (500 L) in 5 min. Figure 5.5a shows an air sampler and Fig. 5.5b shows a plate, after incubation for 5 days, showing numerous colonies of *Aspergillus* (unsatisfactory result). If *Aspergillus* or other fungi are consistently found on air monitoring, the HEPA filter and ducting should be checked as a matter of urgency. Although HEPA filters may generally be expected to last for several months, damage may occur and filters may need to be changed more frequently if there is building work nearby.

Particle counters (set at a level to detect fungal spores) are also useful in HEPA-filtered areas as no airborne particles equates to no fungal spores. A positive reading, however, will not distinguish fungal spores from other airborne particles. Close liaison between ward staff, infection control and the estates department is essential to ensure that a safe environment is maintained.

Water sampling for Legionella

HSCT patients are at greater risk of acquiring and dying from *Legionella* infection. The aim is therefore to supply water to the transplant unit that is free of *Legionella* bacteria. Screening of water samples should therefore be performed and appropriate action taken (e.g. heat disinfection or chlorination) if *Legionella* are found. A continuous dosing system with chlorine dioxide may help suppress growth of *Legionella* in the water system. Close collaboration between infection control and the estates department is essential to maintaining a safe water system. Clinicians should, however, have a high index of suspicion of *Legionella* in an HSCT patient with hospital-acquired pneumonia and should investigate the patient accordingly (see Chapter 6).

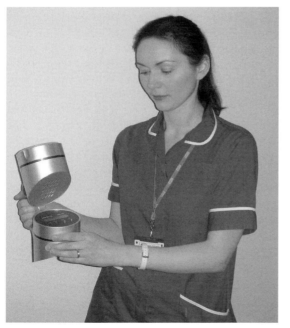

(a)

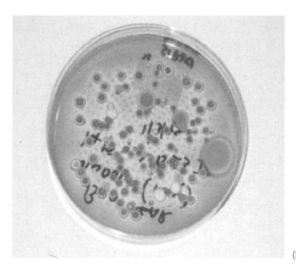

(b)

Fig. 5.5 (a) Hand-held air sampler. Air is drawn in through the top of the instrument onto an agar plate. Large volumes of air can be sampled in a short space of time. (b) Air sampling plate showing multiple colonies of *Aspergillus*.

Prophylaxis for infection

During HSCT the patient is at risk of infection from a wide range of bacterial, viral, fungal and parasitic infections. Many of these can be reduced by the use of prophylactic agents; examples are outlined in Table 5.3. The use and timing of prophylactic agents varies between units. However, treatment is usually started with conditioning and continued at least until engraftment for bacterial and fungal infections, and for 100 days for viral infection. However, prophylaxis does need to be adjusted to the needs of the individual and may need to be continued in patients with complications, e.g. graft-vs.-host disease.

Routine prophylaxis with ciprofloxacin in neutropenic patients is controversial. It does appear to decrease the incidence of Gram-negative septicemia but does not affect mortality. Each unit should have a policy on its use depending on local sensitivity data.

Gut decontamination

Gut decontamination is not routinely performed in the HSCT setting, although some non-absorbable agents, e.g. nystatin, are often used for fungal gut decontamination.

Co-trimoxazole prophylaxis covers a range of organisms, including bacteria, pneumocystis and toxoplasma, and will to some extent affect bacterial gut flora.

Ciprofloxacin and metronidazole taken orally have also been used as bacterial gut decontamination in cases where the gut has been damaged by viral pathogens, to prevent bacterial translocation through the bowel wall causing infection and inflammation that could lead to GVHD.

Table 5.3 Prophylactic agents used during allogeneic HSCT

Antimicrobial	Pathogen
Co-trimoxazole	Bacteria (e.g. pneumococci), *Pneumocystis*, *Toxoplasma*
Aciclovir	*Herpes simplex*, CMV
Itraconazole	*Aspergillus* and *Candida*

Granulocyte-colony stimulating factor (G-CSF), granulocyte-monocyte colony stimulating factor (GM-CSF) and granulocyte infusions

G-CSF and GM-CSF are products that stimulate the progenitor cells in the bone marrow to produce neutrophils (G-CSF) and macrophages and neutrophils (GM-CSF). In practice G-CSF is most commonly used in the HCST setting. Neutrophils are an essential defense mechanism and reduced duration of neutropenia may reduce the risk of infection. G-CSF is indicated to accelerate reconstitution after allogeneic and autologous transplant. The timing of its use varies between centers and it may be started between days 1–8 post-transplant and continued until the neutrophil count is $>1.0 \times 10^9$ L on consecutive days.

The use of granulocyte infusions (which need to be given daily) is controversial but has been used as an attempt to improve the neutrophil count if G-CSF is not effective.

Intravenous immunoglobulin

This may be used to prevent or modify infections, especially viral infections, as it contains antibodies to a range of common viral infections. Use of intravenous immunoglobulin (IVIG), however, varies between different units and tends to be used for allogeneic patients under the following circumstances:
- donor or recipient CMV is seropositive;
- unrelated, haploidentical or other mismatched donor;
- viral infection occurs early post-transplant (before immune reconstitution).

The dose is usually 0.4–0.5 g/kg weekly, continued for up to 100 days, but it may be used less frequently depending on the clinical situation. It may not be continued for longer, especially if there is slow engraftment, chronic GVHD or disseminated viral infection (e.g. adenovirus) post-transplant.

Spirituality

Hematopoietic stem cell transplantation remains a daunting undertaking, which causes many of the patients and families we see to question their mortality. This can lead to a patient seeking or being presented with religious objects, which they bring to hospital with them. Staff will need to use tact, understanding and discretion when determining how best to deal with particular objects.

• Religious texts pose little problem as they can usually be laminated to prevent damage.

• All forms of holy water need to be sterilized if it is to be consumed or applied topically during HSCT. These waters are usually obtained from a well or spring and have usually been bottled in non-sterile conditions. Where the container is intact or leak proof it may be possible to clean the outside of the container to enable the bottle to remain near the patient.

• Baptism will cause no risk for the patients. However, the normal rules for water safety will apply from the onset of reduced immunity.

• Jewellery or amulets can be difficult to clean or made of materials that are not desirable within the transplant patient environment. The patient may wish to have the item placed in a small plastic bag as it can then be taped to the bed or locker.

• Candles, although not an infection control hazard, will always remain a fire hazard. It is possible to obtain battery-operated candle substitutes, which some patients will accept as an alternative.

Alternative treatments and invasive procedures

Herbal treatments and homeopathy

If a patient wishes to use these products alongside the prescribed medications it must be ascertained that the product does not pose a threat, particularly from fungi, or counteract the prescribed medications. It is also to be remembered that the nurse may not wish to be responsible for administration of non-prescribed medicines and this responsibility will need to be assumed by the patient or one of the family carers.

Body piercing, tattooing, circumcision

Body piercing, tattooing and circumcision for religious reasons should not be undertaken around the time of transplant or until the patient is fully recovered.

Further reading

Centers for Disease Control and Prevention (2000) Guidelines for preventing opportunistic infections among hematopoietic stem cell transplant patients. *Morbidity and Mortality Weekly Review* **49** (RR10); 1–128.

Centers for Disease Control and Prevention (2004) Guidelines for preventing health care associated pneumonia, 2003. *Morbidity and Mortality Weekly Review* **53**(RR03), 1–36.

Dykewicz, C.C.A. (2001) Hospital infection control in hematopoietic stem cell transplant recipients. *Emerg Infect Dis* **7**: 263–267.

NHS Estates, Department of Health, TSO (2005) Isolation facilities in acute settings. Health Building Note (HBN) 4. London. www.tso.co.uk/bookshop

Pagliuca, A., Carrington, P.A., Pettengell, R., Tule, S., Keiden, J., Haemato-oncology Task Force of the British Committee for Standards in Haematology (2003) Guidelines on the use of colony-stimulating factors in haematological malignancies. *Br J Haematol* **123**: 22–23.

Shapiro, T.W, Davison, D.B, Rust, D.M. (eds) (1997) *A Clinical Guide to Stem Cell and Bone Marrow Transplantation*. Sudbury, MA: Jones & Bartlett, pp. 81–97.

Stiamsuddin, H.H., Dickema, D.J. (2003) Opportunistic infections in haematopoietic transplant recipients. In: Wenzel, R.P. (ed) *Prevention and Control of Nosocomial Infections*, 4th edn. Philadelphia, PA: Lippincott Williams & Wilkins.

Sub-committee of the Scientific Advisory Committee of the National Disease Surveillance Center (2002) National Guidelines for the Prevention of Nosocomial Invasive Aspergillosis during Construction/Renovation Activities. Dublin, Republic of Ireland: National Disease Surveillance Centre. Available on www.ndsc.ie

Chapter 6
Bacterial, fungal, and parasitic infections in the transplant patient

G. Jones, J. Clark and A. Galloway

Introduction

Infection is a major cause of morbidity and mortality in hematopoietic stem cell transplant (HSCT) patients, increased susceptibility to infection being an inevitable consequence of the associated myelo- and immunosuppression. Factors that cause reduced host immunity making the patient susceptible to infection include:

- neutropenia;
- impaired cell-mediated immunity (T cells);
- impaired humoral immunity (B cells), deficiency in antibody production;
- breakdown of usual skin and mucosal barriers (central lines, mucositis).

Each transplant center needs to work closely with the local microbiologist, virologist and infectious diseases consultants to ensure appropriate and timely diagnosis and treatment of infection in HSCT patients. Infection is caused not only by classical pathogenic organisms, e.g. *Staphylococcus aureus*, *Streptococcus pneumoniae*, but also by commensal organisms that lack specific virulence factors, which in immunocompetent patients would be considered as part of the patients' normal flora, e.g. *Staphylococcus epidermidis*. Opportunistic pathogens, e.g. *Aspergillus* and *Pneumocystis*, are also frequently found. Although most severe infections occur within the first 6 months after HSCT, infective complications can arise many years post HSCT.

Risk periods for infection post HSCT

It is useful to consider the post-transplant period in 3 stages:

- early – starting on the day of transplant, day 0–30 (pre-engraftment phase);
- mid – day 30–100 (early post-engraftment phase);
- late – >day 100 (late post-engraftment phase).

Patients are susceptible to different infections at these different phases of transplant and this reflects their changing immune status over time (Fig. 6.1). There is a significant difference in the degree of immunosuppression engendered by autologous and allogeneic HSCT, rendering the latter patients more susceptible to infection (Table 6.1).

Risk factors for the development of infection

The risk of developing infection in HSCT patients depends on the following factors:

- type of transplant received;
- latent infection in donor cells, e.g. cytomegalovirus (CMV), Epstein–Barr virus (EBV);
- previous latent infections in recipient, e.g. CMV, EBV;

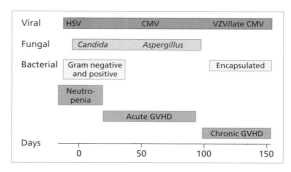

Fig. 6.1 Infectious complications occurring after allogeneic HSCT. Reproduced from Craddock & Chakraverty (2005) with permission.

Table 6.1 Reasons for increased risk of infection in HSCT recipients

Risk factor	Cause	Consequent infection susceptibility	Type of transplant
Neutropenia	Conditioning therapy	Bacteria Fungi	Auto and allo
Damage to mucosal barriers	Conditioning therapy	Bacteria Fungi	Allo > auto
Central venous line	Need for access	Bacteria Fungi	Auto and allo
Reduced cellular immunity	Conditioning therapy GVHD prophylaxis GVHD	*Pneumocystis* Viruses	Allo > auto
Reduced humoral immunity	GVHD (especially chronic GVHD)	Encapsulated bacteria, e.g. *Streptococcus pneumoniae*	Allo > auto

- colonization by microorganisms, e.g. *Candida*;
- condition requiring transplant;
- degree and duration of previous immunosuppressive therapy;
- underlying immunodeficiency.

Allogeneic transplants may take a number of different forms. Donors may be related or unrelated. Stem cells from a matched sibling are associated with faster immune recovery and less graft-vs.-host disease (GVHD) – hence less infection risk – than grafts from unrelated donors. Also the donor graft may be depleted of T cells prior to infusion. T-cell function does not therefore develop for 3 months post HSCT. Whilst this reduces the incidence of GVHD it also increases the risk of graft rejection, CMV reactivation, invasive fungal infection, and EBV-associated post-transplant lymphoproliferative disease (PTLD). In recent years stem cells from umbilical cord blood have been used for allogeneic transplants and, while excellent results can be obtained, immune reconstitution may be slower than after HSCT using bone marrow. Reduced-intensity HSCT using agents such as fludarabine and melphalan can also prolong suppression of lymphocytes and thus carry a greater risk of viral infections.

Prevention of infection and effective prophylaxis are essential if HSCT is to be successful, and these are discussed in Chapter 5.

In this chapter we aim to describe the bacterial, fungal and parasitic organisms commonly responsible for infection in HSCT patients. Viral infections are dealt with in Chapter 7.

Bacterial infections

Patients are at risk of bacterial infections most of the time during HSCT and particularly during the neutropenic phase. Table 6.2 lists the bacteria commonly causing infection in HSCT patients.

Gram-positive organisms
Staphylococci

Staphylococci are the bacteria that most commonly cause infection in HSCT patients. *Staphylococcus epidermidis* or other coagulase-negative staphylococci are the organisms most frequently isolated. They colonize the skin and oropharynx and commonly cause central venous line (CVL) infections. Although a frequent cause of morbidity in HSCT patients, infection with coagulase-negative staphylococci is rarely life threatening. Treatment may not be required immediately if these organisms are recovered from a single blood culture, unless there are signs or symptoms of a CVL infection. Repeated isolation from blood cultures in a patient with a central venous line will warrant further action (see Chapter 8 under Central venous line (CVL) infections).

Staphylococcus aureus, a coagulase-positive staphylococcus, also frequently colonizes the oropharynx and skin, especially the nose, perineum, groin and axillae. Meticillin-resistant *Staphylococcus aureus* (MRSA) is a more antibiotic-resistant variant. Both meticillin-sensitive *Staphylococcus aureus*

Table 6.2 Bacteria commonly causing infection in HSCT patients

	Notes
Gram-positive	
Staphylococci	*Staphylococcus aureus* including MRSA
	Coagulase negative staphylococci including *Staphylococcus epidermidis*
Streptococci	*Streptococcus pneumoniae*
	Viridans streptococci
Enterococci	*Enterococcus faecalis*, *Enterococcus faecium* including GRE/VRE
	All resistant to cephalosporins
Corynebacteria	Diphtheroids – skin organisms
Listeria	Infection may be food related
Nocardia	Can cause abscesses and pulmonary nodules
Gram-negative	
Escherichia coli	Known as coliforms
Klebsiella	Known as coliforms
Pseudomonas aeruginosa	Can rapidly cause serious infection
Acinetobacter	May be multiply resistant
Stenotrophomonas maltophilia	Inherently resistant to meropenem, imipenem
Haemophilus influenzae	Encapsulated bacteria
Neisseria meningitidis	Encapsulated bacteria
Other bacteria	
Clostridium difficile	Anaerobe causes pseudo-membranous colitis
Legionella	Water borne infection causing pneumonia
Mycobacteria	Includes *Mycobacterium tuberculosis*, BCG (vaccine strain) and atypical mycobacteria

(MSSA) and MRSA, however, can result in life-threatening sepsis and require urgent treatment.

Treatment of staphylococcal infections depends on their sensitivity pattern. The following provides a guide.

• *S. epidermidis* and other coagulase-negative staphylococci are often resistant to flucloxacillin but sensitive to the glycopeptides (vancomycin and teicoplanin). Centers that use teicoplanin as a first-line agent for treating Gram-positive infections are finding increasing resistance in *S. epidermidis* and other coagulase-negative staphylococci, and this should be monitored.

• *S. aureus* other than MRSA are sensitive to flucloxacillin/oxacillin and the glycopeptides.

• MRSA is usually sensitive to teicoplanin and vancomycin, although resistance to vancomycin has recently been reported.

• Almost all staphylococci appear to be sensitive to linezolid, a new antibiotic, which has both oral and intravenous (i.v.) formulations. However, a side effect of its use is a possible fall in platelet count, so it should be used with caution in HSCT patients.

• New agents with anti-staphylococcal activity include daptomycin (i.v. formulation only) and fosfomycin (not yet licensed in UK).

Streptococci

Streptococci are classified in the laboratory on the basis of the degree of hemolysis they cause on a blood agar plate.

• Beta hemolytic streptococci produce complete clearing of the blood, e.g. *Strep. pyogenes* (group A streptococci).

- Alpha hemolytic streptococci produce a partial clearing or greening of the plate, hence the term *"viridans streptococci"*, which is used for most alpha hemolytic streptococci other than *S. pneumonia*. *S. pneumonia* (pneumococcus*)* is an alpha hemolytic streptococcus that is encapsulated and is therefore particularly virulent in patients with defective immunity, especially those with anatomical or functional asplenia (see "Encapsulated bacteria" below). Viridans streptococci are part of the normal oral flora but can be the cause of septicemia especially in patients with mucositis. Poor dental hygiene is also a risk factor for infection. Occasionally this is associated with a sepsis syndrome with a high mortality especially in children.
- Non-hemolytic streptococci do not produce hemolysis on a blood agar plate and may occasionally cause infection in HSCT patients.

Useful antibiotics for streptococcal infections may include β lactam antibiotics, such as penicillin, amoxicillin, meropenem, imipenem, piperacillin/tazobactam (Tazocin®), cephalosporins; glycopeptides (vancomycin, teicoplanin) and linezolid. Treatment should be based on antibiotic sensitivity testing.

Enterococci

Enterococci were once classified as streptococci and are closely related to this group of organisms. The main species are *Enterococcus faecalis* and *Enterococcus faecium*. They inhabit the bowel and were previously considered to be of low pathogenicity; however, they can cause serious infection in HSCT patients. Many strains of enterococci are sensitive to amoxicillin and most are usually sensitive to vancomycin and teicoplanin. However, vancomycin-resistant enterococci (VRE) – otherwise known as glycopeptide-resistant enterococci (GRE) – are increasingly seen and have caused outbreaks in hematology units. Although these organisms generally colonize rather than infect patients, serious infection can occur, often central line-related. Linezolid is useful for treating such VRE infections. All enterococci are resistant to all cephalosporin antibiotics (e.g. cefuroxime, ceftazidime, ceftriaxone).

Corynebacteria and Listeria

Corynebacteria, commonly known as diphtheroids, are Gram-positive bacilli that frequently colonize the skin and oropharynx. They are usually relatively slow growing and cause a low-grade infection similar to coagulase-negative staphylococci. Their appearance in blood cultures should not be confused with *Listeria*, which are also Gram-positive bacilli, but are more rapidly growing and can cause serious sepsis. Sensitivities of *Corynebacteria* are difficult to predict but they are usually sensitive to vancomycin and teicoplanin. Occasionally very resistant strains are found, which may be difficult to treat (e.g. *Corynebacteria JK*).

Listeria can grow well at 4°C (refrigerator temperature) and is often found in raw vegetables and soft cheeses. It can cause meningitis and septicemia in immunocompromised patients. Like enterococci, *Listeria* is resistant to all cephalosporin antibiotics and sensitive to amoxicillin.

Other aerobic Gram-positive organisms

Nocardia is a branching Gram-positive bacillus, usually found in decaying matter and soil, which can cause opportunistic infection in HSCT patients. Most commonly *Nocardia* is associated with nodules in the lung or lung infiltrates but can also cause brain abscesses and skin infections. Treatment of choice is with co-trimoxazole.

Leuconostoc (Gram-positive coccus) and *Lactobacilli* (Gram-positive bacillus) are occasionally isolated from HSCT patients and may be part of the normal gastrointestinal flora. Their importance is that most strains are inherently resistant to vancomycin and teicoplanin, so may be detected in VRE screening samples. However, they do not have the same infection control implications regarding spread of infection.

Gram-negative organisms

The bowel is the commonest source of Gram-negative bacilli (coliforms) where they are normal flora e.g. *Escherichia coli*, *Klebsiella* spp.

Antibiotic therapy may result in changes to the normal flora, and patients may become colonized with coliforms and other Gram-negative bacilli such as *Pseudomonas aeruginosa*. *Acinetobacter* is a Gram-negative bacillus, which frequently colonizes the skin and can cause central line infections. Recently highly resistant strains of *Acinetobacter* have been identified, which may cause cross-infection and can be difficult to treat. Although Gram-negative bacilli cause infection less frequently than Gram-positive organisms, they are of major clinical importance as their cell wall structure contains endotoxin, which can trigger septic shock. Antibiotics with activity against Gram-negative bacilli such as *Pseudomonas* include aminoglycosides; piperacillin/tazobactam (Tazocin®); carbapemens (meropenem and imi-

penem); ceftazidime and ciprofloxacin (see Table 6.3). Tigecyline is a new broad-spectrum antibiotic, which may be useful to treat resistant infections (but not *Pseudomonas*).

More unusual Gram-negative bacilli may also cause colonization or infection, and of particular concern is *Stenotrophomonas maltophilia* (previously known as *Pseudomonas* or *Xanthomonas maltophilia*). This organism is usually resistant to many antibiotics and survives well in the environment. It has been found contaminating ice from ice-making machines and has caused outbreaks of infection in immunosuppressed patients. It is always resistant to the carbapenems (meropenem and imipenem), and usually sensitive to co-trimoxazole. A number of environmental Gram-negative organisms occasionally cause line infections, especially in

Table 6.3 Antibiotics useful in the management of infection in HSCT patients

	Agent	Activity
Glycopeptides	Vancomycin Teicoplanin	Gram-positives: *Staphylococci*, MRSA, *Streptococci*, *Enterococci*, VRE. Useful in penicillin allergy Oral vancomycin for *C. difficile*
Broad-spectrum β lactams	Ceftazidime Piperacillin/Tazobactam (Tazocin®)	Gram-negative bacteria Also good anaerobic activity
Carbapenems	Meropenem Imipenem	Gram-negatives and some Gram-positive cover; also good anerobic activity. May be used in patients with suspected penicillin allergy
Aminoglycosides	Gentamicin Tobramycin Amikacin	Gram-negative bacteria, some *Staphylococci* including MRSA. Need to measure levels to avoid toxicity. Amikacin has activity against atypical mycobacteria
Quinolones	Ciprofloxacin Moxifloxacin Levofloxacin	Gram-negatives, *Legionella*, atypical mycobacteria (moxifloxacin>levofloxacin>ciprofloxacin). Moxifloxacin has good anti-pneumococcal activity
Macrolides	Erythromycin Azithromycin Clarithromycin	Staphylococcal or streptococcal infections in penicillin allergy, *Legionella* Azithromycin useful for cryptosporidia Clarithromycin useful for atypical mycobacteria
Miscellaneous	Metronidazole Linezolid	Anaerobes including *C. difficile* Gram-positive including MRSA, VRE. Need to monitor platelet count. Long term use >28 days associated with peripheral neuropathy and optic neuritis
	Co-trimoxazole	Prophylaxis and treatment for *Pneumocystis*; prophylaxis for encapsulated bacteria, toxoplasma
	Co-amoxiclav	May be useful oral antibiotic for non-neutropenic patients

patients who are not in a protected environment. Many of these have interesting or unusual names (see Chapter 8, central line infections).

When Gram-negative bacilli cause septicemia, various potential sources of infection should be considered:
• Bowel – translocation of bacteria from bowel to blood; this is more likely if there is mucosal damage due to mucositis or a gastrointestinal viral infection;
• urine – especially if there is an indwelling urinary catheter;
• respiratory tract;
• skin – especially if there is evidence of perineal infection;
• central line – especially if there is fever or a rigor after line manipulation.

Anaerobic infections

The gastrointestinal tract is the usual source of anaerobes causing infection and, although anaerobes do not usually cause primary infection, they can co-infect with other bacteria. Almost all anaerobes are sensitive to metronidazole. Other antibiotics with good activity against anaerobes included piperacillin/tazobactam, meropenem and co-amoxiclav.

The most common anaerobe causing infection in HSCT patients is *Clostridium difficile*, which can produce an enterotoxin causing antibiotic-related diarrhea and pseudomembranous colitis. If not actively treated this infection may be fatal. Treatment with oral metronidazole or oral vancomycin is usually recommended in the first instance.

Antibiotic resistance

Resistant organisms are now recognized as a significant problem and include:
• meticillin-resistant *S. aureus* (MRSA);
• vancomycin-insensitive *S. aureus* (VISA – a more resistant variant of MRSA);
• vancomycin- or glycopeptide- resistant enterococci (VRE or GRE);
• extended-spectrum lactamase (ESBL) producing Gram-negative bacilli – these confer resistance to all the cephalosporins and other β-lactam antibiot-

ics such as amoxicillin; the treatment of choice is a carbapenem, e.g. imipenem or meropenem;
• carbapenem-resistant *Pseudomonas aeruginosa*;
• multiply resistant *Acinetobacter* spp. (MRAB) – a recently recognized "super bug," resistant to the aminoglycosides (e.g. gentamicin) and cephalosporins (e.g. ceftazidime); a more resistant variant is also resistant to the carbapenems (meropenem and imipenem) known as MRAB-C.

Table 6.3 lists the antibiotics that are particularly useful for treating bacterial infections in HSCT patients.

Encapsulated bacteria

This term refers to bacteria that produce a protective capsule. This includes:
• *Streptococcus pneumonia* (pneumococcus);
• *Haemophilus influenzae* type B (HiB);
• *Neisseria meningitidis* (meningococcus).

These organisms classically cause infection in patients with asplenia or hyposplenism and can cause septicemia, which is rapidly fatal. Patients undergoing HSCT can suffer from hyposplenism due to radiotherapy, chemotherapy and conditioning drugs and are therefore at risk of serious infection. Pneumococcal, meningococcal and HiB vaccines are given to HSCT patients post-transplant (see Chapter 13).

Miscellaneous bacteria
Legionella

Legionnaire's disease was first recognized in 1976 when an outbreak of pneumonia with high mortality occurred among war veterans (legionnaires) in Philadelphia, USA. The organism had not been previously recognized as it was not Gram-stainable in clinical specimens and grew only slowly on special culture media. The commonest *Legionella* causing serious infection is *Legionella pneumophila*. There are also several serotypes of *L. pneumophila* and serotype 1 is the commonest causing infection. Other *Legionella* species can also cause infection especially in immunocompromised patients, e.g. *L. bozemanii, L. micdadei*.
• Patients typically have fever and a non-productive cough.

- Infection can be transmitted by inhalation of aerosols generated from water contaminated with *Legionella*, e.g. from sinks, showers, whirlpool spas, air conditioning units, and cooling towers.
- Maintenance of good water quality is essential for the prevention of infection in a transplant unit (see Chapter 5).
- Person-to-person spread does not occur.
  Diagnosis is made by:
- culture of bronchoalveolar lavage (BAL) or lung tissue;
- urinary antigen detection (for the diagnosis of *L. pneumophila* serotype 1 only) – this is a rapid test and the antigen is excreted in the urine in the first few weeks of infection;
- serology – note that a rise in antibody titer is not useful in patients who are unable to mount an immune response.

Treatment is with a macrolide, e.g. erythromycin or clarithromycin plus ciprofloxacin or rifampicin. A single case on a transplant unit that is thought to be hospital acquired should prompt investigation for a source of infection on the unit.

Mycobacteria

Mycobacteria include *Mycobacteria tuberculosis*, non-tuberculous mycobacteria and bacillus Calmette–Guérin (BCG), the vaccine strain. All may cause severe disseminated disease in the immunocompromised. Although infrequently causing infection in HSCT patients, mycobacterial infection should be considered in patients with a fever not responding to first- or second-line antibiotics or antifungal agents.

Mycobacterium tuberculosis
This is occasionally seen in HSCT patients and usually represents reactivation of disease in adults. Presentation may be atypical with rapid development of lymphadenopathy or overwhelming pneumonia.

Non-tuberculous mycobacteria
Many environmental mycobacteria, including *M. avium complex*, *M. malmoense*, *M. chelonei*, and *M. kansaii*, may cause disseminated disease by hematogenous spread, with patients developing lymphadenopathy or lung, liver, spleen and bone marrow involvement. This appears less frequently

in HSCT patients than in patients with advanced human immunodeficiency virus (HIV) disease, but is generally associated with lymphopenia and may cause fevers, sweats, weight loss and gastrointestinal upset. Like BCG, non-tuberculous mycobacterium may also cause secondary immune reactivation with granuloma formation, as engraftment progresses. Initial treatment options include combinations of clarithromycin, rifabutin and ethambutol.

Fast growing mycobacteria, such as *M. fortuitum* and *M. chelonei*, are well-recognized pathogens of central venous line-associated blood stream and exit site infections. Combinations of appropriate antibiotics to which they are sensitive often include macrolides, ciprofloxacin, and aminoglycosides. Their presence usually requires CVL removal.

BCG
In the UK BCG vaccination is given to neonates at "high risk" of infection just after birth. Disseminated BCG, especially in children with primary immune deficiencies such as chronic granulomatous disease (CGD), is well described and is a risk when young children with primary immune deficiency are further immunosuppressed prior to transplant. Miliary spread to lungs, liver, spleen or bone marrow may occur. Prophylaxis with isoniazid and rifampicin should therefore be given to at-risk children undergoing HSCT.

Locally there may be abscess formation or continuing discharge at the BCG site. As engraftment occurs and an effective immune response develops there is a significant inflammatory reaction with granulomata possibly being produced in the areas of disseminated infection, or at the BCG site and associated lymph nodes, abscess formation may occur.

Fungal infections

Invasive fungal infections (IFIs) are a major cause of morbidity and mortality after HSCT. The vast majority are due to *Candida*, *Aspergillus* spp. and non-*Aspergillus* moulds. The incidence of these infections varies from study to study and is reported to be between 3 and 30%. Partly as a result of progress in the early detection and treatment of CMV infections, invasive aspergillosis (IA) has now become the leading cause of infection-related death after allogeneic HSCT. Patients receiving allogeneic HSCT are 10 times more likely to develop IFI than autologous transplant patients. Mortality from IFIs is high and may approach 100% for cerebral infections

There are 2 main groups of fungi that cause problems post-HSCT.
• yeasts – e.g. *Candida albicans*, *C. glabrata*, *C. krusei*, *Cryptococcus neoformans*;
• moulds – e.g. *Aspergillus*, *Fusarium*, *Mucor*.

Yeasts

Yeasts are unicellular fungi. *Candida* is the most common fungus isolated from HSCT patients and may cause:
• superficial infections – e.g. intertrigo, nappy rash, pharyngitis;
• deep infections – e.g. hepatosplenic candidiasis, abscesses (renal, brain);
• systemic infections – often central line related.

Candida can be isolated from clinical specimens including blood cultures but may need 48 hours to grow. Figure 6.2 shows *Candida* growing on culture media and under the microscope. Specialist media or tests may be used, which allows rapid distinction of *Candida albicans* from other *Candida* species. The importance of this is that *Candida albicans* is usually sensitive to most antifungal agents but other

Candidia spp. may show resistance to some of the azole antifungals, particularly fluconazole. Fluconazole may therefore not be suitable as treatment for all suspected *Candida* infections (*C. krusei* and *C. glabrata* are frequently resistant). Most *Candida* spp. are sensitive to Caspofungin and Amphotericin B.

The epidemiology of systemic candidiasis has changed in the last few years. Fluconazole prophylaxis has decreased the incidence of systemic candidiasis from 10–20% to <5% in HSCT recipients and changed the predominant species from *Candida albicans* to non-*albicans Candida*, e.g. *C. glabrata*.

Cryptococcus neoformans is a yeast that can cause meningitis in immunocompromised patients (see Chapter 8). Rarely other yeasts, including *Saccharomyces*, *Trichosporon*, *Malassezia*, *Rhodotorula*, *Histoplasma* and *Coccidioides*, cause disease in the post-transplant setting. *Histoplasma* and *Coccidioides* are more commonly seen in USA and are not endemic in the UK.

Moulds

Moulds are filamentous fungi. They form branching, cellular filaments, which amalgamate to form a mycelium. The most important in this group in terms of frequency and seriousness of infection is *Aspergillus*. Figure 6.3 shows *Aspergillus* growing on a culture plate and under the microscope. Approximately 10–20% of HSCT recipients will

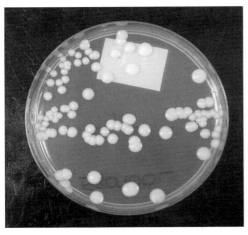
(a)

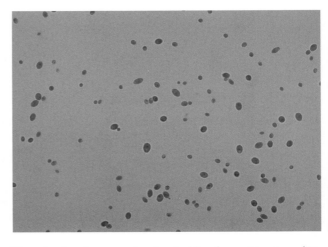
(b)

Fig. 6.2 (a) *Candida* growing on a culture plate. (b) *Candida* under the microscope showing budding forms. (Courtesy of Dr E.M. Johnson, Mycology Reference Laboratory, Health Protection Agency Bristol.)

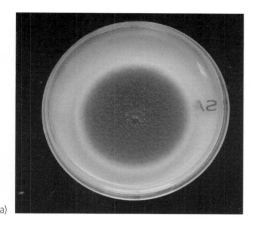
a)

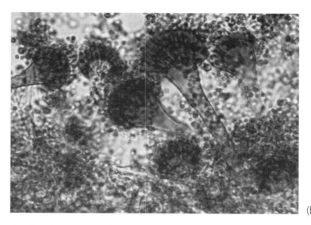
(b)

Fig. 6.3 Aspergillus (a) growing on a culture plate and (b) sporing heads as seen under the microscope (courtesy of Dr E.M. Johnson, Mycology Reference Laboratory, Health Protection Agency Bristol).

develop invasive aspergillosis (IA). Mortality rates due to IA are approximately 50% in patients with hematological malignancies receiving intensive chemotherapy, but the severity of such infections in the post-transplant setting is even higher, with mortality rates of over 80% reported in many studies.

Other moulds that can cause serious infection include the zygomycetes (*Rhizopus, Mucor, Rhizomucor, Absidia*), which cause zygomycosis, and the zygomycetes (*Fusarium* and *Scedosporium*). These may present as infection in the lung or paranasal sinuses and grow rapidly to invade blood vessels and the brain.

Microbiological confirmation of invasive mould infection may be difficult as blood cultures and superficial infections are rarely positive and tissue biopsies or BAL may be required (see below).

Dermatophyte infections

Dermatophytes, which commonly cause infection in skin, hair and nails in immunocompetent patients, may rarely cause severe infection during transplant. A careful examination prior to transplant should be performed and treatment given prior to HSCT if necessary.

Pneumocystis jiroveci

This was previously termed *Pneumocystis carinii*

and deserves special mention. It was formerly considered a parasite but is now classified as a fungus. Although it is a unicellular organism it is more closely related to *Aspergillus* than *Candida*. Unlike other fungi it is exceedingly difficult to culture in the laboratory.

Pneumocystis *pneumonia (PCP)*

This was first recognized in malnourished children in the 1940s after World War II. *Pneumocystis* is now recognized as an important opportunistic pathogen in any patient with lymphopenia and is often a presenting feature in patients with HIV infection or children with severe combined immunodeficiency (SCID). In the HSCT setting it typically causes pneumonia in the early post-engraftment phase (days 30–100). Effective prophylaxis with co-trimoxazole has now markedly reduced the incidence of infection post-transplant. See Chapter 8 for diagnosis and treatment.

Risk factors for invasive fungal infection (IFI)

The main risk factors for invasive fungal infections are shown in Table 6.4.

Taking these factors into account, it is not surprising that autologous HSCT recipients generally develop IFI during the neutropenic period in the first 21 days post-HSCT. In contrast, allogeneic

Table 6.4 Risk factors for invasive fungal infection

Neutropenia
GVHD
Steroids
Broad spectrum antibiotics
Previous invasive infection
Severe mucositis

HSCT recipients are at risk during this early period but also experience a second peak of IFI between days 26 and 95. This coincides with the development and treatment of acute GVHD.

Colonization with yeasts, especially *Candida* spp., is common and may lead to invasive infection. Colonization at several superficial sites including CVL site and detecting *Candida* in the urine should raise suspicion of a more serious invasive infection.

Defining fungal infections

In order to effectively compare clinical studies that have been undertaken in this field, it is essential to have clear criteria for defining invasive fungal infections. Recently an international group has published guidelines clarifying these issues (Ascioglu *et al.*, 2002). In essence, IFI is said to be proven, probable, or possible on the basis of various host factors and microbiological, clinical, and radiological criteria:
• proven fungal infection: microscopic demonstration of fungi in a biopsy or fluid from a normally sterile area or positive culture and clinical or radiological evidence of infection;
• probable fungal infection: demonstration of fungi from other areas that are not usually totally sterile, together with clinical and radiological or microbiological (including antigen testing) features that suggest IFI;
• possible fungal infection: clinical symptoms and signs of infection.

Empirical antifungal therapy is often commenced on suspicion of infection (possible infection) before results of investigation are available as delay in treatment may be fatal.

Antifungal agents

There are a number of agents available for the treatment of fungal infections. These can broadly be divided into:
• Polyenes – nystatin and amphotericin B-based drugs
  • conventional amphotericin B
  • liposomal amphotericin B (AmBisome®)
  • lipid formulation amphotericin B (Abelcet®);
• azoles (fluconazole, itraconazole and voriconazole); newer azoles include posaconazole, ravuconazole;
• echinocandins (caspofungin; newer agents include micafungin and anidulafungin).

The activity of these agents against various fungi is shown in Table 6.5. Several agents are only available as an intravenous preparation. Table 6.6 indicates the preparations that are currently available in UK.

Amphotericin B compounds

Conventional amphotericin B has been available for 40 years. Despite its efficacy, it has significant toxicity. Discontinuation rates of up to 38% are reported due to:
• nephrotoxicity;

	Fluconazole	Itraconazole	Voriconazole	Amphotericin	Caspofungin
Candida	Variable	Variable	Sensitive	Sensitive	Sensitive
Aspergillus	Resistant	Sensitive	Sensitive	Sensitive	Sensitive
Cryptococcus	Sensitive	Sensitive	Sensitive	Sensitive	Resistant
Fusarium	Resistant	Resistant	Sensitive	Sensitive	Resistant
Mucor	Resistant	Resistant	Resistant	Sensitive	Resistant

Table 6.5 Sensitivity of common fungi to the available antifungal agents

Table 6.6 Antifungal agents in common use in transplant patients

Class of agent	Agent	Formulation	Notes
Azoles	Fluconazole	oral, i.v.	Well absorbed
	Itraconazole	syrup	Well absorbed
		capsules	Poorly absorbed
		i.v.	
	Voriconazole	Tablets, syrup	Main side effect visual
		i.v.	disturbances
Amphotericin based	Amphotericin B	i.v., oral (lozenges)	Marked renal toxicity i.v.
	AmBisome®	i.v.	May be used in high doses
	Abelcet®	i.v.	Use with antihistamines
	Nystatin	oral, topical	
Echinocandins	Caspofungin	i.v.	
	Micafungin	i.v.	Not widely available

- infusion-related toxicity, including fevers and rigors;
- electrolyte disturbances, including hypokalemia and hypomagnesemia.

These side effects can be particularly difficult to manage in the transplant setting; patients are often already receiving other significantly nephrotoxic therapies such as gentamicin or ciclosporin A.

AmBisome® and Abelcet®

Lipid-based agents are less toxic than conventional amphotericin B and AmBisome® has been used in high doses (10 mg/kg/day). However, it adds significantly to the cost of therapy.

Amphotericin B has a broad spectrum of activity against yeasts and moulds with few exceptions, which include *Candida lusitaniae*, *Aspergillus terreus*, *Scedosporium* and *Pneumocystis*. Penetration into tissues varies with the different preparations, AmBisome® and Abelcet® having lower penetration into the kidney than conventional amphotericin B.

Azoles
Fluconazole

This has been available since 1989 and replaced ketoconazole as the azole of choice in the HSCT setting. It has:
- good activity against *Candida albicans* and many other *Candida* spp. (but notably excluding *C. krusei* and *C. glabrata*);

- dramatically reduced invasive *Candida* infections when used as a prophylactic agent in the HSCT setting;
- no activity against *Aspergillus* and other moulds, which limits its use as a sole agent for prophylaxis in transplant patients.

Itraconazole

This has activity against yeasts and some filamentous fungi like *Aspergillus*. It is now mainly used for prophylaxis rather than treatment of fungal infections.
- It is available orally as capsules or syrup. The absorption of syrup is superior to capsules and is to be preferred.
- To ensure adequate blood levels (>0.5 mg/L), levels should be measured after 2 weeks of treatment once a steady state has been achieved; this is particularly important if capsules are used rather than syrup. Dosage can be increased as necessary to achieve satisfactory blood levels.
- In patients who cannot tolerate the bitter taste of the syrup, capsules may be used. Keeping the syrup in a fridge may, however, improve its palatability.
- Syrup should be taken after a fast of at least one hour.
- Capsules should be taken with food. Absorption can be increased by taking them with food and an acidic fizzy drink such as cola.
- Grapefruit juice inhibits absorption of itraconazole.

• Treatment needs to be started at least 1 week before transplantation to ensure adequate serum levels.

• During conditioning it may be necessary to change itraconazole prophylaxis to an amphotericin B product because of drug interactions.

• Main complications include gastrointestinal upset and raised liver function tests, which may necessitate stopping its use and switching to an alternative antifungal agent.

Voriconazole

This is the most recent azole antifungal agent to be licensed in the UK and has the advantage of being available in both intravenous and oral preparations. It has the advantage of good central nervous system penetration and is used for the treatment of a range of fungal infections and for empirical therapy. The commonest side effects are:

• visual disturbances – these are common but usually transient and reversible, and patients should be warned of their occurrence;

• hepatotoxicity;

• electocardiograph changes (prolonged QT).

Other new azoles

These include posaconazole and ravuconazole (under development). These have a similar spectrum of activity to voriconazole.

Echinocandins
Caspofungin

This is an echinocandin antifungal which has been available since 2002 in the UK. It works by inhibiting the synthesis of fungal cell walls, which have a completely different structure to mammalian cell walls, and is therefore a relatively non-toxic product. It is used for treatment of *Aspergillus* and *Candida* infections, and is also licensed for the empirical therapy of fungal infections in HSCT patients. Caspofungin covers *Candida* spp. and *Aspergillus* spp., the most common causes of IFI in the post-transplant period, but has a reduced spectrum of antifungal activity, as compared to amphotericin B-based agents (Table 6.5). It does not have activity against non-*Candida* yeast such as *Cryptococcus* or moulds other than *Aspergillus* (e.g. *Mucor*, *Fusarium* or *Scedosporium*). Caspofungin has the advantage of reduced toxicity as compared to the other agents.

New echinocandins – micafungin and anidulafungin

These have a similar spectrum of activity to caspofungin and are also only available as i.v. preparations. Micafungin has been used for prophylaxis in HSCT patients.

Investigation of fungal infections

Given the high mortality associated with IFI in HSCT patients, there is a need to investigate patients with prolonged fever, or suspicious symptoms or signs of fungal infection. Investigations include imaging and laboratory investigations.

Imaging to diagnose fungal infections

Conventional X-rays may be suggestive of fungal infection but the most useful investigation is high-resolution CT scanning. This is particularly useful for suspected chest and sinus fungal infection (see Chapter 8).

Laboratory techniques for the diagnosis of fungal infections

These include:

• microscopy (microbiology and histopathology);

• culture;

• detection of fungal antigens;

• detection of fungal DNA.

Microscopy and culture

Tissue samples and body fluids (e.g. urine, sputum, paranasal sinus aspirate, bronchoalveolar lavage (BAL), cerebrospinal fluid) that are sampled at the time of fever development should be examined directly microscopically and cultured for fungi, which requires prolonged incubation. Microscopy is important as it yields better results than culture alone and can provide a rapid result. Histopathological examination of tissues should include the use of special stains to visualize fungi. *Candida* and other yeasts can usually be grown from blood cultures, urine and swabs; however, isolation of moulds usually requires a biopsy or BAL, i.e. a specimen taken directly from the infected site.

Non-culture techniques

Antibody response cannot be relied on for diagnosis as immunocompromised patients do not generate a normal antibody response. IA may be amenable to early detection using immunological or molecular biological strategies.
* detection of antigens such as:
  * galactomannan, from the aspergillus cell wall;
  * mannan from the candida cell wall;
  * 1,3-β- D-glucan produced by *Candida* and *Aspergillus*;
* detection of fungal DNA in blood, by polymerase chain reaction (PCR).

These methods have been found to be useful for screening for fungal infection in the transplant setting and may be used in combination.

Aspergillus galactomannan

* Negative results with this assay is likely to mean that the patient does not have IA.
* Single positive assay result is less reliable as an indicator of genuine IA and should be repeated.
* Two consecutive positive results are required to make a diagnosis of infection.

Although this seems disappointing, it must be remembered that currently many patients with persistent febrile neutropenia are commenced on antifungal therapy; this test could reduce the need for unnecessary therapy in a proportion of patients. False positive results have been reported from patients receiving piperacillin/tazobactam and with other fungal pathogens. At present there is no standard method of reporting positive results in the UK, Europe and USA. This needs to be addressed.

Candida mannan

* Results do not appear to be as reliable as galactomannan testing for *Aspergillus*.
* False positive results may occur from yeast antigens present in food that may be absorbed.

1,3-β- D-glucan

This is also part of the fungal cell wall of a number of common fungal pathogens causing infection in HSCT patients including *Candida* spp., *Saccharomyces*, *Histoplasma*, *Aspergillus*, and *Fusarium*. The test is not suitable for diagnosing infection with the Zygomycetes (*Mucor* and *Rhizopus*) or *Cryptococcus*, which produce little or no 1,3-β- D-glucan.

Fungal DNA detection by polymerase chain reaction (PCR)

The reported data are variable.
* Negative predictive value of the test appears high.
* Positive predictive value of the test is increased by finding the test repeatedly positive.
* Testing has not been fully standardized.

Although none of these immunological or molecular tests is likely to be sensitive or specific enough to be considered diagnostic when used alone, their use in a rational protocol incorporating clinical and radiological assessments can be helpful. With improvement in techniques, particularly for PCR, it is hoped that these tests will be helpful in diagnosing or excluding fungal infection in HSCT patients.

Parasitic infections

Everyone is susceptible to a number of parasitic infections. In many cases such infections cause minimal symptoms among individuals with functioning immune systems; in patients with reduced host defenses infection can be life threatening. Two parasites are particularly important in HSCT patients:
* toxoplasma;
* cryptosporidia.

Infection/colonization	Management	Table 6.7 Specific infections, which may need treatment pre-transplant
MRSA	Attempt topical eradication prior to transplant	
Aspergillus	Made need pre-transplant resection of affected lung	
	Prophylactic or therapeutic doses of antifungal	
Cryptosporidia	Treatment required during transplant if carriage detected	
Dermatophytes	Careful examination of skin, nails, hair and treatment required	
BCG (previous vaccination)	Prophylaxis with isoniazid and rifampicin to immunodeficient children prior to transplant	

Toxoplasma

Toxoplasma is an intracellular parasite. Infection may be acquired in childhood and cause asymptomatic infection or transient lymphadenopathy. It is common in the UK and Europe; cats are the definitive host. Organisms are usually transmitted from contaminated soil or meat to humans. Infection in HSCT patients is usually due to reactivation and can cause central nervous system infection or pneumonia. Allogeneic HSCT with GVHD is a significant risk factor for infection; typically disease occurs at a median of 62 days post-transplant, but is recognized up to a year after HSCT. Co-trimoxazole prophylaxis may help decrease reactivation.

Cryptosporidia

Cryptosporidium is a common animal parasite and is spread by the feco-oral route both via humans and animals. Transmission is often from farm animals or from fecally contaminated water or food. Outbreaks have been described in association with contaminated swimming pools and drinking water. Rarely lung infection has been described. Prevention is important for the HSCT patient; see Chapter 8, Gastrointestinal infections, for details of diagnosis and management.

Infections pre-transplant

Pre-transplant assessment should identify previous infections and colonization with resistant organisms, e.g. MRSA, VRE. Infections may need specific treatment and attempts to eradicate MRSA may be appropriate especially in high-risk transplant patients. Table 6.7 identifies specific infections that may need treatment pre-transplant. Pre-transplant assessment is dealt with in Chapter 2.

Further reading

Ascioglu, S., Rex, J.H., de Pauw, B., Bennett, J.E., Bille, J., Crokaert F. *et al.* (2002) Defining opportunistic invasive fungal infections in immunocompromised patients with cancer and hematopoietic stem cell transplants: An international concensus. *Clin Infect Dis* **34**: 7–14.

Bowden, R.A., Ljungman, P., Paya, C.V. (eds) (2003) *Transplant Infections*, 2nd edition. Philadelphia, PA: Lippincott Williams & Wilkins.

Centers for Disease Control and Prevention (2000) Guidelines for preventing opportunistic infections among hematopoietic stem cell transplant recipients. *Morbidity and Mortality Weekly Report 2000*; **49**(RR-10): 1–128

Craddock, C., Chakraverty, R. (2005) Stem cell transplantation. In: Hoffbrand, A.V., Catovsky, D., Tuddenham, E.G.D.(eds), *Postgraduate Haematology*. Oxford: Blackwell Publishing.

Leather, H.L., Wingard, J.R. (2001) Infections following hematopoietic stem cell transplantation. *Infect Dis Clin North Am* **15**: 483–520.

Marty, F.M., Rubin, R.H. (2006) The prevention of infection post-transplant: the role of prophylaxis, preemptive and empiric therapy. *Transplant Int* **19**: 2–11.

Pappas, P.G., Rex, J.H., Sobel, J.D. *et al.* (2004) Guidelines for treatment of Candidiasis. *Clin Infect Dis* **38**: 161–189.

Stevens, D.A., Kan, V.L., Judson, M.A. *et al.* (2000) Practice guidelines for diseases caused by *Aspergillus*. *Clin Infect Dis* **30**: 696–709.

van Burik, J., Weisdorf, D. (2000) Infections in recipients of blood and marrow transplantation. In: Mandell, G.L., Bennett, J.E., Dolin, R. (eds), *Principles and Practice of Infectious Diseases*, 5th edn. Philadelphia, PA: Churchill Livingstone, pp. 3136–3147.

Chapter 7
Virus infections in the HSCT patient

C. Taylor and A. Turner

Introduction

Virus infections cause significant morbidity and mortality in hematopoietic stem cell transplant (HSCT) patients. The risks from infection are less for autologous transplants than for other types of stem cell transplants but they are still a major clinical problem. The herpesviruses are the most common cause of virus infections but the importance of respiratory virus infections, and of invasive adenovirus infection, has been increasingly recognized in recent years.

Viral infection can also have indirect effects: cytomegalovirus (CMV) and other herpesviruses have been implicated as causes of graft-vs.-host disease (GVHD) and delayed engraftment or graft failure. Furthermore, they may predispose to bacterial or fungal superinfection, either by depressing immunity directly or because the necessary antiviral therapy does so.

As well as being generally more susceptible to virus infections and associated disease, HSCT patients are more likely to develop persistent, often multiple, virus infections because they are immunocompromised. Multiple virus infections are particularly seen in patients with severe combined immunodeficiency (SCID). HSCT patients may also present with disease manifestations that do not occur in immunocompetent individuals. Infections acquired pre-transplant may persist through the post-transplant period until immunological recovery occurs post; similarly, infections acquired post transplant may be much slower to resolve than in an immunocompetent individual.

There are also difficulties in managing virus infections because of limitations in diagnostic methods and availability of safe and effective antiviral drugs. However, technical developments in recent years, particularly in molecular diagnosis, have led to dramatic improvements in the ability to provide a timely and clinically relevant diagnostic service, which means that virus infections can be diagnosed and treated before they cause fatal damage. In addition, an increasing number of antiviral agents available now are widely used for prophylaxis as well as treatment. However, extensive use of CMV prophylaxis, for example, does not eliminate the risk of CMV disease but instead tends to delay its onset and has led to concerns about the emergence of resistance. This emphasizes the importance of rational protocols for diagnosis, treatment and prevention of virus infections in HSCT patients.

Viruses and diseases

Herpesviruses

These include:
- *Herpes simplex* (HSV);
- *Varicella zoster* (VZV);
- cytomegalovirus (CMV);
- Epstein–Barr virus (EBV);
- human herpes virus types 6 and 7 (HHV6 and HHV7).

Herpesvirus infections are important for several reasons. They are ubiquitous and usually cause life-long infection, commonly acquired in childhood or adolescence. Rates of infection vary according to socioeconomic factors and geographically but, in general, infection prior to transplant is common, particularly in adults. Because herpesviruses cause persistent infection, which can reactivate and may lead to disease, and because the immunosuppression associated with transplantation or with the treatment of GVHD can cause reactivation of latent virus, there is a potential for recurrent infection and consequent disease post transplant. In addition, some herpesviruses, e.g. CMV, may be transmitted by transfused blood or blood products. Figure 7.1 shows the structure of a herpesvirus.

HSV, CMV and VZV are the most important of the human herpesviruses in HSCT patients; active infections with these viruses tend to occur in a characteristic pattern post transplant (Table 7.1).

Herpes simplex virus

HSV may be shed asymptomatically. The commonest clinical presentation of reactivated HSV infection is oral ulceration, which may extend by direct spread to cause esophagitis or pneumonitis. Pneumonitis may also follow viremic spread. Patients with a history of herpes genital infection may experience recurrent genital herpes.

Varicella zoster virus

Primary infection with VZV causes chickenpox; reactivation of latent virus causes shingles (*Herpes zoster*). Chickenpox is uncommon in HSCT patients, particularly in adults, because most of them will have had primary VZV infection prior to transplant. When it does occur, fever and new lesion formation may be prolonged for up to 2

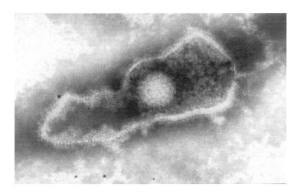

Fig. 7.1 Electron micrograph (EM) of *Herpes* (*simplex*) virus. (reprinted from *Virus Morphology*, 2nd edn, C.R. Madeley & A.M. Field, p. 50, copyright (1988) with permission from Elsevier.)

weeks and there is a high mortality rate, usually because of pneumonitis. In contrast, *Herpes zoster* is common in adult HSCT patients and may either be localized or disseminated; disseminated *Herpes zoster*, as with chickenpox, may be fatal.

Cytomegalovirus (CMV)

In contrast to solid organ transplantation, where CMV can be transmitted by the donor organ, reactivation of the patient's own latent virus is the main source of CMV disease in HSCT patients. However, CMV seropositive patients receiving T-cell-depleted stem cells from CMV seropositive donors appear to be at reduced risk of disease. Active CMV infection may remain asymptomatic; it does not always progress to disease. Progression to disease is predicted by detection of CMV in blood (viremia) and high levels of viremia (high viral loads) detected in the blood, using quantitative polymerase chain reaction (PCR). Disease manifestations include a pyrexia of unknown origin (PUO)-like syndrome, delayed engraftment and pneumonitis, the commonest fatal outcome; retinitis due to CMV is uncommon in HSCT patients but may lead to blindness. CMV disease is associated with GVHD, although it is not clear whether CMV precipitates GVHD or GVHD and its treatment lead to reactivation of CMV.

Epstein–Barr virus (EBV)

Epstein–Barr virus can cause post-transplant lymphoproliferative disease (PTLD), which varies from polyclonal B-cell proliferation to malignant B-cell lymphomas. PTLD is generally uncommon in HSCT patients, except in recipients of T-cell-depleted grafts. Polyclonal B-cell proliferation usually occurs in children, in the first year post transplant, after primary EBV infection; it may be accompanied by fever, sore throat and lymphadenopathy. Monoclonal B-cell lymphomas usually occur in older patients, late after transplant, following EBV reactivation; they tend to present as single or multiple localized lesions, often in the gut, central nervous system or the bone marrow.

Human herpes virus types 6 and 7

Infections with HHV6 and HHV7 are extremely

Table 7.1 Timing of herpesvirus infections after HSCT

Time after transplant	Virus	Disease
1–4 weeks	HSV	Oral/genital ulceration, esophagitis, pneumonia
	HHV6	Encephalitis, pneumonitis and graft failure
1–3 months	CMV	PUO-like syndrome, gastrointestinal symptoms, pneumonia
3–12 months	VZV	*Herpes zoster* (shingles)
0–12 months (children)	EBV	Post-transplant lymphoproliferative disease (PTLD)
> 12 months (adults)	EBV	Post-transplant lymphoproliferative disease (PTLD)

common causes of febrile childhood illnesses, which may be associated with a rash – exanthem subitum (roseola) – or may be asymptomatic. Also asymptomatic reactivation of HHV6 post-HSCT appears to be common, so interpretation of positive PCR results can sometimes be problematic. However, HHV6 infection has been associated with encephalitis, pneumonitis and graft failure. Whether HHV7 causes disease in HSCT patients is currently unclear.

Adenoviruses

Adenovirus infection following HSCT is increasingly recognized as a cause of severe and often fatal disease; the reasons for this are thought to include increasing use of intensive conditioning regimens, and improvements in diagnostic tests. Adenovirus infections are common, especially during early childhood; infection following HSCT is more common and occurs earlier in children than in adults. Adenoviruses replicate in respiratory tract and gut epithelial cells and establish persistent, or latent, infection with periodic shedding in feces and respiratory secretions. Infection following HSCT is thought to be due either to reactivation of latent virus or to the transmission of latent virus with the graft or with transfused blood. Adenoviruses of subgenus C (types 1, 2, 5) and subgenus B (types 7, 14 and 35) are particularly associated with disease in HSCT patients. Clinical manifestations of adenovirus infections include:

- fever;
- pneumonia;
- hepatitis;
- colitis;
- hemorrhagic cystitis;
- disseminated infection.

Risk factors for disease include the type of transplant (allogeneic, T-cell depleted and unmatched donor transplants are high risk); GVHD; viremia and detection of adenovirus at multiple sites. Figure 7.2 shows the characteristic histological changes seen in adenovirus pneumonia.

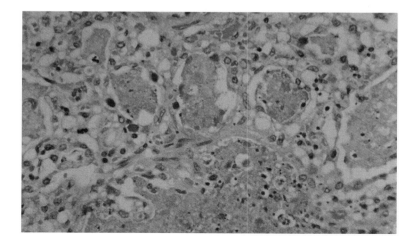

Fig. 7.2 High-power magnification of lung. Several "smudge cells" are seen lining the alveolar spaces containing large, darkly staining inclusions characteristic of adenovirus-associated interstitial pneumonitis.

Respiratory viruses

Respiratory infections are important causes of morbidity and mortality in HSCT patients. They are more likely to follow a complicated, prolonged course with higher mortality than in immunocompetent patients. A wide range of viruses cause disease, not only those that cause upper and lower respiratory tract infections in immunocompetent individuals (Table 7.2). Adenoviruses and herpesviruses can also cause respiratory tract infections; this may be as a complication of a systemic infection. The introduction of community-acquired infections onto HSCT units is an increasingly recognized problem, with the potential for nosocomial spread, leading to significant outbreaks.

Influenza A and B viruses

Influenza viruses may cause severe disease in HSCT patients; they are at risk of pneumonia, bacterial superinfection and, in children, neurological complications. Vaccination post transplant is recommended for all patients (see Chapter 13). In addition, vaccination of healthcare workers who have close contact with HSCT patients is also recommended in many units.

Parainfluenza viruses

Parainfluenza viruses (PIVs) are also important causes of respiratory infection in HSCT patients. Nosocomial spread of community-acquired PIV

Table 7.2 Viruses causing respiratory infections in HSCT patients

Influenza A and B viruses
Parainfluenza viruses 1, 2, 3, & 4
Respiratory syncytial virus (RSV)
Rhinoviruses
Human metapneumovirus
Measles
Adenoviruses
CMV
HSV
VZV

infection introduced onto HSCT units can be a serious problem. Lower respiratory tract infection (LRTI) is usually a consequence of infection with PIV 3 but all four types may be involved; pneumonia is usually preceded by an upper respiratory tract infection (URTI) and is associated with significant mortality. Infection with parainfluenza 3 virus is commonly found at presentation in children with severe combined immunodeficiency (SCID), often associated with other respiratory infections e.g. *Pneumocystis* (see Chapter 6).

Respiratory syncytial virus (RSV)

RSV is an important cause of respiratory infection in HSCT patients; nosocomial transmission of RSV is well described and may be a significant source of infection post-HSCT. Pneumonia is a frequent complication and, as with PIV infection, usually follows URTI; mortality rates are high, particularly if disease occurs pre-engraftment, and may exceed those associated with PIV infection.

Rhinoviruses

Rhinovirus infections are common; they mainly cause URTIs, including the common cold. They also cause LRTIs, which may be fatal in HSCT patients.

Human metapneumovirus

Human metapneumovirus was first described in 2001. It causes an illness similar to RSV; co-infection with RSV appears to be more clinically significant than either alone. Its precise role in HSCT patients is still to be established.

Measles

Measles has become uncommon in countries where there are vaccination programs with high measles coverage but it can cause life-threatening infection in susceptible HSCT patients. Measles giant cell pneumonia is a severe, usually fatal, form of pneumonia in HSCT recipients; patients may present without a rash or any other typical features of measles, so a high index of suspicion is important.

Viral gastroenteritis

The viruses associated with gastroenteritis in HSCT patients are the same as those seen in immunocompetent patients but infection in HSCT patients is more likely to be severe and persistent (Table 7.3). Norovirus infection and, to a lesser extent, sapovirus and astrovirus infection can be associated with outbreaks on HSCT wards, as on other hospital wards. Gastrointestinal tract involvement may also occur with non-enteric adenoviruses and with herpesvirus infections.

Viruses associated with central nervous system infections

The viruses associated with central nervous system (CNS) infections in immunocompetent patients are also seen in HSCT patients (Table 7.4). Enteroviruses comprise a group of viruses that can multiply in the gastrointestinal tract but can also cause CNS diseaes (e.g. poliovirus, Coxsackie A and B). If meningitis is suspected and a CSF sample is not available, a feces sample should be sent for virus culture. Other viruses, e.g. HSV, may be isolated from nose or throat swabs and may be helpful if CSF is not available. CNS disease may also occur with EBV-driven PTLD; with HHV6 infection and as a complication of JC virus infection.

JC virus

JC virus is a human polyomavirus. It is ubiquitous and is generally not associated with disease, but it is the cause of progressive multifocal leukoencephalopathy (PML), a rare neurological disorder seen in HSCT and other groups of immunocompromised patients. PML is characterized by demyelination throughout the central nervous system; it leads to dementia and is almost always fatal.

Viruses associated with rashes and other skin lesions

The virus infections associated with rashes and other skin lesions in immunocompetent patients also occur in HSCT patients but the presentation and duration of disease may differ. Table 7.5 indicates the viruses commonly associated with rashes and skin lesions.

Parvovirus B19

This virus deserves a special mention as it can cause severe hematological problems in HSCT patients. Parvovirus B19 infection is the cause of erythema

Table 7.3 Viruses causing gastroenteritis

Rotavirus
Norovirus*
Sapoviruses**
Astroviruses
Adenovirus types 40 and 41 (enteric adenoviruses)

* Previously termed Norwalk-like viruses or small round structured viruses (SRSVs).
** Previously termed caliciviruses.

Table 7.4 Viruses associated with central nervous system infections

HSV
Enteroviruses
VZV
EBV
HHV6
JC virus
Parvovirus

Table 7.5 Viruses associated with rashes and other skin lesions

Vesicular rashes	Non-vesicular rashes	Nodular lesions
HSV	Adenoviruses	Human papillomaviruses
VZV	Enteroviruses	*Molluscum contagiosum* virus
Enteroviruses	Parvovirus B19	
	Measles	
	Rubella	
	HHV6	
	HHV7	

infectiosum, or fifth disease (slapped cheek syndrome), one of the common childhood rash illnesses, in immunocompetent patients. However, in HSCT patients, B19 infection can lead to red cell aplasia and severe chronic anemia, often without a rash; neutropenia, thrombocytopenia and pancytopenia have also been reported. Nosocomial outbreaks have been described.

Blood-borne viruses

The viruses shown in Table 7.6 are commonly described as blood-borne viruses (BBVs), although sexual transmission and vertical transmission from mother to baby occur in addition to transmission by the blood-borne route.

These infections are uncommon in HSCT patients because of risk assessment and screening of donors and recipients. BBV infection in a potential donor is generally a contraindication to donation. Transplantation of BBV-infected patients is controversial for a number of reasons, including the potential adverse consequences of immunosuppression on the course of BBV infection.

It is possible that vCJD could be transmitted to HSCT recipients from donors who have been exposed to vCJD, and a risk assessment should be made (see Chapter 2).

Other viruses – BK virus

BK virus, like JC virus, is a ubiquitous human polyomavirus. Infection occurs during childhood or early in adulthood and is lifelong; it is generally asymptomatic in immunocompetent individuals. BK virus may reactivate in immunosuppressed patients: urinary excretion is common following

Table 7.6 Blood-borne viruses (BBVs)

Hepatitis B (HBV)
Hepatitis C (HCV)
Hepatitis D – *delta* hepatitis (HDV)
HIV
HTLV 1 and 2

HSCT and may be associated with hemorrhagic cystitis, which may be mild but can also cause severe prolonged bleeding and require surgical intervention.

Laboratory diagnosis of virus infections

Specimen selection, quality and transport

When attempting to make a diagnosis of a virus infection it is vital that appropriate specimens are taken correctly (Table 7.7). One or more specimens may need to be taken depending on clinical signs and symptoms. The virologist will be able to give advice regarding the most suitable samples. The quality of specimen (e.g. a respiratory sample) can be equally important. Otherwise the virus diagnostic technique, however excellent, may yield a false negative result.

• Respiratory secretions collected for diagnosis by immunofluorescence must contain adequate numbers of respiratory epithelial cells and should be taken from the posterior, rather than the anterior, nasal epithelium.
• Respiratory viruses tend to be labile, so respiratory specimens should be transported as quickly as possible to the laboratory. If a delay occurs then the specimen must be kept in a refrigerator.
• If a BAL cannot be performed, testing a blood sample (e.g for CMV or Adenovirus) may be helpful.
• Nose swabs should be collected from the turbinates, not the anterior nares.
• Throat swabs should be taken from the posterior pharyngeal wall, not the tonsils or the palate.
• Swabs from skin lesions should be collected by firmly abrading the base of fresh lesions in order to harvest epithelial cells.
• Specimens (of any type) for virus diagnosis must *never* be frozen as this will either destroy the virus or compromise the effectiveness of diagnosis. Swabs must be placed in virus transport medium and should never be sent dry.
• Specimens should be transported in leak-proof containers placed in plastic bags; packaging must comply with current transport regulations.
• Blood samples for PCR should be sent in a bottle containing EDTA anticoagulant.

Table 7.7 Specimens for investigation of virus infections

Symptoms or illness	Specimen
Respiratory	NS/TS, NPA, ETA, NW, BAL, lung biopsy, EDTA blood
Pyrexial illness	NPA, NS/TS, feces, EDTA blood
Central nervous system	CSF, NS/TS, feces
Gut	Feces, tissue biopsy
Rash, ?infection or GVHD	Tissue biopsy (e.g. skin, gut), EDTA blood
Eye	ES
Liver	Biopsy (if available), EDTA blood
Vesicular lesion	LS
Post-transplant lymphoproliferative disease	EDTA blood, biopsy (if available)
Myelosuppression/anemia	EDTA blood, bone marrow (if available)
Hemorrhagic cystitis	Urine

BAL, bronchoalveolar lavage; NW, nasal washings; CSF, cerebrospinal fluid; ES, eye swab; ETA, endotracheal aspirate; LS, lesion swab; NPA, nasopharyngeal aspirate; NS/TS, nose swab/throat swab.

• Samples of feces and nose and throat swabs should be sent if viral CNS infection is suspected and CSF is not available.

Timing of specimen collection and diagnosis

It is important to diagnose virus infection as early as possible so that treatment, where possible, can be given to limit the spread of the virus before it causes serious organ damage. The earlier treatment is started, the higher the chance of controlling virus infection. Furthermore, early diagnosis will limit the chance of nosocomial spread of virus. Ideally the laboratory should make the diagnosis and notify the result the same day or within 24 hours. The HSCT team needs to be aware that even apparently trivial symptoms may need to be urgently investigated. This is particularly important in profoundly immunocompromised patients, such as those early post-allogeneic HSCT, when respiratory viruses such as RSV or parainfluenza viruses can cause considerable morbidity or mortality.

Diagnostic methods according to symptoms

The modern diagnostic virology laboratory has a spectrum of methods ranging from classic techniques (e.g. virus isolation on cell culture) to modern molecular methods (e.g. PCR). Each have their strengths and weaknesses (see Table 7.8) and the diagnostic virologist will choose one or more methods depending on the clinical signs and symptoms.

Table 7.8 Diagnostic methods and applications

Method	Application	Advantages/disadvantages
Immunofluorescence (IF)	Respiratory infections	Rapid but dependent on specimen type and quality
Electron microscopy (EM)	Virus detection in feces, skin or urine	Rapid, catch-all method but limited availability
Virus culture	Respiratory infections, e.g. rhinoviruses Enteroviruses	Alternatives not widely available but slow May be useful if meningitis is suspected and CSF not available
Serology	Antibody testing in serum	Useful for baseline testing but not useful post-HSCT
Enzyme immunoassay (EIA)	Virus detection in feces	Can differentiate, e.g. rotavirus and adenoviruses; enteric and non-enteric adenovirus infection
Molecular diagnosis	Virus detection in blood, CSF, feces, skin lesions, tissue biopsies and urine; therapeutic monitoring	Rapid, sensitive, can be quantitative but requires expertise and dedicated facilities

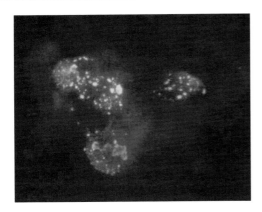

Fig. 7.3 Immunofluorescence of nasopharyngeal secretions showing a positive result for respiratory syncytial virus.

• Immunofluorescence (IF) is still the main method used to detect most respiratory viruses, although PCR is becoming more widely available. IF will give a result the same day (as can PCR). Figure 7.3 shows a specimen positive for RSV using immuno-fluorescence.

• Virus culture tends to be less useful as viruses can take days or even weeks to grow, giving a result too late to contribute to management. However, virus culture is still used – for example to isolate rhinoviruses, as rapid methods for their detection, such as PCR, are not widely available. It is also useful if viral sensitivity testing is required.

• Virus antibody detection in blood is of limited use for diagnosing virus infections in HSCT patients as the immune response is compromised, but it is important pre-HSCT for defining which viruses the patient has previously encountered, including latent viruses such as CMV and EBV, which may reactivate during transplant.

• Molecular diagnosis, e.g. by PCR, is very useful in HSCT patients. It can be used in the immunocompromised because it depends on detection of virus nucleic acid rather than the hosts' immune response (unlike antibody tests) and provides rapidly available results that will influence management. PCR testing can be applied to a range of specimens types, e.g. blood, urine, CSF, nasal washings. Also, quantitative PCR on blood samples, i.e. viral load testing, will give an estimate of the degree of infection, which can be useful when deciding when to treat

CMV infection. CMV PCR testing has thus largely replaced detection of CMV pp65 antigen in leukocytes (CMV antigenemia testing). Viruses associated with pyrexia of unknown origin (PUO) post-HSCT (adenovirus, CMV, EBV, HHV-6 or enteroviruses) can be detected in EDTA blood by PCR.

Gastrointestinal symptoms

• The viruses that can cause gastroenteritis post-HSCT (Table 7.3) can be detected in fecal samples by methods such as electron microscopy (EM), enzyme immunoassay (EIA), and PCR.

• Non-enteric adenoviruses (types other than 40 and 41) may be detected in feces samples by electron microscopy, EIA, or PCR.

• Herpesvirus infections involving the gastrointestinal tract, such as CMV, HSV or EBV, may be detected in tissue biopsies by PCR. To differentiate this from GVHD, a feces sample should be submitted for virology together with a tissue biopsy, where appropriate, for virological investigations and histological examination.

• Outbreaks of diarrhea on an HSCT ward have been associated with norovirus, rotavirus and adenovirus, although sporadic cases can occur with sapovirus and astrovirus. The latter two viruses can also cause outbreaks but this is less common. EIA (and less commonly PCR) techniques can be used for diagnosis, although electron microscopy should be employed when other techniques have given negative results.

Rashes or skin lesions

• Vesicular lesions are generally caused by HSV or VZV, although certain enteroviruses (e.g. Coxsackie type A16) are sometimes responsible.

• Severely immunocompromised patients, when infected with viruses that usually cause a non-vesicular rash in immunocompetent patients(see Table 7.5), may not have a rash at all or it may have an atypical presentation, e.g. a subtle erythematous rash may be significant and due to disseminated adenovirus infection, CMV or HHV6 (diagnosed by blood PCR).

• Measles is diagnosed by obtaining a respiratory sample, e.g. nasopharyngeal aspirate or nasal washings, and using immunofluorescence or PCR.

Table 7.9 Viruses associated with myelosuppression and/or anemia

CMV
HHV6
HHV7
Parvovirus B19

- Virus infections causing nodular lesions, commonly skin warts, may be diagnosed by EM or PCR.

Myelosuppression or anemia

Viruses associated with myelosuppression and/or anemia (Table 7.9) are diagnosed by testing EDTA blood (and bone marrow, if available) by PCR.

Central nervous system symptoms

Table 7.10 indicates the viruses associated with CNS infection.
- HSV and enteroviruses should be the first viruses sought in cases of encephalitis and meningitis, respectively.
- Other viruses are tested for depending on the clinical symptoms, e.g. VZV in cases of chickenpox or shingles, although VZV can on occasions cause neurological disease in the absence of rash.
- EBV is a prime candidate in lymphoproliferative disease and likewise JC virus in cases of PML.
- HHV6 infection should be sought in cases of encephalitis where negative results have been obtained in testing for other viruses.
- CSF samples are tested for virus infection by PCR.

Table 7.10 Viruses associated with central nervous system infections

HSV (encephalitis)
Enteroviruses (meningitis)
VZV
EBV
JC virus
HHV6 (encephalitis)

Table 7.11 Viruses associated with hepatitis, jaundice, abnormal liver function tests

Adenoviruses
CMV
EBV
Hepatitis A virus (HAV)
Hepatitis B virus (HBV)
Hepatitis C virus (HCV)

Hepatitis, jaundice, abnormal liver function tests

- Infection with the hepatitis viruses (Table 7.11) is seldom encountered but, if suspected, a blood sample should be tested for HAV and HCV by PCR (as antibody testing is insensitive and may give false negative results).
- Hepatitis B surface antigen (HBsAg) testing by serology is satisfactory for diagnosing active HBV infection.
- Viral hepatitis post-HSCT is more likely to be due to adenovirus, CMV, EBV, or HHV6 infection and diagnosis is performed by testing EDTA blood samples by PCR and, where available, liver biopsy samples.

Hematuria

Hemorrhagic cystitis can be due to:
- BK virus infection;
- adenovirus.

EM testing of urine samples can provide rapid results; alternatively, PCR can be used.

Prevention of virus infections

Prevention of virus infections in HSCT involves a range of measures, including immunization, infection control (see Chapter 5 for details), antiviral prophylaxis, and pre- and post-HSCT monitoring for infection (surveillance). Prevention is important because:
- After receiving chemo- and radiotherapy pre-HSCT, viral infections are more difficult to eradicate than bacterial infections. Consequently patients can get very ill and may even die.

• Virus infection can complicate diagnosis and management, e.g. it can sometimes be difficult to differentiate between virus infection and GVHD. Furthermore, if a patient with GVHD were to acquire a virus infection nosocomially due to inadequate infection control, then the increased immunosuppression required to treat GVHD could exacerbate virus infection with the risk of dissemination.

Immunization

Viral vaccines are included among the vaccines given post-HSCT, following immune recovery; for a full account of immunizations the reader should consult Chapter 13.

A live VZV vaccine has been available in the UK since December 2003 and is also available in other European countries. The vaccine can be used in seronegative family members to protect patients with severe cell-mediated immunodeficiency post-HSCT (i.e. prior to marrow engraftment). Use of the vaccine in HSCT patients themselves is contraindicated due to the possibility of disseminated infection with the vaccine strain of virus.

Screening blood and blood products

CMV-negative patients are commonly given CMV-negative blood and blood products, from screened donors, to reduce the risk of acquiring CMV infection.

Prophylaxis

Prophylaxis, particularly against herpesvirus infections, is essential during the period from conditioning up to engraftment, when the patient is extremely vulnerable to infection. Prophylaxis may not always prevent virus infection but it may delay it, thereby allowing some degree of engraftment with resultant control and clearance of virus infection. Aciclovir is commonly used; it is an effective prophylaxis against HSV and there is some evidence of a prophylactic effect against CMV. However, the antivirals used and the dose, route of administration, and duration of prophylaxis will vary according to local protocols.

Surveillance of virus infections

Surveillance is instituted as soon as the patient is admitted to hospital for HSCT for the following reasons.

• To allow antiviral therapy to be given as early as possible in order to gain maximum effect. Although complete clearance of virus infection is rarely achieved prior to successful engraftment, it may restrict the extent of the infection or prevent spread to other organs.

• To reduce the risks of nosocomial transmission of infection to other patients or staff. Sometimes surveillance will detect virus infection before it causes disease and early treatment may prevent progression to disease.

Surveillance is carried from admission until after the patient is discharged from hospital with a functioning graft. Protocols are generally designed to detect herpesvirus and adenovirus infection but each center must have a protocol that details the types of specimens to be taken and the frequency of sampling; the details depend on the characteristics of the patient populations, the type of transplant performed and the particular infections they experience, e.g. screening for CMV (by PCR) once or twice weekly in allogeneic HSCT patients who were known to be CMV positive.

Antiviral therapy

Although relatively few antiviral drugs are currently available to treat virus infections in HSCT patients (see Table 7.12), treatment can still be a complex process and a number of factors need to be taken into consideration.

• Treatment needs to be started as soon as possible in order to achieve maximum control.

• Early detection of virus infection by taking surveillance specimens may allow pre-emptive treatment, i.e. before infection has progressed to disease. Consequently, treatment may be started during the period leading up to HSCT as well as early and late post-HSCT.

• Prior to engraftment, clearance of virus infection may be difficult or even impossible. The rationale is to limit virus replication even if the virus

Table 7.12 Antiviral drugs used in therapy

Virus	Drugs
CMV	Ganciclovir, valganciclovir, foscarnet
HSV	Aciclovir, valaciclovir, famciclovir
VZV	Aciclovir, valaciclovir, famciclovir
HHV-6/7	Ganciclovir, valganciclovir, foscarnet
EBV	Ganciclovir
Adenoviruses	Cidofovir, ribavirin
RSV	Ribavirin
Parainfluenza viruses	Ribavirin
Measles	Ribavirin
Influenza A and B	Oseltamivir, zanamivir
Parvovirus B19	Intravenous immunoglobulin

cannot be eliminated. This is necessary to reduce the amount of later damage that occurs when cells from the donor immune system destroy virus-infected cells in a tissue following successful engraftment.

• Drug dosage, route of administration, and duration of therapy should be according to national guidelines or local protocols. Effectiveness of therapy is monitored by sampling for virus by an appropriate method (often quantitative PCR testing). In practice the duration of therapy is often prolonged and may be as long as months. After the virus has been eradicated, a period of maintenance therapy (at a lower dose) may be used in order to limit the risk of rebound of infection.

• With the exception of aciclovir, famciclovir and valaciclovir, antiviral drugs are toxic and the dosage may need to be reduced if adverse events (e.g. myelosuppression) occur.

• A prolonged period of therapy, combined with sub-optimal dosage due to toxicity, increases the possibility that antiviral resistance may occur. Awareness of the possibility of resistance is essential and, if suspected, testing should be carried out with a change of therapy if anti-viral resistance is detected.

Developments for the future

• Use of PCR assays for respiratory virus infection will replace or complement immunofluorescence to give improved detection. These PCR assays will improve the detection of rhinoviruses and allow the detection of respiratory coronaviruses.

• Discovery of new viruses. Currently on occasions no pathogen is found in patients with, for example, lower respiratory tract infection or encephalitis. Some of these cases may be due to virus infection. New viruses are being discovered, e.g. human metapneumovirus in 2001 and a new human respiratory coronavirus in 2004 (previously known as SARS – severe acute respiratory syndrome virus). Also viruses that do not usually cause human disease, e.g. avian influenza virus, have recently been reported as being transmitted to humans, causing serious infection.

• Development of antivirals with little or no toxicity. Currently only members of the aciclovir class of antiviral drugs fall into this category. There is also a need for new antivirals with proven efficacy, e.g. against adenoviruses.

• New technologies for improved laboratory diagnosis of virus infection, e.g. nucleic acid microarrays. Such technologies may give a very rapid diagnosis of a broad spectrum of viruses.

Further reading

Richman, D.R., Whitley, R.J., Hayden, F.G. (eds) (2002) *Clinical Virology*, 2nd edn. Washington, D.C: American Society for Microbiology.

Walls, T., Shankar, A.G., Shingadia, D. (2003) Adenovirus: An increasingly important pathogen in paediatric bone marrow transplant patients. *Lancet Infect Dis* **3**; 79–86

Working Party Report (2000) Management of herpesvirus infections following transplantation. *J Antimicrob Chemother* **45**; 729–748.

Yoshikawa, T. (2004) Human herpesvirus 6 infection in haemopoietic stem cell transplant patients. *Br J Haematol* **124**; 421–432.

Chapter 8

Management of febrile neutropenia and system-specific infections

G. Jones, J. Clark and A. Galloway

Management of febrile neutropenia

This is the most common clinical situation encountered during hematopoietic stem cell transplantation (HSCT). This section details a clinical approach to the management of a patient who is neutropenic post-HSCT and has become pyrexial. Figure 8.1 shows an algorithm for the management of febrile neutropenia. The presence of fever (≥38°C) lasting more than one hour or any spike of temperature >38.5°C in a patient with severe neutropenia (neutrophils <0.5 × 10⁹/L) constitutes a medical emergency. Prompt administration of broad-spectrum antibacterial agents to this group of patients has been shown to reduce mortality and is considered a standard of care. Mortality rates of 70% have been observed when broad-spectrum antibiotics are delayed.

Initial clinical assessment

Figure 8.1 shows the principle components of an initial assessment in patients with febrile neutropenia. Particular attention should be given to the intravascular catheter sites, mouth, and perianal region. Digital rectal examination should be avoided due to the risk of infection secondary to damage of the rectal mucosa. Note in particular the following.

• All neutropenic patients who are hypotensive and/or tachycardic should be assessed for infection and promptly started on intravenous antibiotics with circulatory support.

• Some neutropenic patients (especially older patients and those on steroids) fail to develop a fever even in the presence of severe infection.

• Clinicians need to have a low threshold for commencement of broad-spectrum antibiotics.

• The absence of inflammation does not constitute the absence of infection as the patient is often unable to mount a significant inflammatory response.

• Neutropenic patients are unable to develop abscesses.

Initial investigations

These should include:

• blood cultures [from each lumen of the central venous line (CVL) and peripherally, if possible];
• full blood count;
• serum C-reactive protein (CRP);
• chest X-ray;
• urine for culture;
• swabs, sputum, and feces for microbiology and virology as clinically indicated.

Empirical antimicrobial therapy

Rapid administration of broad-spectrum antibiotics is essential. Each transplant unit should have an agreed, and regularly reviewed, antibiotic regimen for use in this situation, dependent upon local infection rates and antibiotic resistance profiles.

• There are several different antibiotics that may be used. Those commonly used include an antipseudomonal antibiotic [e.g. ceftazidime, piperacillin/tazobactam (Tazocin®), and meropenem or imipenem]. These can also be used alone or in combination with an aminoglycoside. The potential nephrotoxicity and ototoxicity of aminoglycosides in conjunction with the need to monitor levels are drawbacks. Recently the use of combination ther-

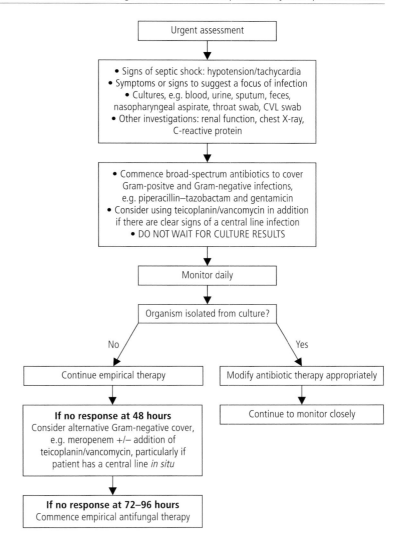

Fig. 8.1 Management of febrile neutropenia in HSCT patients.

apy for neutropenic patients has been questioned. Locally our unit policy in adults circumvents some of these problems by using a single dose of gentamicin (5 mg/kg) along with an antipseudomonal beta-lactam (piperacillin/tazobactam). Gentamicin has the advantage of also being active against staphylococci, including MRSA and some coagulase staphylococci. Gentamicin is only continued on a regular basis if culture results suggest that this would be advantageous, e.g. if septicemia with *Pseudomonas aeruginosa* is confirmed.

• In children the other issue of practical concern is the fluid volume required for administration of certain antibiotics: meropenem can be administered in relatively small volumes and may be favored in this situation.

• Vancomycin or teicoplanin should be considered for first-line use in patients with an obvious CVL infection or in patients in whom infection with MRSA is likely (e.g. prior colonization). Teicoplanin is a glycopeptide antibiotic, which has fewer negative side-effects than vancomycin and does not require routine monitoring. With increasing use of teicoplanin, a growing number of teicoplanin-resistant, vancomycin-sensitive coagulase-negative staphylococci are reported; sensitivities require review locally.

• Vancomycin or teicoplanin are also used in some units, especially in children with primary immunodeficiencies who may be at special risk of life-threatening Gram-positive sepsis including *Staphylococcus epidermidis*. This provides additional empirical coverage against Gram-positive organisms.

• There are concerns regarding the emergence of drug resistance (especially VRE), so many units do not include either vancomycin or teicoplanin as first-line empirical therapy in neutropenic fever but use these when there are specific indications (as above).

Subsequent management: a good clinical response
Positive culture

Treatment is continued with appropriate antimicrobial therapy for 10–14 days minimum. If there is evidence of ongoing sepsis, treatment should be prolonged accordingly. If the patient is well, organisms isolated are sensitive and CRP is falling, it is possible to convert patients from IV to oral antibiotics before the neutrophil count has recovered. It is important to consider additional factors that may reduce the efficacy of oral agents, such as vomiting or gastrointestinal graft-vs.-host disease (GVHD).

No positive cultures or obvious focus of infection

If the fever resolves for at least 48 hours on the initial antibiotic regimen, and CRP is not significantly raised and not rising, empirical antimicrobial therapy may be discontinued, especially if fever is suspected as being due to a non-infective cause. Each patient does need to be individually assessed.

Subsequent management: persistent pyrexia or poor clinical response
Antibacterial agents

The management of patients who remain pyrexial despite first-line empirical antibiotic therapy is more difficult.

• Close monitoring is vital, repeatedly examining the patient specifically for localizing signs of infection, which may help to guide further investigation and treatment; regular serum CRP estimation may help give a pointer as to whether infection is responding or not. Specific infections, their investigation and management are discussed later in this chapter.

• Antibiotic therapy should be modified in the light of any positive culture results obtained. In persistently pyrexial patients, there is no evidence that repeating blood cultures more than once per 24 hours provides any additional benefit.

In approximately 70% of patients with febrile neutropenia no positive culture results are obtained and ongoing management is with empirical antimicrobial therapy. Unit protocols differ with respect to second- and third-line therapeutic strategies. In broad terms, if there is no response to antibiotics after 48 hours it is reasonable to consider a change of agent with activity against Gram-negative organisms and to consider the empirical addition of vancomycin or teicoplanin to the regimen, if not already used.

Treatment may need to be continued until neutrophil recovery (neutrophils >0.5 × 10⁹/L).

If there is no response and CRP remains raised, after switching antibiotic therapy, an antifungal agent needs to be added to replace any antifungal which may have been used for prophylaxis (see below). In the absence of any evidence of a fungal infection and persisting fever with a high CRP, atypical infection should be considered and it has been our practice to use antibiotics such as ciprofloxacin and amikacin that have activity against atypical organisms, e.g. *Mycobacteria* spp. These may be added or substituted for other antibiotics depending on the clinical condition of the patient. In allogeneic transplant recipients GVHD should also be considered as a cause of unresolving fever even in the absence of typical signs and symptoms; it should be noted that GVHD may also be the cause of a raised CRP.

Empirical antifungal therapy

Persistent fever, unresponsive to broad-spectrum antibiotics after 72–96 hours of therapy, can be the first sign of an underlying invasive fungal infection (IFI) in transplant patients and empirical antifungal therapy should be considered.

There are a number of symptoms and signs that should alert the clinician to the possibility of IFI in

Table 8.1 Symptoms and signs of invasive fungal infection

Hemoptysis or epistaxis – when hemostasis is otherwise secure
Pleural pain
Pleural rub
Maxillary tenderness
Periorbital swelling
Meningism
Focal neurological signs
Nodular skin lesions

any neutropenic patient. These are given in Table 8.1.

These features are indications for immediate investigation and commencement of antifungal therapy. An amphotericin-based product, caspofungin or voriconazole may be used.

Other supportive measures
Use of colony-stimulating factors

Granulocyte-colony stimulating factor (G-CSF) and granulocyte macrophage-colony stimulating factor (GM-CSF) are designed to promote granulocyte (+/– macrophage) development, both of which are important in fighting infection. G-CSF is more commonly used in HSCT patients.

• In the immediate post-transplant period the use of G-CSF appears to be associated with a reduction in the total duration of neutropenia and reduced hospitalization, although the long-term effects are unknown.

• The American Society of Clinical Oncology recommends that, for neutropenic patients, G-CSF should be used in patients with infection-related complications such as: pneumonia, hypotension, multi-organ dysfunction (sepsis syndrome) or invasive fungal infection.

Granulocyte infusions

Another potential method of supporting transplant recipients through periods of neutropenia is the administration of granulocytes derived from normal donors, although their use is controversial.

• Because of the potential hazards associated with any apheresis procedure, granulocyte transfusion is not part of routine practice for the maintenance of neutrophil counts during the cytopenic post-transplant phase.

• Granulocyte infusions may be used in the setting of severe infections in patients who are not expected to recover neutrophils for ≥7 days.

Central venous line (CVL) infections

Almost all patients undergoing HSCT have an indwelling CVL. The majority of the lines used are tunneled, fully implantable lines; the line is tunneled subcutaneously such that the exit point of the line from the vein is distant from the skin exit point. Portacaths, where the port is implanted subcutaneously, are also often used in the pediatric setting, though not usually for HSCT patients. Hickman or Broviac lines are most commonly used. These may have single, double or triple lumens. Multiple-lumen lines are preferred for HSCT patients as a number of agents and blood products can be given simultaneously. CVL infections can be considered in three categories:

• line infection;
• exit site infection;
• tunnel infection.

While scrupulous line care can reduce the risk, these devices commonly become infected. If infection is localized in the CVL (line infection) and not systemic, serum CRP may be normal and the patient may have few or minimal clinical signs (mild pyrexia). Occasionally infection may occur subcutaneously (tunnel infection) and this may only be suspected by persistently positive cultures from the line site (pure, heavy growth of an organism). A course of antibiotics is still warranted in neutropenic patients after line withdrawal, especially if a new line is inserted; duration of treatment depends on the organism isolated and the patient's immune status.

Clinical features

There are several features that may suggest a CVL infection:

• fever +/– rigors a short time after the line has been used (line infection); culture results demonstrate an organism in blood drawn from the central line but not from blood taken simultaneously from a peripheral vein (the likelihood of demonstrating an organism on blood culture from a line is increased if "first pull" blood is sent for culture);

• erythema and tenderness around the catheter exit site +/– discharge (exit site infection);
• inflammation and tenderness along the subcutaneous tunnel of the line (tunnel infection).

Exit site and tunnel infections may not be associated with positive blood culture initially. If a multiple-lumen line is *in situ* it is essential to take cultures from each lumen (clearly identified as from which lumen) so that antibiotic therapy may be preferentially infused or locked, if necessary, into the infected lumen. However, if possible all lumens should be treated as there is a high chance of seeding infection to other lumens. In children and patients with poor venous access, taking peripheral cultures may prove difficult and probably will not change management as, whenever detected, infection will be aggressively treated.

Likely pathogens

Central line infections can be due to a variety of bacteria and fungi, from organisms with relatively low pathogenicity such as the coagulase negative staphylococci and corynebacteria (diphtheroids) to more virulent organisms such as *Staphylococcus aureus*, *Pseudomonas aeruginosa* and *Candida*. A wide rage of environmental Gram-negative bacteria with fascinating names may be isolated from patients, especially those not in a protective environment, pre-transplant or post engraftment. These include *Chryseomonas luteola*, *Brevundimonas vesicularis*, *Leclercia decarboxylata*, and *Pantoea agglomerans*.

Management of CVL infections

This depends on the pathogen found and the extent of the infection (e.g. fever only as opposed to sepsis and raised CRP). Removal of infected intravenous lines should be considered, particularly when patients are neutropenic during the early post-transplant phase. However, good venous access is also critical to patient care post transplant; many patients have poor peripheral venous access due to

previous chemotherapy and many have had several previous central lines. Thus the risks and benefits of not removing the line need to be carefully balanced.

Treatment options include:
• antibiotic treatment without CVL removal;
• catheter removal, in addition to appropriate antibiotic therapy.

Antibiotic therapy without CVL removal may be considered for infection due to coagulase-negative staphylococci and other skin organisms, as it may be possible to eliminate infection from the line. As a high proportion of coagulase-negative staphylococci are resistant to beta-lactam antibiotics, a systemic glycopeptide (vancomycin or teicoplanin) is recommended. These may also be used locally as CVL locks (see below). Treatment should be given for 10–14 days using intravenous antibiotics and these must be given at least daily down the affected lumen. In practice, as often more than one lumen is affected and there is a risk of spreading infection to other lumens, it is advisable to split the dosage of intravenous antibiotics between the lumens and the use of antibiotic locks should be considered. Use of oral antibiotics for CVL infections will not be successful with the line *in situ* as they will not penetrate the plastic of the CVL.

Indications for CVL removal

CVL removal in addition to antibiotic therapy is recommended for:
• infections with skin organisms that are not responding to antimicrobial therapy;
• tunnel infections;
• infections with *Candida* spp., coliforms (e.g. *E. coli*, *Klebsiella*, *Enterobacter*), *Staphylococcus aureus*, *Pseudomonas aeruginosa*, and non-tuberculous mycobacteria;
• significant hemodynamic instability in a patient with any documented line infection.

The decision to remove any line should be taken by a senior doctor on the transplant team, weighing up the advantages and disadvantages of line removal. Occasionally it may be considered that positive blood cultures from the CVL represent a septicemic process (e.g. bowel translocation with Gram-negative organisms) rather than an infection in the line. However, once septicemia occurs, infection in the line is likely to follow.

Antibiotic and antiseptic locks

These may help eradicate infection locally in the line. Potentially any antibiotic may be used, but commonly use is restricted to vancomycin for Gram-positive infections or aminoglycosides (e.g. gentamicin, amikacin) for Gram-negative infections. An antibiotic solution of 10 mg/mL should be used and enough antibiotic given to fill the line (approximately 2 mL in adult). These should be left *in situ* for at least 2 hours and can be left for 24–48 hours if necessary in outpatients. We recommend that the antibiotic lock should be removed and discarded prior to reusing the line. Other strategies include line locks of taurolidine (an antiseptic with antimicrobial activity); alcohol or hydrochloric acid alongside systemic antibiotics. In units where resistant organisms, e.g. VRE, have been a problem the use of glycopeptides locks may be discouraged.

Respiratory tract infections

Pneumonia and pulmonary infections

Non-infective pulmonary complications are common after HSCT and are dealt with in Chapter 11. Lower respiratory tract infections do need to be excluded, if possible, as treatment of non-infective complications usually involves high-dose corticosteroid therapy.

Pulmonary infections mostly occur late in the course of transplantation, but up to 35% may occur prior to transplant and these are usually fungal in etiology. Infections in the post-engraftment period (day 30–100) are often viral (see Chapter 7). Opportunistic pathogens are usually responsible for pulmonary infections in HSCT recipients.

Bacterial infections

Bacterial pneumonias occur with an incidence of approximately 12–15% in the first 100 days post-HSCT and occur more frequently in allogeneic recipients than those receiving autologous transplants. Although it seems logical that bacterial pneumonia should be most common in the early neutropenic phase post-HSCT, because of the profound myelosuppression, relatively few bacterial pneumonias are confirmed at this time. It is more common for neutropenic patients to develop a febrile illness and bacteremia during this period. The use of empirical broad-spectrum antibiotics probably accounts for the relatively infrequent confirmation, by positive cultures, of a bacterial pneumonia.

Persistent deficits in cellular and humoral immunity, however, increase susceptibility to infection by encapsulated organisms (e.g. *Streptococcus pneumoniae*) and intracellular pathogens (e.g. *Listeria*). The importance of anti-infective prophylaxis and immunization after HSCT is described in Chapters 13 and 14.

Atypical pneumonias, caused by *Legionella* or *Mycoplasma* for example, are unusual post-HSCT. In the absence of specific clinical or environmental concerns about these organisms, it is reasonable to omit agents such as clarithromycin from initial therapy. Infection with *Mycobacteria* is rare in patients undergoing HSCT in developed countries.

Fungal infections

Fungi are the commonest cause of pulmonary infections post-HSCT.
- *Aspergillus* is the causative organism in around 90% of these infections.
- *Aspergillus* pneumonia is associated with mortality rates as high as 80%.

Pneumocystis was commonly seen late post-HSCT but is uncommon now except in severe immunodefiency conditions and as diagnosis and treatment differ from other invasive fungal infections, it will be considered separately (see below).

Patients may not develop significant clinical abnormalities until the disease is well established but antibiotic-resistant fever, dry cough, pleuritic chest pain, falling oxygen saturations, reduced exercise tolerance, and hemoptysis raise the clinical suspicion and require urgent investigation in the post-HSCT setting.

Pulmonary *Aspergillus* infections can be defined as follows.

• *Angioinvasive* – occurs in 70% of cases. Fungus invades blood vessels and causes lung damage by hemorrhagic infarction. This condition is associated with hemoptysis, which can be catastrophic.
• *Airway invasive* – occurs in 30% of cases. Aspergillosis causes bronchitis, bronchiectasis and pneumonia.

Investigations for fungal infection

Chest X-ray
Parenchymal opacification and pulmonary nodules +/– cavitation are well described in fungal lung infections. Whilst the chest X-ray may be of some use in monitoring response to treatment, it may be normal in the early phases of the disease and cannot be relied upon for diagnosis. This is a problem given the proven benefit of early intervention in this disease. High-resolution CT scanning is therefore essential.

High-resolution computed tomography (HRCT)
This is a more sensitive and specific than a plain chest X-ray. In addition, CT scanning may assist in the differential diagnosis of infection post-HSCT. The following specific changes may be seen in IFI.

• Early signs of angioinvasive aspergillosis include a pulmonary nodule surrounded by a halo of ground glass known as the "CT halo sign." Figure 8.2 shows a CT scan of a patient with invasive pulmonary aspergillosis. The halo represents areas of hemorrhagic infarction around the fungal infection.
• Pulmonary infarction +/– segmental and subsegmental consolidation may be seen.
• Cavitation is a late sign often associated with a recovery in the patient's neutrophil count.
• In airway-invasive aspergillosis the HRCT typically shows patchy peribronchial or peribronchiolar consolidation.
• There is evidence of infection spreading across tissue planes, as shown in Fig. 8.3.

Bronchoscopy and bronchoalveolar lavage (BAL)
BAL fluid can be examined microscopically, cultured for bacteria, fungi and viruses and used for other investigations such as *Aspergillus* antigen and CMV PCR. BAL is a more sensitive technique for detection of airway-invasive aspergillosis than for angioinvasive aspergillosis. If possible lung biopsy may be performed, although this may be hazardous in the post-transplant setting because of

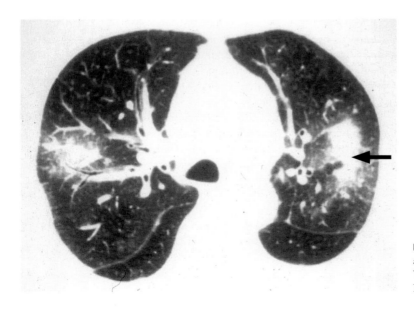

Fig. 8.2 HRCT showing invasive aspergillosis. (Courtesy of Dr S. Worthy, Department of Radiology, Newcastle Upon Tyne Hospitals.)

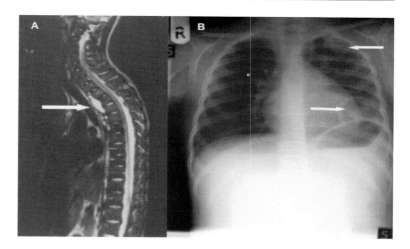

Fig. 8.3 CT scan and chest X-ray showing pulmonary invasive aspergillosis associated with spinal abscess due to direct spread of fungus.

a low platelet count and compromised pulmonary function.

Treatment of pulmonary fungal infections

Aspergillus infection in the lung can be treated with amphotericin B or its lipid alternatives. The use of alternative agents may be considered (caspofungin or voriconazole), on the basis of known toxicities and likely drug interactions. Patients who had fungal pneumonia prior to transplant may be considered for a pneumonectomy prior to transplant and should receive secondary prophylaxis during HSCT (voriconazole or an amphotericin B product).

Pneumocystis

The incidence of *Pneumocystis* pneumonia (PCP) has fallen markedly since the introduction of routine prophylaxis with co-trimoxazole, which is usually given for 6–12 weeks post-transplant. Formerly, *Pneumocystis* pneumonia was seen in the first 100 days post-HSCT but now it is more commonly found in the late post-HSCT phase when prophylaxis has been discontinued. Prophylaxis does need to be continued in patients with chronic GVHD.

Typical features of PCP are:
- fever;
- dry cough;
- reduced exercise tolerance;
- reduced oxygen saturation;
- clinical signs may be minimal.

Chest X-ray findings:
- are usually more florid than the clinical signs;
- most commonly show diffuse bilateral reticular shadowing +/– alveolar consolidation;
- can be variable in appearance with nodular infiltrates and focal consolidation.

Diagnosis

Infection is often suspected from chest X-ray changes (Fig. 8.4) and, if possible, induced sputum or BAL fluid should be sent for PCP immunofluorescence. However, treatment should not be delayed and empirical therapy with high-dose co-trimoxazole is warranted in high-risk patients. Figure 8.5 demonstrates typical pneumocystis cysts seen on immunofluorescence of BAL fluid. Steroids are beneficial in moderate to severe PCP for the first 5 days with a tapering dose to complete 3 weeks of treatment.

Alternatives to co-trimoxazole include dapsone, atovaquone, pentamidine, and clindamycin with primaquine.

Likely pathogens – viral

Viral respiratory tract infections are more common in the post-engraftment period and include those viruses which may have reactivated (CMV and HHV6) and those community-acquired infections such as respiratory syncytial virus (RSV), influenza and parainfluenza, which may be acquired when

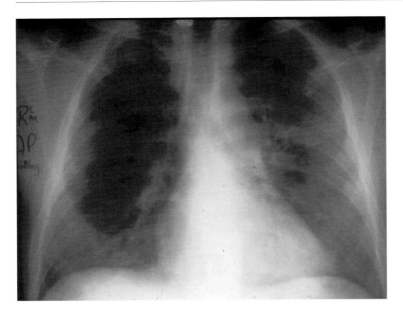

Fig. 8.4 Chest X-ray showing diffuse shadowing due to Pneumocystis pneumonia. (Courtesy of Dr S. Worthy, Department of Radiology, Newcastle Upon Tyne Hospitals.)

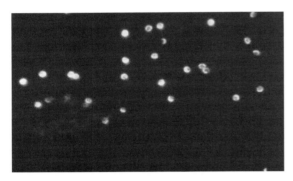

Fig. 8.5 Pneumocystis cysts in bronchoalveolar fluid stained using immunofluoresence.

the patient is not in protective isolation. See Chapter 7 for details of viral infections.

Paranasal sinus infections

These may present with typical symptoms of sinusitis such as:
- frontal headache;
- facial pain and tenderness;
- fever;
- mucopurulent nasal discharge;

- unilateral nasal blockage of new onset.

However, symptoms may be non-specific and CT scanning may be required to exclude infection. Antibiotics as well as antifungal therapy should be started if sinus infection is suspected post-HSCT.

Fungal infection

Acute fulminant invasive fungal sinusitis is much commoner in transplant recipients and has the highest mortality of all fungal infections in the post-HSCT period, particularly among recipients of allogeneic grafts. Most common causative organisms are *Aspergillus* spp., the zygomycetes, *Fusarium* spp. and *Scedosporium* spp. It is vital that such infections are recognized and treated promptly in order to reduce the risk of disseminated fungal infection and/or local bony invasion with subsequent cerebral abscess development.

Bacterial infections

The usual bacterial pathogens may be found infecting the sinuses, e.g. *Haemophilus influenzae*, *Streptococcus pneumoniae*, *Moraxella catarrhalis*, *Staphylococcus aureus*.

Management

• Careful assessment for sinus symptoms must be part of the assessment of any febrile HSCT patient.
• If symptoms are detected, radiological investigations should be performed.
• Plain sinus X-rays are generally not helpful, although they may reveal an air fluid level in the affected sinus, though this is a relatively non-specific finding.
• CT scanning of the sinuses is essential to detect more subtle and specific abnormalities, or signs of infection destroying bone and crossing tissue planes, particularly into the intracerebral cavity, as this is a particularly ominous sign.
• In patients with a demonstrable abnormality on sinus CT scan or persistent sinus symptoms, urgent ENT assessment is essential.
• Sinus washouts with bacterial and fungal culture of aspirated fluid along with surgical debridement and biopsy of the affected sinus mucosa can be therapeutic as well as diagnostic.

Treatment

Antifungal therapy in proven or probable invasive fungal sinusitis is essential. Caspofungin does not have activity against moulds such as *Mucor* and *Fusarium*, which may be the cause of infection. Useful agents include liposomal amphotericin and voriconazole. Antibacterial agents may also be needed unless fungal infection has been proven.

Central nervous system (CNS) infections

Neurological signs or symptoms are not uncommon after HSCT, particularly in the allogeneic setting. Whilst metabolic derangements and the complications of drug therapy, e.g. ciclosporin toxicity, are important causes of such problems, CNS infections account for approximately 40% of these neurological events. Such infections can be divided into:
• focal infections;
• meningoencephalitis/meningitis.

Focal infections
Fungal infections

Fungal infections account for almost all brain abscesses in the post-transplant period. *Aspergillus* is the most common pathogen. Figure 8.6 shows an *Aspergillus* brain abscess on CT scan. Brain abscesses due to more unusual fungi are increasing in incidence and broad-spectrum antifungals should be used for treatment of suspected fungal brain abscesses, in combination if necessary.

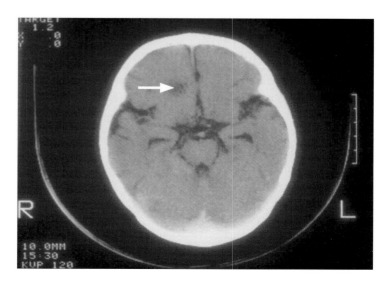

Fig. 8.6 High-resolution CT scan of brain showing fungal brain abscess in frontal lobe.

Candida endophthalmitis may occur with disseminated infection and the eyes should always be examined to look for typical *Candida* "cotton wool" infiltrates in the retina.

Clinical features

Aspergillus brain abscesses occur at a median of 70 days after allogeneic HSCT (range 6–300 days). Infection may be limited to the brain but more commonly occurs in association with another focus of infection, most often the respiratory tract.

• In any patient found to have a brain abscess, the respiratory tract should be imaged for signs of fungal infection.

• In the absence of a respiratory tract fungal infection, biopsy of the cerebral lesion should be considered, to clarify the diagnosis and guide treatment.

Patients typically present with an alteration in mental status, which may initially be very subtle but typically deteriorates rapidly. Seizures, often focal, are reported in up to 40%. Meningism is unusual but can occur due to secondary subarachoid hemorrhage or fungal mycelium rupture into the subarachnoid space. Radiologically, *Aspergillus* brain abscesses are typically multifocal lesions. They usually form in the cerebral hemispheres rather than the cerebellum or brain stem and may be associated with tissue infarction as a result of angioinvasion.

Candida infection is a rare cause of brain abscesses post-HSCT, accounting for <5% of CNS lesions. Radiologically, lesions caused by *Candida* are typically multiple but much smaller than those caused by *Aspergillus* and are located in the gray or deep white matter.

Management

No antifungal agent has been shown to be more efficacious in the therapy of proven *Aspergillus* infection than amphotericin B or liposomal derivatives. Voriconazole penetrates the brain and CSF, and is likely to be useful in treatment of yeast and mould CNS infections. Given the very high mortality associated with fungal brain abscesses (approaching 100% in many studies), many clinicians currently utilize a combination of antifungal agents.

Bacterial infections

Brain abscesses secondary to bacterial infections are rare after allogeneic HSCT. Organisms shown to cause this type of infection include: *Nocardia*, *Klebsiella*, *Staphylococcus aureus* and *Pseudomonas aeruginosa*.

Like fungal infections, bacterial brain abscesses often develop as a secondary event after failure to control infection at a primary site.

Protozoal infections

Toxoplasma

Toxoplasmosis may affect up to 1 in 300 allogeneic HSCT recipients; this increases to 1 in 100 when autopsy data are taken into account. New infection, but more usually reactivation of existing cysts, typically occurs within the first 100 days post transplant. As with many other infections, ongoing GVHD, steroid therapy and use of other immunosuppressants increase the risk of disease developing.

Toxoplasma seems to have a predilection for the CNS and causes infection either by local invasion or hematogenous spread to the brain. In the brain cysts may form with surrounding calcification, which produce typical CT changes. Prognosis is often poor with mortality rates of 40–66%. Clinical symptoms are usually those of a space-occupying lesion with some of the following features:

• focal neurological signs such as hemiparesis;

• cranial nerve palsies;

• visual fields defects;

• less specific features such as seizures or drowsiness;

• pulmonary involvement with respiratory symptoms may also be seen.

Imaging such as CT and MRI are very helpful and can give characteristic but not diagnostic changes. Lesions are typically multiple, periventricular and demonstrate ring enhancement. Ring enhancement may be reduced or absent in HSCT patients due to their reduced ability to generate an effective inflammatory response to the infection.

Management

Reaching a definitive diagnosis in the immunocompromised patient is difficult. Histology of biopsied areas is suggestive, and tissue and CSF cultures are diagnostic but not sensitive. Obtaining a tissue diagnosis may require overly invasive procedures; hence PCR of CSF and blood is increasingly useful.

Treatment is with pyrimethamine and sulfadiazine; with clindamycin and pyrimethamine as an alternative. Folinic acid should also be added. Steroids may be useful to prevent pressure effects. Treatment should be continued for at least six weeks and maintenance considered whilst immunosuppression continues.

Meningoencephalitis and meningitis
Viral infections

Most cases of meningitis or meningoencephalitis in the post-transplant setting are caused by viruses, e.g. CMV, adenovirus, parvovirus, HHV6. These infections are discussed in Chapter 7. Although rarer, bacterial and fungal infections can also occur.

Bacterial infections

As with bacterial brain abscesses, it is more common for bacterial meningitis to occur on a background of a systemic infection rather than *de novo*. The most common causative bacteria are *Klebsiella*, *Haemophilus influenzae*, *Pseudomonas aeruginosa* and *Staphylococcus aureus*. Tuberculous meningitis is rare. *Listeria* has also been documented to cause meningitis, typically in the late post-HSCT period. Trimethoprim–sulfamethoxazole prophylaxis, used to prevent *Pneumocystis* pneumonia, should also prevent *Listeria* meningitis.

Fungal infections

While fungal brain abscesses can result in meningitis or meningoencephalitis, as described above, the most common fungus to cause meningitis is *Cryptococcus.*
- Onset of symptoms is generally slower than in meningitis due to other infections.
- A typical headache of raised intracranial pressure may be described.

- Diagnosis is by visualization of cryptococci by microscopy, detection of cryptococcal antigen in the CSF and/or positive culture of the organism from that site.
- Treatment is usually a combination of amphotericin B and either fluconazole or flucytosine for 2 weeks or until the CSF is sterile, with at least 6 weeks, total completed treatment with amphotericin B or fluconazole.

Gastrointestinal infections

Among HSCT recipients, the gastrointestinal (GI) tract is both a very common portal of entry for pathogens and a site of infection. Loss of integrity of the mucosal barrier within the gut predisposes to both local and systemic infections with both bacterial and viral pathogens.

Bacterial infections

Organisms causing food poisoning (e.g. *Salmonella*, *Campylobacter*) may be seen in the transplant patient mostly in the post-engraftment or late transplant phase. Attention to food hygiene in any immunocompromised patient is important to prevent these infections.

Clostridium difficile

Clostridium difficile is a relatively common infection in this group of heavily antibiotic-treated adult patients, but surprisingly rare in children. Fecal carriage of *Clostridium difficile*, as detected by culture, is not necessarily always associated with significant infection. However, detection of *Clostridium difficile* toxin in the stool in transplant patients would usually warrant treatment with oral vancomycin or metronidazole, especially if the patient has a fever, diarrhea, or abdominal pain. If oral agents cannot be tolerated then intravenous metronidazole should be used. Relapsing cases may require repeated prolonged courses of vancomycin or metronidazole. Intravenous immunoglobulin (given as two doses) has been used with some success in these cases.

Table 8.2 Symptoms and signs of typhlitis

Severe right iliac fossa pain
Nausea and vomiting
Diarrhea or constipation
Abdominal tenderness
Abdominal distension
Guarding
Absent bowel sounds

Typhlitis

During the neutropenic period, patients are at risk of developing neutropenic enterocolitis (also called typhlitis). This is more common in adults and rarely seen in children. Symptoms and signs are given in Table 8.2. CT scanning shows edema of the bowel mucosa, most commonly in the cecum and terminal ileum. Rarely, typhlitis may be due to fungal infection.

Laparotomy and bowel resection in this highly vulnerable group of patients is extremely dangerous and conservative management is the best approach. Treatment should include broad-spectrum antibiotics to cover Gram-negative bacilli including *Pseudomonas aeruginosa* and anerobes. G-CSF is generally administered to minimize the duration of the neutropenic phase and to help improve mucosal defenses. Typhlitis occurs most frequently among patients who have had a previous episode; vigilance is required when patients who have had typhlitis during previous periods of neutropenia are transplanted. Given the high mortality associated with this condition, it may be worth considering antibiotic prophylaxis in this group of high-risk patients.

Viral infections

These will include rotavirus, norovirus, sapovirus and adenovirus, especially type 40/41. Infection may persist until engraftment. Further details of viral infections are given in Chapter 7.

Fungal infections

The most common fungal infection to affect the GI tract is candidiasis. Other yeasts, e.g. *Saccharomy-* *ces*, can cause a similar clinical picture to candidal infections. Moulds, e.g. *Aspergillus*, rarely affect the gut but may do so with disastrous consequences as diagnosis is usually made very late. Candidiasis most commonly affects the esophagus but the stomach and small intestine can also be involved. Patients typically complain of pain on swallowing and often describe the sensation of "food sticking." Diagnosis is often made clinically with endoscopy and cultures or biopsies where appropriate. Patients with extensive localized candidal infection are at risk of developing disseminated disease.

Hepatosplenic candidiasis

This may be difficult to diagnose and should be considered in patients with a fever not responding to antibiotics, and who have worsening liver function tests for no other obvious reason; the liver may also be tender to palpation. Ultrasound imaging and a positive serum mannan may be suggestive of infection. Antifungal may need to be used on suspicion of infection if liver biopsy cannot be performed.

Protozoal infections
Cryptosporidium

In the immunocompetent *Cryptosporidium* causes a self-limiting but acute illness with diarrhea and vomiting, abdominal pain, fever and malaise. In the face of a T-cell immune deficiency, cryptosporidia are not cleared from the gut and symptoms persist. In certain primary immune deficiencies such as CD40 ligand deficiency, prolonged infection may also be associated with ascending cholangitis and liver disease. Infection may be occult, and only present after pre-HSCT conditioning treatment when unexplained fevers are seen.

Diagnosis
Oocytes may be seen on direct feces microscopy; however, more sensitive methods, e.g. immunofluorescence or PCR, may be needed to detect low numbers of organisms. Patients at high risk of infection, e.g. with T-cell immune defects, should have feces screened by PCR prior to transplant. *Cryptosporidia* may also be detected in jejunal or rectal biopsies by histology or PCR.

Treatment

Cryptosporidia infection is difficult to treat and treatment will not be fully successful until immune recovery; however, treatment may limit progression of infection. Paromomycin has been used and there is a suggestion that azithromycin may be beneficial. Recently nitazoxanide has been shown to decrease symptoms in the immunocompetent and may have a role in controlling symptoms in the immunocompromised. Although no treatment has proven benefit in the HSCT patient, it is suggested that specific treatment should be given for patients undergoing transplant if they are found to be colonized prior to transplant, as fatal infection can occur. It has been our practice to use azithromycin sometimes in combination with nitazoxanide during transplant in these patients.

Strongyloides

The nematode *Strongyloides stercoralis* needs to be considered as a cause of diarrhea among patients who have lived in areas of the world where this infection is endemic: the tropics and some parts of Europe and North America. Immunosuppressed patients may develop hyperinfection, during which time larvae migrate into the lungs and intestine but can also be found in the CNS, liver, kidneys, and other organs. Bowel involvement may cause significant abdominal pain, vomiting and diarrhea. Ulceration of the colonic mucosa can be associated with secondary bacteremia and massive hemorrhage. For diagnosis fresh stool specimens should be sent for microscopy, and possibly duodenal fluid and respiratory secretions. Ivermectin, thiabendazole or albendazole are curative, though an infectious diseases specialist should be consulted regarding treatment.

Other parasites

These include *Microsporidia*, *Cyclospora*, *Balantidi coli*, *Blastocystis* and *Isospora*, which are uncommon parasites that also cause diarrhea, both in the immunocompetent and immunocompromised. Diagnosis requires special stains on feces.

Skin and soft tissue infections

The most common infective lesions in HSCT patients are due to:
- central line exit site or tunnel infections;
- primary or secondary bacterial infections;
- fungal infections;
- *Varicella zoster*.

The most common bacteria to cause skin or soft tissue infections include *Staphylococci* and *Streptococci*. Gram-negative organisms such as *E. coli*, *Klebsiella* and *Pseudomonas* are less commonly responsible. Similarly fungal skin infections, e.g. intertrigo and nappy rash, commonly occur. Superficial fungal infections are usually due to *Candida* or other yeasts, like *Saccharomyces*, and should be treated with topical agents in the first instance, after sending appropriate swabs to the laboratory. Although *Candida albicans* is the most common yeast causing these infections in the general population, in the immunocompromised other *Candida* species and other yeasts may be responsible. Sensitivity, especially to azole antifungal, cannot be predicted. Rarely skin lesions are due to disseminated yeast infection (*Candida* or *Cryptococcus*). Mould infections of skin, other than dermatophytes, are usually as a result of invasion from deep-seated invasive infections.

In many cases the cause of a skin or soft tissue infection is clear. Generally the skin has been directly compromised, for example by an indwelling central venous line or a biopsy needle. Folliculitis is also relatively common, though often much more extensive than that seen in patients who are immunocompetent. Antibiotic therapy may be chosen empirically, particularly if the patient is profoundly neutropenic, but treatment should be guided by cultures of the particular lesions.

Ecthyma gangrenosum

- Ecthyma gangrenosum is a skin disorder specific to neutropenic patients, which occurs as a result of infection within deep subcutaneous veins.
- It is most often due to bacteria such as *Pseudomonas aeruginosa* (Fig. 8.7) but can also occur secondary to fungal infection such as aspergillosis or mucormycosis.

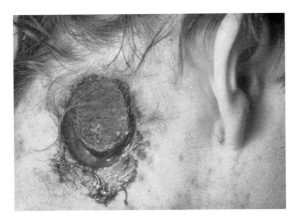

Fig. 8.7 Ecthyma gangrenosum causing severe skin and tissue necrosis.

• Clinically the lesions are painful, well circumscribed, bright red and usually just palpable with a ring or surrounding pallor. Over a relatively short time (24 hours) the center becomes darker and may be raised into a bulla. Eventually the sharply demarcated central portion becomes black.

• These lesions are best treated by isolating the organism responsible and biopsies may be necessary.

Urinary tract infections

The urinary tract may be a source of sepsis in the HSCT patient and cultures should be sent from all patients with a fever. During transplantation the patient will be neutropenic; therefore pyuria is unlikely to be present. The absence of pyuria should not be taken as a guide to the significance of any microbial growth.

• Catheterization increases the risk of UTI and should be avoided if possible.

• Treatment with antibiotics should not be withheld because of lack of pyuria.

• Children with a UTI should be managed and investigated as in any child, although imaging may need to be delayed until after the transplant period.

• Urine should always be cultured for *Candida* as well as bacteria, as candiduria may be the first indication of a systemic *Candida* infection.

• Viruses, e.g. polyoma, may also cause urinary symptoms and in particular hematuria. Urine needs to be sent for polyoma PCR in patients with gross hematuria. There is no specific treatment, other than encouraging hydration to prevent the development of clots obstructing the urinary tract.

• On isolation of a significant bacterial count from urine, antibiotics should be started without delay. During neutropenia the standard neutropenic sepsis antibiotics should be used initially.

• Treatment of UTI in patients who are not neutropenic (post-transplant) may be with standard antibiotics that produce good serum and urinary levels, e.g. cefalexin, trimethoprim, co-amoxiclav, and ciprofloxacin. Nitrofurantoin is only a urinary antiseptic and should not be used.

Use of the microbiology laboratory

Throughout this chapter the specimens required to make a diagnosis have been highlighted. However, some general principles do need to be stressed:

• Ensure the patient's details are correct and the name on the samples matches that on the request forms. The wrong result on the wrong patient can have disastrous consequences.

• Precise clinical details should be given to guide the laboratory. For example, "transplant patient" will not be sufficient – indicate symptoms.

• If fungal infection is suspected, prolonged fungal culture may need to be specifically requested.

• If specimens are taken that are not easily repeated, e.g. biopsies, brain aspirate, always telephone the laboratory to warn them in advance that the specimen is on its way.

• Ensure that biopsies and tissues for culture are not placed in formalin.

• Contact the laboratory if in any doubt about which specimens to take and when.

• Automated runs of certain tests, e.g. CMV PCR, may only be carried out on certain days of the week. To maximize obtaining timely results make sure that you take specimens in time for a particular run.

• Some tests may need to be sent away to a reference laboratory and take longer to get a result.

Know what your local laboratory can and cannot do.

• Have an agreement about what results will be telephoned through to the ward.

• Make sure that specimens are taken where possible during the working day.

Close collaboration between the laboratory staff and the HSCT unit is essential for the timely diagnosis and management of infection in HSCT patients.

Future developments

As the range of conditions for which patients receive a transplant increases, so does the variety of pathogens to which patients may be exposed pre- and post-transplant. Antimicrobial resistance is increasing worldwide and presents a further challenge to treatment. Molecular diagnostic techniques, such as PCR, are improving and rapid diagnosis is essential to ensure appropriate antimicrobial therapy is delivered promptly, to minimize patient morbidity and mortality.

Further reading

Apperley, J., Carreras, E., Gluckman, E. *et al.* (eds) (2004) Infections after HSCT. In: *Hematopoietic Stem Cell Transplantation: EBMT Handbook*. Paris: European School of Haematology, pp. 147–160.

Baddley, J.W., Stroud, T.P., Salzman, D., Pappas, P.G. (2001) Invasive mould infections in allogeneic bone marrow transplant recipients. *Clin Infect Dis* **32**: 1319–1324.

Bishton, M., Chopra, R. (2004) The role of granulocyte transfusions in neutropenic patients. *Br J Haematol* **127**: 501–508.

Bowden, R.A., Ljungman, P., Paya, C.V. (eds) (2003) *Transplant Infections*, 2nd edn. Philadelphia, PA: Lippincott Williams & Wilkins.

Craddock, C., Chakraverty, R. (2005) Stem cell transplantation. In: Hoffbrand, A.V., Catovsky, D., Tuddenham, E.G.D. (eds), *Postgraduate Haematology*. Oxford: Blackwell Publishing.

Hovi, L., Saarinen-Pihkala, U.M., Vettenranta, K., Saxen, H. (2000) Invasive fungal infections in pediatric bone marrow transplant recipients: single center experience of 10 years. *Bone Marrow Transplant* **26**: 999–1004.

Hughes, W.T., Armstrong, D., Bodey, G.P. *et al.* (2002) Guidelines for the use of antimicrobial agents in neutropenic patients with cancer. *Clin Infect Dis* **34**: 730–751.

Kruger, W., Russmann, B., Kroger, N. *et al.* (1999) Early infections in patients under going bone marrow or blood stem cell transplantation – a 7 year single centre investigation of 409 cases. *Bone Marrow Transplant* **23**: 589–597.

Leather, H.L., Wingard, J.R. (2001) Infections following hematopoietic stem cell transplantation. *Infect Dis Clin North Am* **15**: 483–520.

Mermel, L.A., Farr, B.M., Sherertz, R.J. *et al.* (2001) Guidelines for the management of intravascular catheter–related infections. *Clin Infect Dis* **32**: 1249–1272.

Ninin, E., Milpied, N., Moreau, P. *et al.* (2001) Longitudinal study of bacterial, viral and fungal infections in adult recipients of bone marrow transplants. *Clin Infect Dis* **33**: 41–47.

Pagliuca, A., Carrington, P.A., Pettengell, R., Tule, S., Keidan, J., Haemato-Oncology Task Force of the British Committee for Standards in Haematology (2003) Guidelines on the use of colony-stimulating factors in haematological malignancies. *Br J Haematol* **123**: 22–33.

Viscoli, C., Castagnola, E. (2005) Prophylaxis and empirical therapy for infection in cancer patients. In: Mandell, G.L., Bennett, J.E., Dolin, R. (eds) *Mandell, Douglas and Bennett's Principles and Practice of Infectious Diseases*. Philadelphia, PA: Elsevier Churchill Livingstone, pp. 3442–3461.

Chapter 9

The role of intensive care in the management of hematopoietic stem cell patients

B. Fulton and A. Gascoigne

Introduction

Hematopoietic stem cell transplantation (HSCT) is now a widely accepted technique in the treatment of hematological and solid organ malignancies as well as in primary immunodeficiency and other nonmalignant congenital disorders. The intensive care unit (ICU), both for adults and children, may become involved in patient care at many stages. This includes the early presentation and management of the underlying disorder and any associated problems, but more importantly post-HSCT in the management of complications related to the disease or the transplant process.

The role of the ICU is to provide supportive care and organ support to allow sufficient time for specific therapies to work. The specific details of individual organ support are beyond the remit of this book and general principles are discussed. ICU protocols follow standard practices and are available in ICU textbooks.

The admission of any patient to ICU should be after careful consideration of the reversibility of the underlying conditions in combination with the predicted survival. The power to do good should be carefully considered and balanced with the chances of harm. In conditions where the prognosis is poor and the predicted survival is less than 6 months, ICU care should be questioned.

The admission of a patient to ICU after HSCT is a highly significant indicator of mortality. It is therefore vital that the ICU and transplant teams work closely to manage these patients from the outset to allow the maximum chance of survival and also to recognize the possible futility of admission, allowing for palliative care. In a number of studies the rate of admission to ICU following HSCT is 10–40% and the need for mechanical ventilation 6–33%.

Recently there has been an attempt to move away from the traditional terms of ICU and high-dependency unit (HDU), recognizing that patients require different levels of care (Table 9.1), not necessarily being governed by the need to be managed in a specific unit. The presence of a comprehensive critical care service within a hospital performing HSCT is mandatory; this includes an outreach service providing both specialist nursing and medical input to the HSCT unit, traditionally only delivered in the ICU setting.

Table 9.1 Different levels of patient care

Level 0	Patients whose needs can be met through normal ward care in an acute hospital
Level 1	Patients at risk of their condition deteriorating, or those recently relocated from higher levels of care, whose needs can be met on an acute ward with additional advice and support from the critical care team
Level 2	Patients requiring more detailed observation or intervention, including support for a single failing organ system or postoperative care, and those stepping down from higher levels of care
Level 3	Patients requiring advanced respiratory support alone or basic respiratory support together with support of at least two organ systems. This includes all complex patients requiring support for multiple organ failure

Pre-transplant issues

In children with primary immune deficiency syndromes the early clinical presentation includes general deterioration, failure to thrive, skin problems, and recurrent infections. A number of infants will present to the pediatric ICU with respiratory infections requiring assisted ventilation. Often the child may have opportunistic/atypical infections including *Pneumocystis jiroveci* pneumonia (PCP).

Children undergoing chemotherapy for malignancy may also present with respiratory failure secondary to opportunistic infection. It is important that appropriate diagnostic tests including bronchoalveolar lavage (BAL) are considered at the earliest opportunity. This is the best investigation to identify pneumocystis but it is also important to recognize other concomitant infections. PCP requiring assisted ventilation is more difficult to manage successfully if there is other infection, e.g. cytomegalvirus (CMV).

In the ICU patient or those considered at risk of requiring ventilatory support there may be concern that bronchoscopy with BAL may be hazardous and worsen respiratory failure, leading to the need for endotracheal intubation and ventilation. The need to establish a diagnosis may exceed the need to avoid ventilation but should be carefully considered. The role of pre-emptive nasal (non-invasive) ventilation or continuous positive airway pressure (CPAP) can be considered. CPAP is a means whereby positive pressure is applied via a face mask so as to assist in lung recruitment by preventing small airways from collapsing at closing volume, thus increasing functional residual volume. This is akin to pursed lipped breathing.

In children BAL may be performed during anesthesia for central line insertion or other procedures. Nonbronchoscopic saline lavage (1–2 mL/kg) performed at intubation or under general anesthetic (GA) for other procedures is felt to be satisfactory in identifying respiratory pathogens and has minimal risk of precipitating assisted ventilation.

The need for either an individual to be admitted to the ICU prior to HSCT or acceptance onto the program should be guided by the treatability of the condition leading to the deterioration. The fact that a HSCT is technically possible should not confuse the issue; if the clinical picture appears futile and death is inevitable, ICU-type care should not be considered.

Prior advice and information as to the feasibility of ICU in a patient's care has been advocated in the HSCT transplant consent process.

Preparation for transplant

The individual will need long-term IV access and usually will undergo surgical placement of central lines. This is our opportunity to perform saline lavage (nonbronchoscopic BAL) and obtain other biopsies that will help diagnosis and management. Most children will tolerate the anesthesia for these procedures without significant deterioration. However, additional care should always be taken with aseptic preparation of drugs and infusions to minimize infection risks for the central lines once inserted.

Post-transplant issues

Serious complications occurring after HSCT that may require admission to the ICU include:
- toxicity of conditioning regime;
- severe prolonged marrow suppression – with hemorrhagic and infective risks;
- graft-vs.-host disease (GVHD);
- veno-occlusive disease (VOD) – hepatic and renal impairment;
- respiratory impairment –infection, hemorrhage, inflammation;
- systemic inflammatory response syndrome;
- septic shock.

General ICU care issues
ICU isolation

When HSCT recipients are admitted to ICU, where possible they should be cared for in single cubicles, with high-efficiency particulate air (HEPA) filtration and positive pressure. The need for preparation of drugs aseptically and general isolation precautions mean that these individuals have a very high nursing dependency. When requiring multiple organ system support in ICU these patients may require at least two nurses to deliver their care.

Skin

Infants with primary immune deficiency often have severe problems with dry or damaged skin, and careful protection is required with tapes used to secure tubes and IV lines. Pressure areas are also at risk and special mattresses are often required. In others the presence of extensive tissue edema or the frequent problem with diarrhea makes caring for these patients challenging.

Sedation and analgesia

Appropriate drugs to maintain comfort and alleviate distress are part of any ICU care package. The drugs used will usually be a mixture of sedative and analgesic agents. Table 9.2 indicates the common agents used.

Common regimes used

In occasional instances where a localized pain problem exists, then local anesthetic and regional blockade may be helpful, e.g. epidural analgesia for severe hemorrhagic cystitis. Advice from the hospital acute pain team and specialists in chronic pain should be sought when there is additional concern.

Respiratory support in ICU

Respiratory complications that require assisted ventilation post-HSCT are associated with a high

Table 9.2 Commonly used agents for sedation and analgesia

Analgesia	Sedation	Oral sedatives
Morphine infusion	Propofol (adults only)	Vallergan
Fentanyl infusion	Midazolam	Triclofos
	Lorazepam	Chloral hydrate
		Chlorpromazine
		Diazepam
		Lorazepam

mortality. Respiratory deterioration is therefore often an early trigger for referral to ICU.

Increased oxygen requirement and work of breathing should alert the clinician to investigate likely causes – infection, inflammation, hemorrhage, and pulmonary edema.

Clinical features to note:
- increased work of breathing:
  - tachypnea;
  - recession – intercostals and subcostal;
  - accessory muscle use;
  - alar flaring;
  - grunting respiration;
- tachycardia;
- hypoxia;
- acidosis;
- apneas.

Chest radiograph (CXR) appearances are frequently indistinguishable, whether the deterioration is as a result of infection, inflammation or even pulmonary hemorrhage, and the common picture is of "fluffy white lungs" due to diffuse air space shadowing. Sputum or tracheal aspirates (once intubated) should be sent for microbiological and virological investigations. When infection is suspected, formal BAL or non-bronchoscopic BAL should be performed to identify respiratory pathogens. These cases are often complicated and in many clinical situations no organisms may be isolated and treatment must be empirical.

Initially the individual may simply need humidified oxygen with empirical antimicrobial chemotherapy or other specific interventions as indicated. If clinical deterioration occurs then early referral for ICU assessment should be requested and outreach services utilized. Careful fluid management is essential to minimize additional respiratory deterioration from fluid overload.

Techniques of respiratory support in ICU
CPAP

CPAP can be achieved by connecting the airway to a high-flow gas supply at constant positive pressure. This prevents alveolar collapse at end expiration and can help maintain oxygenation. This can be applied via nasal prongs in small infants, short endotracheal (ET) tube or even with nasal or full face mask in older children and adults. CPAP may be sufficient to improve oxygenation and provide support, with the specific therapies introduced, to prevent the need for tracheal intubation and ventilation. Some individuals with respiratory failure may be managed with non-invasive ventilation (NIV) from suitable ventilators and breathing circuits with a well-fitting nasal or full face mask.

Children requiring CPAP or NIV should be managed in the PICU in the event of rapid deterioration requiring intubation and mechanical ventilation. However, familiarity with these techniques in the adult HSCT unit may prevent the need for transfer to the ICU.

Intubation and ventilation

Intermittent positive pressure-controlled or -assisted ventilation will be required in many infants and children with respiratory distress after HSCT. This is delivered by appropriate ITU ventilators, which can support both the small 3-kg infants and the older transplant patients who are adult sized. The severity of the pulmonary problems may require high pressures and high fractional-inspired oxygen (FiO_2).

The development of a severe acute lung injury picture is not uncommon and, when encountered, requires lung recruitment strategies adopted with acute respiratory distress syndrome (ARDS). The role of prone ventilation in patients with profound hypoxia is now a recognized method to improve recruitment and thus oxygenation. Its role in conferring survival advantage remains controversial. When high inspired oxygen is needed, protective lung strategies of ventilation are used with high levels of positive end expiratory pressure (PEEP) and low tidal volumes to reduce the risk of further lung injury by volu-trauma. This desired under-ventilation leads to an accepted rise in arterial carbon dioxide termed permissive hypercapnia. Nitric oxide therapy and high-frequency oscillation are occasionally used in severe lung injury that is unresponsive to conventional ventilation, although in most circumstances these will be part of an end-stage management. Other unproven interventions include surfactant therapy and immunological interventions.

Where the diagnosis of the respiratory deterioration remains uncertain there may be indications for more aggressive investigations, such as open lung biopsy, to identify any treatable cause. This may help influence the decision to limit or withdraw treatment in the face of untreatable pulmonary GVHD or fibrosis. On rare occasions the diagnosis may be an indication for prolonged respiratory support.

Fluid management

The large volumes of fluid required in these individuals (notably infants) for delivery of daily drugs, blood products and immunological support mean that if modest fluid restriction is imposed in the ICU there is very little fluid left each day for nutrition. It is preferred that they remain enterally fed. If feeds are not tolerated in the ICU then parenteral nutrition will be required.

Regular review of drugs and medications should be undertaken with the ICU and transplant teams to minimize fluid overload from treatment regimes along with advice from pharmacy regarding absolute minimal volumes, compatibility of drugs and infusions, and preparation of drugs aseptically where possible.

Blood product support is often required post-HSCT – in order to maintain hemoglobin and platelets at acceptable ICU levels this may require supplementation on a daily basis. If invasive procedures are needed then the platelets should be maintained at higher levels. This will frequently require daily transfusions in many of these patients on the ICU. Local arrangements should be sought to ensure the ready availability of platelets on this basis with laboratories and transfusion services.

Transfusion-related acute lung injury (TRALI) has been reported. It produces a massive acute deterioration in respiratory function with fatal consequences. In particular this complication appears to be related to fresh frozen plasma (FFP) transfusion where the donor of the plasma was female. This problem should now be recognized and can be avoided by sourcing FFP from male donors.

Renal support

Nephrotoxicity due to either interstitial nephritis or

acute tubular necrosis may result from numerous insults during the transplant process. Renal failure may be precipitated by hepatocellular dysfunction and in some children with solid organ tumors, e.g. neuroblastoma, there may have even been a previous nephrectomy.

Damage can result from:
- toxic drugs during transplant and conditioning;
- ciclosporin;
- reduced perfusion in sepsis and VOD;
- injudicious use of diuretics.

The need to provide renal support in adults post-HSCT is recognized as being an adverse predictor of outcome and in many centers is invariably thought to be fatal.

In clinical situations where there is increasing renal dysfunction with electrolyte disturbance, acidosis, and fluid overload then renal support may need to be instituted. In ICU this is currently done with continuous veno-venous hemofiltration (CVVH). A double-lumen vascath is sited percutaneously in an appropriate central vein once platelets and clotting factor support has been given. Ultrasound control may help to localize the vein to assist in successful puncture. CVVH has a major advantage of managing fluid balance yet allowing appropriate nutrition and drugs, while the machine can be adjusted to achieve fluid removal as necessary for the daily care.

Principles of CVVH

The traditional methods of renal replacement therapy, such as intermittent hemodialysis and peritoneal dialysis, are unsuitable for the critically ill and continuous methods have taken over.

CVVH is a process of continuous ultra-filtration, removing a directed amount of water from the circulation hourly, which can be replaced by a sterile isotonic electrolyte and bicarbonate solution. The technique requires suitable venous access – usually a double-lumen line – connected to an extracorporeal circuit. An adjustable peristaltic pump will drive the blood around the circuit. The blood passes through a filter with a semi-permeable membrane allowing filtration and diffusion before being returned to the venous circulation.

Newer equipment is available for use in children >6 kg and adults. The volume of the extracorporeal circuit – lines and filter – must be taken into consideration when choosing equipment for small children needing renal support. Blood flow rates and fluid volume exchanges per hour should be set according to generally accepted age and weight guidelines. Fluid balance each day can be set to meet the targets of drug and nutrition requirements. Input will therefore be fixed but the desired rate of fluid removal per hour can be adjusted to achieve an overall negative or positive balance per day. Any extracorporeal circuit use will require the addition of heparin or prostacyclin or both as anticoagulant regimes and these must be carefully monitored with regular coagulation screening.

Caring for a patient on CVVH requires an experienced ICU nurse trained in operating the equipment, and in understanding the procedure and associated risks. Fluid balance should be checked regularly and any additional losses or unexpected fluid problems readily corrected.

Coagulation within the extracorporeal circuit will require the circuit and filter to be replaced; this will often mean additional transfusion requirements in the smaller infants and children. The filter life is usually a maximum of 72 hours and it may be possible to change the circuit with minimal blood loss when this is done electively.

Septic shock

Infection is often considered to be the major cause of acute deterioration in these patients. Sites include line infection, lung infections and GI sites. A high index of suspicion is required and treatment should be commenced empirically. The severity of illness can progress rapidly from sepsis to septic shock and multiple organ dysfunction syndromes (MODS).

The definitions for sepsis, severe sepsis, septic shock and MODS have recently been revised by the 2001 SCCM/ESICM/ACCP/ATS/SIS International Sepsis Definitions Conference and are in regular use in ICUs. Clearly the presence of a low white cell count and low platelet numbers is more likely to be the norm post-HSCT.

Diagnostic criteria for sepsis (see Table 9.3)

Initial resuscitation should begin as soon as the clinical picture is suspected. The patient should be discussed with ICU. Where possible, monitoring of CVP and direct arterial pressure should be instituted.

Fluids are the first line of therapy and include crystalloids or colloids. If required, blood and blood products (FFP, platelets) should be used. Large amounts of fluid may need to be given in the early phase and, if there is ongoing capillary leak, fluids may continue to be required over a pro-longed period. In children standard resuscitation calculations are used with volumes given in boluses of 20 mL/kg. Up to 60 mL/kg may be required over the first few hours. This is usually given as a mixture of crystalloid and colloid or blood products.

Inotropes should be considered early and may include a combination of agents.

Where there is continued low cardiac output despite fluid resuscitation, dobutamine is the first-choice agent but may need to be changed to epinephrine. When hypotension continues, vasopressors may be needed to increase blood pressure and organ perfusion, and norepinephrine or dopamine are recommended.

Monitoring of response should include cardiac output monitoring where possible and a reflection of end organ tissue perfusion including lactate, bicarbonate, and base deficit on regular blood gas analysis.

Refractory shock despite fluid resuscitation and high doses of conventional inotropes and vasopressors may respond to vasopressin infusions, although its precise role has to be defined and may simply act to spare the dose of norepinephrine.

Intravenous hydrocortisone may be added in severe cases – if steroids have not already been part of the treatment regimes – for a period of 7 days. This may be preceded by a synacthen test – and therapy can then be discontinued if results return later as normal.

Table 9.3 Diagnostic criteria for sepsis (taken from Levy *et al.*, 2003, with permission)

Clinical features
Fever >38.3°C or hypothermia <36°C
Heart rate >90 bpm
Tachypnea >30 breaths per minute
Altered mental state
Edema
Hyperglycemia

Inflammatory parameters
Leucocytosis >12,000
Leucopenia <4000
Normal white count with 10% immature forms
CRP >2 SD elevated
Elevated plasma pro-calcitonin

Hemodynamic parameters
Arterial hypotension <90 mmHg mean arterial pressure <75 mmHg
Age appropriate levels of BP for infants <5th percentile for age, or
    systolic BP < 2 SD below normal for age
Mixed venous oxygen saturation <70%
Cardiac index >3.5 L/min/m^2

Signs of organ dysfunction
Arterial hypoxemia
Acute oliguria
Creatinine increase
Coagulation abnormalities
Ileus
Thrombocytopenia
Hyperbilirubinemia
Hyperlactatemia
Decreased capillary refill

Specific therapies

Inflammatory lung injury–idiopathic pneumonia syndrome–pneumonitis

This is a descriptive clinical picture where there is acute lung injury but no identifiable pathogens. Treatment includes supportive therapy but, in addition, immunological interventions such as high-dose steroids, IV immunoglobulin, and anti-TNF (see Chapter 11) may be given where there is suspicion that inflammatory responses may be encouraging lung injury. With such interventions and support the inflammatory picture may improve with resolution of respiratory signs within 5–7 days. Where persistent respiratory deterioration occurs despite all treatments then there should be consideration of open lung biopsy in an attempt to target a group with treatable conditions. Open lung biopsy in a poorly oxygenated immunocompromised patient, however, has serious potential complications and should be only carried out after full and frank discussions with all teams and the patient or their carers.

Diagnosis from open lung biopsy may include:

- unrecognized viral and fungal pneumonias;
- pulmonary GVHD;
- pulmonary VOD;
- persistent inflammatory infiltrates.

Veno-occlusive disease

The child with severe veno-occlusive disease (VOD) may be referred to PICU for respiratory support. They may often present with respiratory distress related to the increased abdominal distension from ascites or from associated infection or inflammation within the lungs themselves. The need for respiratory support may be reduced by inserting a peritoneal catheter to permit drainage of the ascites allowing stabilization on CPAP, for example. The child should be commenced on VOD treatment regimes (see Chapter 11) and other organ system failures supported. If there is progression of renal failure then CVVH may need to be introduced.

Outcomes in ICU

Admissions to ICU/PICU following HSCT have been reviewed for many years, with a reported dismal survival rate The decision to offer ICU support to a patient needs careful consideration by both the referring and accepting teams in addition to an understanding of the patient's view along with their family – adult ICU survival rates are 12–46%, or 0–19% if ventilated; ICU survival rates for children are 27–55% and 9–44% if mechanically ventilated. The 6-month survival rate of ventilated adult patients post-HSCT is of the order of 5%; survival for longer than one year is rare. Patients ventilated late on post-HSCT for chronic GVHD have a much worse outcome and the general consensus would be that they should not be offered ventilatory support.

Attempts have been made to identify admission characteristics to predict outcome and none has been clearly identified.

Discussions surrounding the justification of ICU resources for this group have flourished. Many clinicians are reluctant to institute ICU care or consider withdrawing support in this group, and some have advocated strict time-limited ICU admissions. Groups have tried to identify clinical or disease patterns to predict those with poor outcome.

The overriding philosophy of intensive care is to provide technological support to patients whilst therapies or surgery are pursued to control disease processes, such that the patient has a chance of survival. Provision of futile therapy within ICUs may be supported for a short period as an appropriate opportunity to review the severity of the clinical situation with the family and discuss withdrawal of such treatment.

Many deaths in ICU are the result of withdrawal of treatment. In many instances the preparation for HSCT should include discussions about failure and how the complications of the HSCT process should be managed. It may be an opportunity to discuss ICU plans with patients and families along with opportunity for treatment-limiting decisions or advance directives ("living will") to be expressed.

Predictors of mortality include:

- mechanical ventilation;
- multiple organ failure;
- overwhelming infection;
- GVHD.

The dying process in ICU

Heroic measures have often been described within the literature to support these challenging patients and are often offered. The survival of ICU patients with multiple organ failure has improved, and the survival for HSCT patients may be low but is not hopeless for all patients. However, our progress in managing these patients must be such that we can recognize when our efforts are in vain, and guide our patients and their families through this difficult time. Many will refuse to give up – they have fought their illness and disease for too long to give up without a fight. However, there are situations where the doctors must make the difficult decision to withdraw treatment. Most PICU deaths are as a result of withdrawal or limitation of treatment and this is particularly so in this group of patients. Treatment withdrawal in PICU involves a switch to palliative care and comfort measures for the patient, recognizing that our technology is not prolonging life but delaying death. This is a difficult challenge, and it is important that the parent HSCT teams and the ICU medical and nursing teams are in agreement and can support the patient and family through this time.

Conflict can arise between family and medical teams and within the medical teams involved. National and local specialist advice may be available in dealing with this. Guidance from national bodies has been produced – RCPCH and GMC. Teamwork is essential. Medico-legal support may be required if difficulties remain in resolving the conflict – an increasing development in today's ICU.

Conclusion

The challenge of the post HSCT patient who is deteriorating and referred to ICU will continue. Progress with technological support for the failing organ systems in the ICU has given us a wide range of techniques to manage these patients. However, many of these patients still die – but not all. Careful identification of high-risk patients and evolving treatment regimes may see further progress in targeting our scarce resources to those most likely to benefit.

Further reading

Afessa, B., Tefferi, A., Hoagland, H.C., Letendre, L., Peters, S.G. (1992) Outcome of recipients of bone marrow transplants who require intensive-care unit support. *Mayo Clin Proc* **67**: 117–122/992.

Al-Saidi, F., Diaz-Granados, N., Meesner, H., Herridge, M.S. (2002) Relationship between premortem and postmortem diagnosis in critically ill bone marrow transplantation patients. *Crit Care Med* **30**: 570–573.

Bojko, T., Notterman, D.A., Greenwald, B.M., DeBruin,

W.J., Magid, M.S., Godwin, T. (1995) Acute hypoxemic respiratory failure in children following bone marrow transplantation: An outcome and pathologic study. *Crit Care Med* **23**: 755–759.

Crawford, S.W., Petersen, F.B. (1992) Long-term survival from respiratory failure after bone marrow transplantation for malignancy. *Am Rev Respir Dis* **145**: 510–514.

Crawford, S.W., Schwartz, D.A., Petersen, F.B., Clark, J.G. (1988) Mechanical ventilation after marrow transplantation – Risk factors and clinical outcome. *Am Rev Respir Dis* **137**: 682–687.

Dellinger, R.P., Carlet, J.M., Masur, H. *et al.* (2004) Surviving sepsis campaign: guidelines for management of severe sepsis and septic shock. *Int Care Med* **30**: 536–555.

Faber-Langendoen, K., Caplan, A.L., McGlave, P.B. (1993) Survival of adult bone marrow transplant patients receiving mechanical ventilation: a case for restricted use. *Bone Marrow Transplant* **12**: 501–507.

Garland, A., Paz, H.L. (1997) Outcome of marrow transplantation recipients requiring intensive care. *Semin Respir Crit Care Med* **17**: 359–363.

Goldstein, B., Giroir, B., Randolph, A. *et al.* (2005) International pediatric sepsis consensus conference: Definitions for sepsis and organ dysfunction in pediatrics. *Pediatr Crit Care Med* **6**: 2–8.

Hallahan, A.R., Shaw, P.J., Rowell, G., O'Connell, A., Schell, D., Gillis, J. (2000) Improved outcomes of children with malignancy admitted to a paediatric intensive care unit. *Crit Care Med* **28**: 3718–3721.

Hayes, C., Lush, R.J., Cornish, J.M. *et al.* (1998) The outcome of children requiring admission to an intensive care unit following bone marrow transplantation. *Br J Haematol* **102**: 666–670.

Jacobe, S.J., Hassan, A., Veys, P., Mok, Q. (2003) Outcome of children requiring admission to an intensive care unit after bone marrow transplantation. *Crit Care Med* **31**: 1299–1305.

Lamas, A., Otheo, E., Purificacion, R. *et al.* (2003) Prognosis of child recipients of hematopoietic stem cell transplantation requiring intensive care. *Int Care Med* **29**: 91–96.

Letourneau, I., Dorval, M., Belanger, R., Legare, M., Fortier, L., Leblanc, M. (2002). Acute renal failure in bone marrow transplant patients admitted to the intensive care unit. *Nephron* **90**: 408–412.

Levy, M.M., Fink, M.P., Marshall, J.C. *et al.* (2003) 2001 SCCM/ESICM/ACCP/ATS/SIS International Sepsis Definitions Conference. *Crit Care Med* **31**: 1250–1256.

Massion, P.B., Dive, A.M., Doyen, C. *et al.* (2002) Prognosis of hematologic malignancies does not predict intensive care unit mortality. *Crit Care Med* **30**: 2260–2270.

Rano, A., Agusti, C., Jimenez, P. *et al.* (2001) Pulmonary infiltrates in non-HIV immunocompromised patients: a diagnostic approach using non-invasive and bronchoscopic procedures. *Thorax* **56**: 379–387.

Scott, P.H., Morgan, T.J., Durrant, S., Boots, R.J. (2002) Survival following mechanical ventilation of recipients of bone marrow transplants and peripheral blood stem cell transplants. *Anaesth Intensive Care* **30**: 289–294.

Shemie, S.D. (2003) Bone marrow transplantation and in-tensive care unit admission: What really matters? (Editorial.) *Crit Care Med* **31**: 1579.

Shorr, A.F., Susla, G.M., O'Grady, N.P. (2004) Pulmonary infiltrates in the non-HIV infected immunocompromised patient – etiologies, diagnostic strategies and outcomes. *Chest* **125**: 260–271.

Chapter 10

Graft-vs.-host disease and post-transplant lymphoproliferative disease

M. Abinun and J. Cavet

Introduction

Graft-vs.-host disease (GVHD) develops when donor lymphocytes recognize the recipient as "foreign" and may occur at any time from about 10 days following hematopoietic stem cell transplantation (HSCT). GVHD is the commonest serious TRC, occurring in 30–80% of patients, the risk depending on various factors. GVHD strongly influences outcome, mainly because it suppresses immunity and is treated by immunosuppression, therefore significantly increasing the risk of infection.

Acute GVHD (aGVHD), by definition, occurs in the first 100 days after HSCT; typical features include skin rash, diarrhea, and disordered liver function. Pneumonitis (idiopathic pneumonia syndrome) can also be regarded as a manifestation of aGVHD. aGVHD may coincide with the appearance of neutrophils, the so-called "engraftment syndrome," but this has little to do with neutrophil engraftment, rather the action of activated lymphocytes, and it may be seen in the absence of a stable graft. Mild aGVHD is associated with long-term, relapse-free survival, but more severe aGVHD, particularly when resistant to steroid treatment, has a poor prognosis.

Chronic GVHD (cGVHD) occurs after 100 days. cGVHD can cause late morbidity and mortality, but causes more problems to adults than children, particularly because of associated secondary infections.

Immunobiology and pathophysiology

GVHD was recognized as soon as the first HSCTs were performed and Billingham postulated that for GVHD to develop there should be:

- donor graft containing immunologically competent cells;
- host antigens recognized as "non-self" by the donor graft;
- insufficient host-vs.-graft-reaction to reject the graft.

The second point had to be modified when GVHD was seen after autologous HSCT. Autologous HSCT may provoke a clinical picture where immunomodulatory drugs allow dysregulated self-reacting T cells to cause skin reddening, fever, and pulmonary infiltrates (rarely also diarrhea, hepatitis, or auto-immune cytopenias). Autologous GVHD is more common after HSCT performed for breast cancer, in patients with only one prior chemotherapy schedule, and with administration of GCSF.

Another special circumstance is transfusion-associated GVHD (TAGVHD), where lymphocytes in the transfused blood are not rejected by the patient because they are heavily immunosuppressed; TAGVHD is almost uniformly fatal. GVHD also occasionally occurs in solid organ transplantation when "passenger" lymphocytes in the transplanted organ attack the recipient.

Donor T cells, either within the graft or derived from engrafted stem cells, are critical to GVHD pathophysiology, as shown by the striking reduction in GVHD seen after efficient T-cell depletion (TCD), even with mismatch at three HLA loci. Normally T cells bearing self-reactive receptors are eliminated in the thymus, whereas in HSCT donor T cells that react against the host are not deleted, and are activated via interaction with host antigen-presenting cells (APC). Antigens recognized in GVHD reactions include major histocompatibility complex (MHC) class I and II antigens in HLA-mismatched HSCT, together with non-MHC minor histocompatibility antigens (mHags), viral and tissue-specific antigens in both HLA-matched and -mismatched HSCT.

A second signal from costimulatory molecules regulates the T cell/APC interaction, determining whether there is full reaction, partial reaction, non-reaction (tolerance/anergy), or programmed cell death (apoptosis). Activated T cells release lymphokines such as interleukin (IL)-2, which promotes T-cell expansion, increases CD8 cytotoxicity, and stimulates natural killer (NK) and B cells. Activated T cells upregulate IL-2 receptor (CD25) expression, and hence can self-stimulate via an autocrine loop. Activated T cells also produce interferon-gamma (IFNγ), which upregulates MHC Class II on epithelial cells and macrophages, further stimulating T- and NK-cell responses. Activated donor T cells can thereby expand, either developing into cytotoxic T cells or recruiting additional effector cells, such as NK and mast cells. These effectors initiate and sustain tissue damage, in conjunction with cytokines, leading to GVHD.

The "cytokine storm" model of GVHD postulates three phases: host cytokine release due to conditioning-induced tissue damage; cytokine-enhanced recognition and response by donor T cells; and subsequent cytokine-potentiated/cytokine-based effector mechanisms. Initial host cell damage by cytotoxic drugs, irradiation and underlying disease including infection(s), together with lipopolysaccharide from gut bacteria or other infections, leads to release of proinflammatory cytokines including tumor necrosis factor-alpha (TNFα) and IL-1. Such cytokines, together with IFNγ and IL-2, cause enhancement of donor T-cell interactions with host APCs, and upregulation of adhesion and costimulatory molecules, leading to increased immune-stimulation. The efferent phase amplifies and potentiates tissue damage via proinflammatory cytokines, increasing cell-mediated cytotoxicity and also causing cytokine-mediated direct tissue damage (especially TNFα in gut aGVHD).

Graft-vs.-leukemia (GVL)

Donor cells attack host malignant cells, which contributes to leukemia relapse-free survival after allogeneic HSCT, an effect known as graft-vs.-leukemia; patients with aGVHD are less likely to relapse. However, clinically apparent GVHD is not necessary for GVL, and some patients with GVHD still relapse. Identical twin HSCT has a higher relapse incidence than sibling HLA-matched HSCT, even in the absence of GVHD. T cells given in donor lymphocyte infusions (DLI) reinduce remission in over 60% of CML patients in early relapse, with lower rates in other malignancies. In those unresponsive to unmanipulated DLI, T-cell activation with cytokines (e.g. IL-2 or IFNα) can produce responses. It is due to the recognition of the GVL effect that reduced-intensity stem cell transplant is gaining favor, but the main complication of such allogeneic immunotherapy remains GVHD.

aGVHD risk factors

Major and minor histocompatibility antigens (HLA)

HLA disparity, both major and minor, is a key risk factor for GVHD. A single HLA-mismatch in sibling HSCT increases aGVHD, although it may not reduce survival. However, incompatible partially matched unrelated donor HSCT does not always lead to aGVHD, and aGVHD still develops in a proportion of fully genotypically HLA-matched sibling HSCT recipients, confirming influences other than HLA-matching.

Studies of the antigenic determinants that provoke aGVHD in HLA-matched HSCT have allowed the definition of a number of minor histocompatibility antigens (mHags). mHags are non-HLA peptides presented on recipient MHC molecules, and recognized by donor lymphocytes. mHag incompatibility is responsible not only for GVHD, but also GVL and graft rejection in HLA-matched sibling HSCT, and contributes to these phenomena in HLA-mismatched HSCT. Many mHags are found in all tissues but some are restricted to hemopoetic or myeloid tissues. Gender mismatch is thought to increase aGVHD via gender-related mHags, such as the HY antigen encoded on the Y chromosome. Cells from female donors who have had several pregnancies may have increased immunoreactivity to mHags due to repeated exposure to fetal antigens.

Non-histocompatibility antigen-related factors

Factors including graft T cell and CD34-positive cell dose, age of recipient and donor, viral status (both for CMV and other herpes viruses), gender mismatch (particularly multiparous female donor to male recipient), inadequate prophylaxis, advanced underlying disease, increased TBI and/or chemotherapy conditioning, rapid engraftment/ use of GCSF post graft-infusion, pre-existing infection, and failure of gut decontamination have all been shown to increase aGVHD incidence and/or severity. Peripheral blood hematopoieitc stem cell (PBHSC) generally causes greater aGVHD than bone marrow, with reduced GVHD after cord blood HSCT. Recently a genetic predisposition to aGVHD has been demonstrated in individuals with certain cytokine polymorphisms (in particular IL-10) in both related and unrelated HSCT.

Predicting GVHD

There is no universally accepted method for predicting GVHD in an individual, although functional tests may correlate with subsequent GVHD. Mixing donor and recipient lymphocytes and measuring their reactivitiy (mixed lymphocyte reactivity – MLR) forms the basis of the mixed cytotoxic T-lymphocyte precursor frequency (CTLpf) assay, and the helper T-lymphocyte precursor frequency (HTLpf). High levels of reactivity in each of these correlates with severe aGVHD, cGVHD, and GVL. However, these assays do not predict GVHD as accurately as high-resolution molecular HLA-typing for matching of unrelated donors, or T-cell-depleted HSCT. Moreover, CTLpf and HTLpf assessments are technically demanding, expensive and time consuming. Thus the MLR, CTLpf and HTLpf assays are now much less often used than previously, with increasing reliance placed on high-resolution tissue typing of donor and recipient.

MHC- and/or mHag-mismatched recipient skin biopsies cultured with allogeneic donor T cells sensitized by MLR provide an *in vitro* GVHD model. This skin explant model can be used to predict clinical aGVHD, allowing adjustment of prophy-laxis, but may be difficult to standardize between different histopathologists. Biopsies of skin and oral mucosa around day 100 post-HSCT have been used for prediction and pre-emptive treatment of cGVHD in certain centers, but have not been widely adopted.

Acute GVHD (aGVHD)

aGVHD usually arises shortly after engraftment but can occur later, particularly following reduced-intensity conditioning (RIC), or on withdrawal of immunosuppression. Generally donor engraftment precedes aGVHD, but clinically aGVHD can occur before white cells are seen in peripheral blood.

aGVHD mainly affects the skin, liver and gut, although mucosae, conjunctivae, exocrine organs and bronchi can be affected, and marrow suppression is not uncommon when GVHD is severe. The first sign is usually an itchy or painful maculopapular rash, typically involving the palms, soles of the feet, face, ears, neck and/or upper thorax. Occasionally this can progress to erythroderma of the entire skin, with blistering, epidermal necrolysis and fever, with marked fluid and protein losses similar to those seen in burns. Skin aGVHD is usually diagnosed clinically, but biopsy helps to confirm the diagnosis and may be done before starting significant immunosuppression treatment.

Gut aGVHD causes diarrhea and abdominal pain. When severe, the fluid and electrolyte losses may be very debilitating; the severity is best assessed by measuring the large volume of liquid stool. Occasionally it is accompanied by bleeding and/or ileus. Upper gastrointestinal aGVHD can present as nausea, anorexia, or upper abdominal pain with histological evidence of GVHD at endoscopic biopsy.

Hepatic aGVHD is least common and usually accompanies skin and gut GVHD. Jaundice and an enlarged, hard liver are accompanied by a raised conjugated bilirubin and alkaline phosphatase/ gamma-glutamyl transpeptidase, due to immune damage to the bile canaliculi resulting in cholestasis; transaminases rise to a lesser degree. Many other early post-HSCT complications can cause jaundice, including veno-occlusive disease (VOD), drug toxicity, infections, and hemolysis. Hence liver aGVHD is ideally diagnosed histologically, but biopsy is rarely performed due to the risk of hemorrhage; transjugular biopsy is safer, but still has risk even after correction of thrombocytopenia and coagulopathy.

aGVHD is often accompanied by thrombocytopenia and sometimes neutropenia, and rarely can also cause hypogammaglobulinemia. Immunosuppression from GVHD and its treatment, associated with damaged mucosal barriers, can lead to superadded infection which is often the cause of death in severe aGVHD.

aGVHD severity can be staged for each organ according to area of skin involved and the intensity of involvement, depth of jaundice for liver, volume of diarrhea and pain intensity for gut, and these stages are summated with histological grading of biopsy specimens to produce an overall grade, which correlates with outcome. The most widely used system is that of Glucksberg (Tables 10.1 and 10.2), although recently the International Bone Marrow Transplant Registry has devised an index with improved correlation to mortality. Estimates of skin involvement and bowel actions must be well documented if these systems are to be applied accurately.

Table 10.1 Grading of aGVHD: staging of aGVHD in individual organs (after Glucksberg *et al.* 1974)

	Organ stage	Grading
Skin	<25%	+
% surface area affected	25–50%	++
	>50%	+++
	Bullae	++++
Liver	34–50	+
Bilirubin	51–102	++
(mmol/L)	103–255	+++
	>255	++++
Gut	>500	+
Diarrhea	>1000	++
(ml/day)	>1500	+++
Severe pain/ileus		++++

Table 10.2 "Maximum stage wins" grading of aGVHD

Skin		Liver		Gut	Grade
1–2					I
3	or	1	or	1	II
		2–4	or	2–3	III
4		or		4	IV

Maximum stage wins avoids the inherent contradictions and confusions associated with the original grading when there is dissociation of the stages between organs. For example, a patient with skin stage 3, liver stage 2 and no gut GVHD is either II, III or 0, respectively. According to the maximum stage rule, stage 2 liver disease incurs the highest overall grade of III.

Treatment of aGVHD

Mild aGVHD may require no immediate treatment, especially if confined to the skin, but progressive disease, particularly involving liver/gut, or causing constitutional symptoms, should be treated. aGVHD occurring during tapering of prophylaxis may respond to reintroduction, and steroid-responsive aGVHD that flares during dose reduction is likely to respond to increasing the dose of steriod. Supportive measures are very important when treating GVHD, including ensuring adequate nutrition (as this is a hypercatabolic state), fluid and electrolyte replacement, analgesia and prophylaxis/treament of infection.

Corticosteroids, with their broad anti-inflammatory and immunosuppressive activities, are first line treatments. Starting treatment is usually 2 mg/kg/day of methylprednisolone, with gradual tapering in responders after at least 1 week, or in more severe cases 250–500 mg/m^2 for a few (usually 3) days and tapering by halving the dose every 48–72 h. Children usually respond to steroids, and overall around 50% of adult patients respond to steroids. Skin involvement is more likely to respond than liver or gut GVHD. Progression after 3 days or no response after 7 days equates to steroid-refractoriness. Steroid-refractory patients have a poor prognosis, and many survivors develop cGVHD. If there is gut GVHD or diarrhea, ciclosporin should be given intravenously. Second-line aGVHD therapies include functional TCD, either via anti-thymocyte globulin (ATG), or monoclonal antibodies vs. CD3, CD52 (Alemtuzumab) or the IL-2 receptor (daclizumab/basiliximab). Tacrolimus substitution for CsA in combination with mycophenylate mofetil has been employed. Phototherapy shows some promise, particularly in cutaneous GVHD, as does topical application of tacrolimus. Cytokine antagonists, including TNFα antagonists, and IL-1 receptor antagonist, are also used. During such intense immunosuppressive treatment, antimicrobial prophylaxis (antibacterial, antiviral and antifungal) is mandatory. Age is one of the major predisposing factors to GVHD, and children are as a rule less likely to relapse after initial response once the agent is stopped.

Chronic GVHD (cGVHD)

cGVHD occurs more than 100 days after HSCT, sometimes much later, either directly continuing from aGVHD or more commonly after a quiescent phase. cGVHD occurs in up to 50% of HLA-matched sibling HSCT recipients in adults and is more frequent after PBHSCT, but is rare in children, accounting for less than 5% of cases. Increased collagen deposition leads to atrophy and sclerosis, with skin, mucous membranes, liver, lachrymal and salivary glands, gut, joints, esophagus, and other internal organs being affected. Late lung inflammation (e.g. bronchiolitis obliterans) may be a manifestation of cGVHD.

Skin cGVHD presents with papules, areas of reddening or hyper-/hypo-pigmentation. Biopsy shows epidermal atrophy and dermal fibrosis, with destruction of sweat glands and hair follicles. Skin and mucous membranes become thickened and scarred, leading to fixed contractures if untreated. Nails can become dystrophic and there may be alopecia.

Dry eyes and ocular irritation are also common, (keratoconjunctivitis sicca). Lichen planus-like striae, ulcers and atrophy can be seen in the mouth with dryness due to damaged salivary glands (particularly post-TBI). Lichenoid changes can also affect the genital tract, leading to dryness, dyspareunia, erythema and atrophy/stenosis. Nausea/vomiting, dysphagia secondary to esophageal stenosis, diarrhea, weight loss and malabsorption are seen in gut cGVHD. Hepatic cGVHD often manifests

as raised liver function tests alone (particularly alkaline phosphatase), but patients can develop obstructive jaundice or even cirrhosis.

Musculoskeletal involvement can manifest as weakness and cramps/spasms, together with tendonitis, arthralgia, and joint thickening/contracture. Pulmonary involvement can cause cough, wheeze, and breathlessness, with both restrictive and obstructive patterns seen on lung function testing.

cGVHD has autoreactive features including the presence of autoantibodies and/or hypergammaglobulinemia in some patients. Clinically cGVHD has similarities to the autoimmune connective tissue disorders systemic sclerosis, systemic lupus erythematosus (SLE), Sjögren's syndrome, primary biliary cirrhosis, polymyositis, and eosinophilic fasciitis.

The immune system is compromised by cGVHD, and immunosuppressive treatments exacerbate this, leading to high incidence of bacterial, fungal and viral infections. As infection is the leading cause of cGVHD-related death, appropriate antibacterial, antiviral and antifungal prophylaxis is mandatory (e.g. pencillin, co-trimoxazole, aciclovir, fluconazole, itraconazole) (Table 10.3).

cGVHD is graded as limited or extensive disease, although subclinical disease only apparent upon screening biopsies is also reported. Limited cGVHD constitutes localized skin/oral/other mucosal involvement with or without hepatic dysfunction, provided liver histology is not aggressive. Extensive disease includes generalized skin lesions, aggressive liver disease with chronic active

Table 10.3 Common infectious prophylaxis in GVHD

Infection	Prophylaxis
Pneumocystis pneumonia	Pentamidine; co-trimoxazole; azithromycin
Varicella zoster virus	Aciclovir
Cytomegalovirus[1]	Ganciclovir; foscarnet
Fungal[2]	Itraconazole; voriconazole; fluconazole

[1] CMV prophylaxis has been tested in a number of trials but is not routinely used except in high-risk procedures such as T depletion for haplo-transplants.
[2] Some centers continue anti-fungal prophylaxis after neutrophil engraftment, if the patient is on steroids.

hepatitis, bridging necrosis or cirrhosis, or multiple organ involvment, such as mouth, eyes, joints, and esophagus. Grading of cGVHD has been shown to be reproducible in an IBMTR study.

Assessment also involves Karnofsky performance score, an index of capacity for activities of daily living. Prognosis from cGVHD is worse in thrombocytopenic patients, those with early and progressive onset of aGVHD and when there is extensive skin involvement.

GVHD as a rule is significantly less frequently seen in young children than in adults.

cGVHD risk factors

Previous moderate/severe aGVHD is the best predictor of cGVHD. Increasing recipient age is the major risk factor for *de novo* cGVHD and children are less often affected. Other cGVHD risk factors include female donor to male recipient, inadequate prophylaxis, busulfan conditioning, graft T-cell dose, and use of buffy coat or DLI.

Treatment of cGVHD

Limited cGVHD is much easier to treat than extensive cGVHD. Localized mucosal/skin involvement often responds to topical steroids, azathioprine, CsA, and tacrolimus. Ocular involvement is treated with regular preservative-free artificial tears, and sometimes topical immunosuppression; ophthalmic follow-up is advisable for any patient with sicca syndrome. Artificial saliva can aid xerostomia, but is not always tolerated by patients.

Extensive cGVHD is much more difficult to treat; CsA and steroids are used first line. Initially patients respond better to CsA and steroids given together compared to steroids alone, but little difference is seen in long-term survival, and side effects are greater with prolonged combination treatment. Hence cGVHD occurring after recent taper/cessation of CsA prophylaxis can be treated with reintroduction of CsA, but severe or extensive manifestations will require prednisolone (usually 1 mg/kg/day initially, eventually tapering to alternate days regimen to minimize side effects). Often therapy will be needed for at least 6–12 months.

Those on immunosuppressive treatment should receive antifungal prophylaxis with fluconazole or itraconazole, together with aciclovir antiviral prophylaxis, in addition to antibacterials. Monitoring for CMV reactivation is important for those on systemic immunosuppression. Other supportive treatment needed may include nutritional supplementation, immunoglobulin replacement in hypogammaglobulinemia, and hormone replacement/osteoporosis prophylaxis. Vigorous skin hydration/emollients are important to lubricate skin, and exacerbants such as perfume and sun exposure should be avoided. Regular dental follow-up is important for those with oropharyngeal involvement as caries are increased by a dry mouth. Quinine may be helpful for muscle cramps, but dantrolene or other muscle relaxants may be needed.

Other cGVHD therapies include tacrolimus, MMF (often used in combination), ATG or other monoclonal antibodies against (activated) T cells and cytokines or their receptors, lymphoid irradiation, phototherapy (either PUVA or extracorporeal, both more effective in cutaneous disease), retinoids, penicillamine, azathioprine, and thalidomide. Retinoids may be useful as adjunctive treatment to immunosuppression in severe refractory sclerdermatous cGVHD, although mucosal and skin drying together with potential teratogenecity are issues. Ursodeoxycholic acid can be used for cholestasis; the high liver concentrations of tacrolimus make this agent useful in liver cGVHD, although in severe isolated hepatic cGVHD liver transplant has been necessary.

Preventing GVHD

A major goal of transplant therapy is to prevent or at least limit the severity of aGVHD. Prednisolone, ciclosporin or tacrolimus, methotrexate, and mycophenelate mofetil (MMF) are all given to patients after HSCT either singly or in combination to prevent GVHD; using these agents in this way is referred to as "GVHD prophylaxis." Drug treatment may also be supplemented by removing T cells to a greater or lesser degree by T-cell depletion (TCD). This is achieved prior to HSCT by positively selecting stem cells (CD34-positive) and so infusing a much smaller number of T cells, or by adding a

T-cell-killing monoclonal antibody to the bag of marrow or peripheral blood cells *in vitro* before it is infused. Alternatively it can be done within the patient (*in vivo*) by giving a T-cell-killing antibody such as ATG to the patient at the time of HSCT. There is general agreement that unrelated donor transplants require some degree of T-cell depletion supplemented with one- or two-drug GVHD prophylaxis. When T-cell depletion is used for sibling transplants it is usual to use only single-drug prophylaxis. Common regimes are summarized in Table 10.4. Tacrolimus is sometimes substituted for ciclosporin as it has similar actions.

Prophylaxis delays immune reconstitution post-HSCT, increasing the risk of infection and also diminishing the GVL effects, so the risk–benefit ratios of different regimens need to be carefully considered.

Ciclosporin-A (CsA), methotrexate (MTX), and/or corticosteroids, given individually or in combination, are most often used. Combined CsA/MTX is associated with greater survival. Adding steroids to combined CsA/MTX can further reduce aGVHD, but produces little survival advantage and may increase cGVHD.

Dose-adjusted CsA (3–5 mg/kg/day initially; usually continued to day 180) and "short course"

MTX (15 mg/m^2 day 1, and 10 mg/m^2 days 3, 6 and 11) remain the most widely used regimen worldwide, particularly for HLA-matched sibling HSCT. There may be less mucositis and neutropenia if the fourth MTX dose is omitted, with only a slightly increased risk of moderate/severe aGVHD. CsA side effects include hirsutism, renal and hepatic impairment, hypertension, tremor, and more rarely neurotoxicity or thrombotic microangiopathy. MTX can exacerbate mucositis or interstitial pneumonitis, cause hepatic impairment or delay engraftment.

Recently tacrolimus (FK506) and sirolimus (rapamycin) have been used instead of CsA in unrelated-donor HSCT protocols, due to their more potent inhibition of T-cell activation/proliferation. Tacrolimus side effects include renal impairment, neurotoxicity and cardiomyopathy. Mycophenylate mofetil (MMF) blocks both T- and B-cell proliferation, downregulates adhesion molecules, and has been mainly used in conjunction with CsA in reduced-intensity stem cell transplantation (RISCT). MMF's main side effects are gut ulceration and myelosuppression.

TCD by monoclonal antibodies, *in vitro* and/or *in vivo*, or by *in vitro* positive CD34-positive stem cell selection, is used when donor marrow is significantly mismatched. The decreased risk of GVHD has to be set against the increased risk of graft rejection caused by the removal of T cells, which facilitate engraftment. The profound immunosuppression caused by selectiveTCD (i.e. anti-T lymphocyte globulin [ATG] vs. Alemtuzumab) also causes increased risk of opportunistic infections, particularly Epstein–Barr virus (EBV)-related post-transplant lymphoproliferative disease (see PTLD). The increase in graft failure, infection and relapse means there is little overall survival benefit demonstrated for TCD over drug prophylaxis in matched sibling or matched unrelated donor HSCT, despite a reduction in GVHD.

Table 10.4 Common GVHD prophylaxis regimens

Type of transplant	GVHD prophylaxis
Sibling	*Full intensity:*
	Ciclosporin + pulsed methotrexate
	Reduced intensity:
	Ciclosporin + pulsed methotrexate
	Ciclosporin + MMF
	Alemtuzumab *in vivo* + ciclosporin
	ATG + ciclosporin
Unrelated	*Full and reduced intensity:*
	CD34 selection + ciclosporin
	Alemtuzumab *in vitro* + ciclosporin
	Alemtuzumab *in vivo* + ciclosporin
	ATG + ciclosporin
	(All these have been described + pulsed methotrexate)
Cord blood	Ciclosporin + MMF

Post-transplant lymphoproliferative disease (PTLD)

Several forms of malignancy occur more frequency

after HSCT. EBV-driven PTLD occurs after both HSCT and solid organ transplantation and is related to post-HSCT immunosuppression. The overall incidence of PTLD is around 1% at 10 years post-HSCT, most cases occuring within 6 months. The abnormal cells are usually derived from donor B lymphocytes, but rare T-cell lymphomas can develop. Usually EBV drives B-cell clones to proliferate, in the setting of marked reduction in T-cell immunosurveillance (analogous to NHL in HIV-related immunosuppression).

The risk of PTLD relates to the degree of immunocompromise and time to immunoreconstitution; PTLD is more likely after *in-vivo* or *ex-vivo* selective T-cell depletion (TCD), treatment of aGVHD with either anti-CD3 antibodies or ATG, unrelated and/or mismatched donor HSCT (risk increasing with degree of mismatch), and to a lesser extent after TBI conditioning and in association with moderate to severe aGVHD. TCD strategies that also deplete B cells (e.g. alemtuzumab or elutriation) are less likely to cause PTLD than those that selectively target T cells.

Late PTLD is rare, and is usually seen in patients with extensive cGVHD and its associated delayed and aberrant immune reconstitution. Late PTLD is less likely to be EBV driven, and includes most of the T-cell disease reported.

The severity of PTLD varies greatly, ranging from early polyclonal expansions to aggressive multi-site lymphomas with diffuse large-cell or sometimes Burkitt-like features. Tissue biopsies display EBV proteins and EBV is usually detected in the peripheral blood by PCR. Higher levels of EBV in blood probably correlate with a greater risk of PTLD. Oligoclonal or monoclonal disease can progress rapidly with substantial mortality, so clinical and virological vigilance are most important.

The most common presenting features of PTLD are fever with or without night sweats, together with palpable or occult nodal enlargement, less frequently with marrow or other extranodal site infiltration. Of these, gastrointestinal and neurological features can occasionally be overwhelming.

Early effective treatment of PTLD is associated with a much better outcome. Reduction of immunosuppression is very important, although this is not possible when anti-T-cell antibodies have been previously administered. The recent introduction of rituximab (anti-CD20 monoclonal antibody) is a major advance, with potential of curing previously untreatable patients even when it is given as monotherapy. Combination chemotherapy or immunochemotherapy is still required for those not showing complete response. Cellular therapy with anti-EBV cytotoxic lymphocytes (either generated *in vitro* culture from donor cells, or "off-the-shelf" from established CTL "banks") shows promise and can lead to complete remissions in otherwise non-responsive PTLD. However, the investment in biotechnology and technical expertise required is substantial, and exacerbation of GVHD is possible if non-specific CTLs are infused.

Some centers have used pre-emptive therapy with rituximab in those with high EBV load, and suggest that PTLD can be prevented, although as yet there is no consensus as to level of EBV DNA which should trigger treatment with rituximab.

Further reading

Cavet, J., Middleton, P.G., Segall, M., Noreen, H., Davies, S.M., Dickinson, A.M. (1999) Recipient tumor necrosis factor-alpha and interleukin-10 gene polymorphisms associate with early mortality and acute graft-vs.-host disease severity in HLA-matched sibling bone marrow transplants. *Blood* **94**: 3941–3946.

Cavet, J., Dickinson, A.M., Norden, J., Taylor, P.R., Jackson, G.H., Middleton, P.G. (2001) Interferon-gamma and interleukin-6, gene polymorphisms associate with graft-vs.-host disease in HLA-matched sibling bone marrow transplantation. *Blood* **98**: 1594–1600.

Curtis, R.E., Travis, L.B., Rowlings, P.A. *et al.* (1999) Risk of lymphoproliferative disorder after bone marrow transplantation: a multi-institutional study. *Blood* **94**: 2208–2216.

Glucksberg, H., Storb, R., Fefer, A. *et al.* (1974) Clinical manifestations of graft-versus-host disease in human recipients of marrow from HLA-matched sibling donors. *Transplantation* **18**: 295–304.

Jacobsohn, D.A., Vogelsang, G.B. (2004) Anti-cytokine therapy for the treatment of GvHD. *Curr Pharm Des* **10**: 1195–1205.

Ringden, O., Deeg, H.J. (1997) Clinical spectrum of graft-versus-host-disease. In: Ferrara, J.M.L., Deeg, H.J., Burakoff, S.J. (eds), *Graft-versus-host-disease.* New York: Marcel Dekker, pp. 525–560.

Rowlings, P.A., Przepiorka, D., Klein, J.P. *et al.* (1997) IBMTR Severity Index for grading acute graft-versus-host disease: retrospective comparison with Glucksberg grade. *Brit J Haem* **97**: 855–864.

Socie, G., Loiseau, P., Tamouza, R. *et al.* (2001) Both genetic and clinical factors predict the development of graft-versus-host disease after allogeneic hematopoietic stem cell transplantation. *Transplantation* **72**: 699–706.

Vogelsang, G.B. (2001) How I treat chronic graft-versus-host-disease. *Blood* **97**: 1196–1201.

Chapter 11

Gastrointestinal, respiratory and renal/urogenital complications of HSCT

M. Abinun and J. Cavet

Veno-occlusive disease

Veno-occlusive disease of the liver (sinusoidal obstruction sydnrome)

Veno-occlusive disease (VOD) of the liver, recently renamed as "sinusoidal obstruction syndrome," is a clinical syndrome characterized by painful hepatomegaly, jaundice, ascites, fluid retention, and weight gain. It is one of the most common and important conditioning regimen-related complications following hematopoietic stem cell transplantation (HSCT), with reported incidence up to 70%.

Pathophysiology

VOD occurs usually in the first 2 (up to 3–4) weeks after HSCT as a result of damage to the endothelial cells lining the veins in the liver as well as direct hepatocyte damage. Recently it has been suggested that the sinusoidal endothelial cells are the primary site of toxic injury.

Following the initial damage, impairment of microcirculation and progressive venous occlusion leads to widespread liver failure. Low plasma levels of antithrombin III and protein C, consumption of factor VII, and increased levels of plasminogen activator inhibitor-1 are features of a procoagulant state throughout this process, and increased levels of von Willebrand factor multimers and refractoriness to platelet transfusion suggest ongoing endothelial damage.

Histological features at early stage are deposition of fibrinogen and factor VIII within venular walls and liver sinusoids, with later changes including deposition of collagen in the sinusoids, sclerosis of venular walls, and fibrosis of venular lumens. Finally, hepatocellular necrosis and vascular occlusion lead to hepatorenal pathology, multiple organ failure (MOF) and death.

Risk factors

The most consistently described risk factors for developing VOD include pre-existing liver dysfunction (infection, inflammation, cirrhosis), previous abdominal irradiation, use of higher-dose preparative regimens, especially alkylating agents such as busulfan, or total body irradiation (TBI).

Other reported risk factors include advanced disease status at the time of HSCT, HLA-mismatched or unrelated donor transplants (particularly second myeloablative transplant), previous therapy with gemtuzumab ozogamicin, and several mainly pediatric disorders such as inborn errors of metabolism (osteopetrosis, hemophagocytic lymphohistiocytosis, adrenoleukodystrophy), and neuroblastoma, as well as very young age at the time of HSCT.

Clinical features

The clinical features of VOD are non-specific and may be mimicked by a number of other conditions common in patients undergoing HSCT. These are sepsis with renal insufficiency, cholestatic liver disease (due to total parenteral nutrition), hemolysis, congestive heart failure (due to chemotherapeutic agents), and acute graft-vs.-host disease (aGVHD).

Often more than one of these conditions is involved in the liver toxicity, making the differential diagnosis really challenging. In such cases liver biopsy

Table 11.1 VOD – Criteria for diagnosis

	McDonald (Seattle) (2 of 3)	Jones (Baltimore) (hyperbilirubinemia and 2 out of 3)
Hepatomegaly or right upper quadrant pain	+	+
Weight gain (>2% from pre-transplant baseline)	+	+
Hyperbilirubinemia (>2 mg/dL or 34 μmol/L)	+	+
Ascites	−	+

can be very useful, as besides obtaining liver tissue for histopathology, the measurement of hepatic venous pressure gradient gives a good correlation to the clinical parameters of VOD severity. However, due to the very high risk of life-threatening hemorrhage in patients undergoing HSCT, it has a limited role.

Criteria for diagnosis were established independently by McDonald and Jones in the mid-1980s (Table 11.1) and remain essential in clinical practice.

Another very helpful diagnostic parameter is the demonstration of normal portal venous flow by Doppler ultrasound before HSCT, with flow reversal within 3 weeks after HSCT, as this is highly suggestive but still a relatively insensitive marker for VOD.

VOD is usually arbitrarily subdivided into clinically mild, moderate and severe disease (Table 11.2), although there are no clear criteria and consensus regarding this. In general, the outcome of

Table 11.2 VOD – clinical disease staging

Mild	No apparent adverse effect from liver disease
	Occasionally symptomatic treatment (analgesics, diuretics)
	Complete resolution of symptoms and signs
Moderate	Adverse effects from liver dysfunction
	Requires symptomatic and specific treatment (defibrotide, r- tPA/heparin)
	Eventual complete resolution (no progression to MOF)
Severe	Severe adverse effects from liver dysfunction
	Requires symptomatic and specific treatment
	Fails to resolve despite treatment – progression to MOF
	Mechanical ventilation, dialysis, inotropes, drainage of ascites
	Death (before day 100) of ongoing VOD

patients with mild and moderate VOD is usually good, with a predicted survival of 77–91% at day 100. However, severe VOD, especially when associated with MOF, has a high mortality exceeding 90%, and in established severe VOD the death rate is close to 100% by day 100 post-HSCT.

To predict severity of VOD, Bearman *et al.* developed a very useful model in the early 1990s. The serum bilirubin level is plotted against percent weight gain, forming graphs with contour lines to estimate the probability of developing severe VOD as >30%, >40%, >50%, and >60% at six time intervals within the first 2 weeks post-transplant. If the plotted point was 0.3 on the contour lines, then the probability of developing severe VOD was 30%. This model seems to be in use in most of the centers reporting their experience in treating VOD.

The aim of the staging is to identify high-risk patients at an early stage and so start treatment before MOF develops. However, because of a lack of consensus regarding both the classifications of the different stages of the disease and the criteria for timing of initiation of specific treatment, the interpretation of studies on prophylaxis and/or therapeutic drugs remains problematic.

The scoring system developed in our unit (Table 11.3) incorporates the features from Jones and McDonald diagnosis criteria, and includes raised prothrombin time (PT), the need to regularly transfuse platelets, risk factors for VOD (such as raised alanine aminotransaminase [ALT] pre-HSCT), and associated organ system failure at diagnosis of VOD. Each parameter is assigned a score of 1 or 2 and a total score is calculated on a daily basis. A score of 4 suggests early or impending VOD, a score of 5–7 moderate VOD (at which stage initiating of specific treatment is suggested), and a score of 8–10 indicates severe VOD and a poor prognosis (Bajwa *et al.*, 2003).

Table 11.3 Scoring system for VOD (adapted from Bajwa *et al.*, 2003, *Bone Marrow Transplantation*)

1 Progressive and persisting increase in bilirubin	• SBR ≥34 but <75 µmol/L or	1
	• SBR ≥75 µmol/L	2
2 Persisting hepatomegaly (>2 cm from baseline)		1
3 Ascites		1
4 Persisting weight gain (from baseline)	• ≥5% but <15% or	1
	• ≥15%	2
5 Raised prothrombin time (T) or need to transfuse platelets regularly		1
6 Risk factors (one or more present)	• Age <6 months and/or	1
	• Raised alanine aminotransferase pre-BMT	
7 Associated organ system failure[1] (excluding liver failure)	• Each system failure	1
	• Maximum	2
Maximum total score		10

[1] Respiratory failure needing ventilation, or circulatory failure needing inotropes, or renal failure needing dialysis, or need for abdominal paracentesis.

Treatment

Until relatively recently, therapy of VOD has largely been disappointing.

1 Supportive measures, such as maintaining careful fluid and electrolyte balance, judicious use of diuretics, analgesics, platelet transfusions and correction of clotting derangements, have been the mainstay of conservative treatment.

2 Use of antithrombotic and thrombolytic agents, including prostaglandin E1 and recombinant tissue plasminogen activator (r-tPA) with or without concurrent heparin, have been limited by significant toxicity such as fatal hemorrhage. In spite of that, r-tPA has been shown to be effective and was the treatment of choice for severe VOD until recently.

3 Antithrombin III, a naturally occurring anticoagulant protein made by the liver (and as a recombinant product) and a potent inhibitor of the clotting system, is of potential benefit. Given with the goal to achieve the AT-III levels at >120%, it was reported to be effective in small series and, very importantly, with no major side effects.

4 Defibrotide (DF), a single-stranded polydeoxyribonucleotide derived from mammalian tissue, is currently the most promising agent. DF has antithrombotic, anti-ischemic, anti-inflammatory and thrombolytic properties without significant systemic anticoagulant effect. It is bound to vascular endothelium, and stimulates fibrinolysis by increasing endogenous tPA function while decreasing activity of PAI-1. Several studies reported that DF, given i.v. in a dose of 5–60 mg/kg/day during 2–3 weeks (sometimes longer) to patients (adults and children) with severe VOD post-HSCT, showed beneficial effect on both the complete resolution (10–40%) and survival at day +100 (30–50%) without significant DF-associated toxicity. Results of a larger randomized trial are awaited.

5 Other options, such as use of N-acetylcysteine, nitric oxide, transhepatic shunts and liver transplantation, have been reported.

Prophylaxis

The efficacy of different agents used in prophylaxis of VOD has not been clearly demonstrated or confirmed (prostaglandin E1, heparin and low molecular weight [LMW] heparin, pentoxifylline, ursodeoxycholic acid). However, most centers are still using ursodeoxycholic acid and/or heparin.

More recently, defibrotide was given from day −1 to day +20 (in a dose of 10–25 mg/kg/day) together with low-dose heparin (5000–10,000 IU continuously i.v. over 24 hours) in a non-randomized series of 100 patients undergoing allogenic HSCT. None of these patients developed VOD in comparison to 10/52 patients from the historical control series receiving only heparin, of which 3 died (Chalandon *et al.*, 2004).

In another study, a strategy of two-step therapy was explored. DF was given "early" to all patients diagnosed with VOD based on Jones criteria, and only if a reversal of portal flow was detected subsequently on daily Doppler ultrasound monitoring (suggestive of progression to a "severe" stage), was r-tPA commenced (Cesaro *et al.*, 2005).

Other gastrointestinal complications

Gastrointestinal (GI) and hepatic complications represent a major cause of morbidity and significant mortality following HSCT.

- Clinically demonstrable jaundice is only a symptom of multiple underlying processes (hemolysis, biliary obstruction, hepatocellular injury). Hepatic VOD, aGVHD and medication-related injury, as well as infections, are main underlying conditions.
- Biliary sludging, often associated with abdominal (right upper quadrant) pain, hepatomegaly and vomiting, and diagnosed by ultrasound, is seen with use of total parenteral nutrition. Ursodeoxycholic acid is used in prevention of this complication.
- Acute pancreatitis is a rare complication.
- Mucositis, dysphagia/odynophagia, vomiting and abdominal pain are the most common GI complications impairing adequate nutritional oral intake. Preventive measures (soft toothbrush/sponges post-feed), infection prevention, daily careful observation, and adequate and timely pain control are usually helpful.
- Neutropenic enterocolitis (typhlitis) is diagnosed radiologically (pneumatosis intestinalis) and managed conservatively. Causes of diarrhea are usually either infectious (viruses, *Clostridium difficile*) or graft-vs.-host disease (GVHD). Melena and hematochezia are occasionally of serious nature when associated with intestinal inflammation, ulcerations or coagulation derangement during infections, GVHD or hepatic VOD and vasculopathy.

Pulmonary complications

Pulmonary complications, including infections and GVHD, are a major cause of morbidity and mortality in recipients of HSCT.

Pulmonary vasculopathies are rare but often life-threatening complications. On the other hand, interstitial pneumonitis accounts for over 40% of HSCT-related deaths in most large series of patients; almost half of these are non-infectious idiopathic pneumonias.

The "classical" infectious agents, such as cytomegalovirus, adenovirus, parainfluenza, respiratory syncytial virus (RSV), *Pneumcystis jiroveci*, as well as human herpes virus (HHV)-6, *Varicella zoster*, BK polyoma viruses and toxoplasma, have been reported to cause life-threatening interstitial pneumonia at different stages post-HSCT. Recurrent viral infections and chronic, low-grade GVHD are recognized factors for the development of bronchiolitis obliterans, one of the common late complications post-HSCT with significant morbidity. Supportive and conservative treatment options with anti-inflammatory agents such as corticosteroids and hydroxychloroquine have been generally disappointing. Promising results with anti-TNFα agents have been reported recently.

Pulmonary vasculopathies

Pulmonary veno-occlusive disease (PVOD) is a very rare complication of HSCT, and is almost universally fatal. Unfortunately, the diagnosis of PVOD is often reached only post mortem.

The criteria for clinical diagnosis are even less well defined than those for hepatic VOD. Most common clinical features are dyspnea, cardiomegaly and infiltrates on chest radiography, tachycardia, congestive hepatomegaly, ascites, edema, cough and metabolic acidosis. Open lung biopsy can be diagnostic, but patients are usually too unstable for the procedure. Histopathology shows characteristic veno-occlusive lesions involving small pulmonary veins, as well as partial or complete arterial occlusions due to intimal fibrosis.

High index of suspicion and clinical observation remain essential in identifying patients with early PVOD who may benefit from early initializing treatment, preventing further progression to life-threatening disease. Although there has been no consistently effective treatment for this condition, some response to high-dose steroids has been reported and defibrotide is a possible option.

Patients with PVOD often present with pulmonary hypertension (PH), another potentially life-threatening disorder of the lung vasculature. The presenting symptoms are usually subtle, such as lethargy, non-productive cough, and poor appetite and vomiting. Progressive dyspnea/desaturation, tachypnea, tachycardia or bradycardia, chest pain, and effort-related syncope are more specific features of PH. Cardiopulmonary evaluation is crucial with chest radiography (cardiomegaly, increased pulmonary vascular/interstitial marking), ECG (right axis deviation) and Doppler echocardiography (right ventricle dilatation, increased systolic pulmonary artery pressure).

The underlying mechanism of the vasculopathy affecting small muscular arteries (in lung as well as in gastrointestinal tract) is unknown. It was observed that HSCT-related PH occurs more frequently in children with malignant osteopetrosis.

Potential treatment options include a range of vasodilators such as prostacyclin and its derivates, sildenafil, nitric oxide, calcium channel blockers, and methylprednisolone.

Idiopathic pneumonia syndrome

Idiopathic pneumonia syndrome (IPS) is a term used to describe diffuse lung injury after either autologous or allogeneic HSCT for which an infectious etiology is not identified. The reported incidence is ~15% with mortality from respiratory failure ~30%.

IPS after autologous HSCT most likely represents the result of myeloablative conditioning-related toxicity including irradiation. The syndrome of diffuse alveolar hemorrhage (DAH) due to lung damage can progress to respiratory insufficiency, leading to death. In a murine model of IPS after high-dose chemotherapy and syngeneic HSCT (mimicking the human autologous situation), the oxidative stress due to the conditioning regimen initiated the inflammation promoted by alveolar macrophages in the lung epithelium, secreting chemokines such as monocyte chemotactic protein-1 (MCP-1) and macrophage inflammatory protein-1α (MIP-1α). This lung injury was partially attenuated by administration of antioxidant N-acetylcysteine.

In IPS after allogeneic HSCT, the toxic effects of conditioning regimens, infection (particularly viral) and acute GVHD all play important roles in immunologic cell-mediated injury via activated T cells and inflammatory cytokines.

The clinical spectrum of IPS is broad, ranging from acute respiratory distress to incidental radiographic infiltrates. The classical, although non-specific, presentation includes breathlessness, nonproductive cough and hypoxemia; chest X-rays show bilateral or unilateral multilobar infiltrates and pleural effusion. Two major histological findings seen on lung biopsy are interstitial pneumonitis and diffuse alveolar damage.

Signs and symptoms of fluid overload responding to diuretics, as well as finding of infectious etiology on bronchoalveolar lavage or lung biopsy, exclude the diagnosis of IPS.

There is no established therapy for IPS post-HSCT except for supportive care combined with the prevention and treatment of infections. High-dose corticosteroid therapy is generally advocated, and, more recently, combination of aggressive anti-inflammatory (TNFα blockade) and immunosuppressive agents seems promising.

Hemorrhagic cystitis

Painful hematuria due to hemorrhagic inflammation of the urinary bladder mucosa or hemorrhagic cystitis (HC) occurring post-HSCT is a serious complication and can be life threatening. Direct bladder mucosa injury by chemotherapy in the conditioning regimen, including irradiation, is playing a role, as do virus reactivation (polyoma BK virus [BKV] most commonly, but adenovirus and cytomegalovirus as well) and possibly the recovery of the immune system post-HSCT and GVHD.

MESNA (2-mercaptohethane sulphonate) and hyperhydration are useful in preventing HC due to cyclophosphamide in the conditioning regimen. If it develops, this pre-engraftment HC is of transient nature and usually mild. However, post-engraftment HC is more serious and a major complication, and may last for several months. This is closely related to the reactivation of BKV, as the viruria is usually present. It has been noticed that HC is more likely to develop after allogeneic than autologous HSCT, highlighting the possible role for alloimmune reaction and GVHD in its pathophysiology.

Anti-viral agent cidofovir could theoretically be used for virus neutralization, but serious side effects (myelo- and nephrotoxicty) are the limiting factor. There are reports that quinolone antibiotics (cip-

Table 11.4 Hemorrhagic cystitis (HC) – clinical grading

I	microscopic hematuria
II	macroscopic hematuria
III	II + blood clots in urine
IV	III + renal impairment (urinary obstruction)

rofloxacin, levofloxacin) may suppress BKV replication and that retinoic acid derivatives (nalidixic acid) inhibit BKV activity, but their role in prophylaxis during the conditioning and engraftment process (4–5 weeks post-allo-HCST) is questionable.

Intensive intravenous hydration and forced diuresis, analgesia (systemic opoids often needed), and spasmolytics are used for grade I and II patients (see Table 11.4), as well as platelet and clotting factor transfusions for correcting underlying deficiencies. Bladder irrigation is indicated in cases of macrohematuria with blood clots, and beneficial effects of orally administered estrogen are well documented in mild/moderate cases. The severe HC associated with urinary tract obstruction is a potentially life-threatening complication, and more invasive measures are usually needed, such as cystoscopic examination for cauterization, allum or formalin instillation, and cystectomy with urinary diversion.

Renal complications and thrombotic microangiopathy

Early and late renal complication post-HSCT include acute (occurring in 5–15% of patients undergoing HSCT) and chronic renal failure (5–20%), and, less frequently, hemolytic uremic syndrome (HUS), crescentic and membranous glomerulonephritis, and nephrotic syndrome.

The typical acute renal failure is seen within the first 30 days following either allogeneic (more commonly) or autologous HSCT. The etiology is multifactorial, related to acute tubular necrosis, sepsis, concurrent liver disease (e.g. VOD), and use of nephrotoxic drugs (e.g. antibiotics and calcineurin inhibitors), while fluid overload is a recognized bad prognostic factor. Chronic renal failure is related to nephrotoxic effects of calcineurin inhibitors (ciclosporin; tacrolimus), or it can be caused by the effects of TBI conditioning (radiation nephropathy) presenting as HUS up to 12 months post-HSCT. The classical features are hypertension, hematuria, proteinuria, anemia, azotemia; pathological characteristics are mesangiolysis, focal thickening and splitting of the glomerula basal membrane, and thrombotic microangiopathy in severe cases.

Nephrotic syndrome following allogeneic HSCT is a very rare complication, and is thought to be a part of the chronic GVHD process with TNFα playing a major role in its pathogenesis. Reintroduction of immunosuppression (e.g. ciclosporin) most often results in remission.

Thrombotic microangiopathy, with its clinical syndromes, thrombotic thrombocytopenic purpura (TTP) and hemolytic uremic syndrome, is a well known and serious complication of HSCT, especially from an allogeneic donor (with variable incidence ~0–75%). TTP is defined by simultaneous occurrence of red cell fragmentation on the blood film, laboratory features of hemolysis, need for red blood cell transfusions, *de novo* or prolonged thrombocytopenia caused by consumption, and negative laboratory tests for disseminated intravascular coagulation (DIC). Endothelial injury and use of ciclosporin and/or steroids, as well as administration of norethisterone to prevent menstrual hemorrhage, are the presumed factors in pathogenesis. VOD of the liver, nephropathy and neurological manifestations are commonly associated features, and patients with increased serum creatinine levels have significantly poorer outcome. The mortality rate is reported to be from 25 to 100%, and there is no consistently effective treatment available (discontinuing ciclosporin, plasma exchange), although recently trials with defibrotide were more promising.

Central nervous system dysfunction

Encephalopathy, manifesting with the concurrent liver, renal and/or lung disease (as part of the metabolic or multiple organ dysfunction – systemic inflammatory response syndrome), has been reported earlier as a frequent finding, occurring in ~30% of patients. More recently, changes in mental status such as lethargy or confusion, have been reported to occur in ~11% of patients as isolated single-organ (i.e. CNS) dysfunction, with over 50% of these patients progressing further to second organ dysfunction with ~40% surviving to day 100 post HSCT. Use of TBI, non-bacteremic infections, and platelet transfusions are thought to be the initial stimulus, with subsequent involvement of cytokine network, complement, hemostatic and kinin-generating cascades, and vascular endothelium damage. Another well-recognized cause of transient and reversibile neurotoxicity (hypertension, visual symptoms, seizures, mental status changes, coma) associated with occipital lobe density changes on imaging (MRI/NMR more sensitive than CT) is the use of ciclosporin and to a somewhat lesser extent tacrolimus (FK506). As mentioned above, the underlying mechanism is thought to be endothelial damage related to microangiopathic hemolytic anemia (thrombotic microangiopathy), TBI, and chemotherapy (steroids, etoposide, etc.).

Further reading

Bajwa, R.P.S., Cant, A.J., Abinun, M. et al. (2003) Recombinant tissue plasminogen activator for treatment of hepatic veno-occlusive disease following bone marrow transplantation in children: effectiveness and a scoring system for initiating treatment. Bone Marrow Transplant 31: 591–597.

Barker, C.C., Anderson, R.A., Sauve, R.S., Butzner, J.D. (2005) GI complications in pediatric patients post-BMT. Bone Marrow Transplant 36: 51–58.

Bredius, R.G.M., Ouachee, M., van Brempt, R. et al. (2004) Pulmonary hypertension in two severe combined immunodeficiency disease patients post haematopoietic stem cell transplantation. Br J Haematol 125: 405–406.

Cesaro, S., Pillon, M., Talenti, E. et al. (2005) A prospective survey on incidence, risk factors and therapy of hepatic veno-occlusive disease in children after hematopoietic stem cell transplantation. Hematolofica 90: 1396–1404.

Chalandon, Y., Roosnek, E., Mermillod, B. et al. (2004) Prevention of veno-occlusive disease with defibrotide after allogenic stem cell transplantation. Biol Blood Marrow Transplant 10: 347–354.

Chopra, R., Eaton, J.D., Grassi, A. et al. (2000) Defibrotide for the treatment of hepatic veno-occlusive disease: results of the European compassionate-use study. Br J Haematol 111: 1122–1129.

Cohen, E.P. (2001) Renal failure after bone-marrow transplantation. Lancet 357: 6–7.

Crooks, B.N., Taylor, C.E., Turner, J. et al. (2000) Respiratory viral infections in primary immune deficiencies: significance and relevance to clinical outcome in a single BMT unit. Bone Marrow Transplant 26: 1097–1102.

Fukuda, T., Hackman, R.C., Guthrie, C.A. et al. (2003) Risks and outcomes of idiopathic pneumonia syndrome after nonmyeloablative and conventional conditioning regimens for allogeneic hematopoietic stem cell transplantation. Blood 102: 277–285.

Fullmer, J.J., Fan, L.L., Dishop, M.K., Rodgers, C., Krance, R. (2005) Successful treatment of bronchiolitis obliterans in a bone marrow transplant patient with tumor necrosis factor-alpha blockade. Pediatrics 116:767–770.

Gordon, B., Lyden, E., Lynch, J. et al. (2000) Central nervous system dysfunction as the first manifestation of multiple organ dysfunction syndrome in stem cell transplant patients. Bone Marrow Transplant 25: 79–83.

Heath, J.A., Mishra, S., Mitchell, S., Waters, K.D., Tiedemann, K. (2006) Estrogen as treatment of haemorrhagic cystitis in children and adolescents undergoing bone marrow transplantation. Bone Marrow Transplant 37: 523–526.

Ibrahim, R.B., Peres, E., Dansey, R. et al. (2004) Antithrombin III in the management of hematopoietic stem cell transplantation associated toxicity. Transplantation 38: 1053–1059.

Leung, A.Y.H., Yuen, K.-Y., Kwong, Y.-L. (2005) Polyoma BK virus and haemorrhagic cystitis in haematopietic stem cell transplantation: a changing paradigm. Bone Marrow Transplant 36: 929–937.

Michael, M., Kuehnle, I., Goldstein, S.L. (2004) Fluid overload and acute renal failure in pediatric stem cell transplant patients. Pediatr Nephrol 19: 91–95.

Ruutu, T., Hermans, J., Niederwieser, D. et al. (2002) Thrombotic thrombocytopenic purpura after allogeneic stem cell transplantation: a survey of the European Group for Blood and Marrow Transplantation (EBMT). Br J Haematol 118: 1112–1119.

Sandler, E.S., Aquino, V.M., Gos-Shohet, E., Hinrichs S., Krisher, K. (1997) BK polyoma virus pneumonia following hematopoietic stem cell transplantation. Bone Marrow Transplant 20: 163–165.

Seconi, J., Watt, V., Ritchie, D.S. (2003) Nephrotic syndrome following allogeneic stem cell transplantation associated with increased production of TNF-alpha and interferon-gamma by donor T cells. Bone Marrow Transplant 32: 447–450.

Steward, C.G., Pellier, I., Mahajan, A. et al. (2004) Severe pulmonary hypertension: a frequent complication of stem cell transplantation for malignant infantile osteopetrosis. Br J Haematol 124: 63–71.

Trobaugh-Lotrario, A.D., Greffe, B., Detering, R., Deutsch, G., Quinones, R. (2003) Pulmonary veno-occlusive disease after autologous bone marrow transplantation in a child with stage IV neuroblastoma: case report and literature review. J Pediatr Hematol Oncol 25: 405–409.

Chapter 12

Follow up in the first year after hematopoietic stem cell transplantation

A.R. Gennery and M.P. Collin

Blood product support

Myeloablative or lymphoablative chemotherapy prior to hematopoietic stem cell transplantation (HSCT) will leave most patients dependent on blood product support, usually red blood cells and platelets, for a period of 2–3 weeks post-HSCT until engraftment has been achieved. Neutrophil recovery may be aided by the giving of neutrophil growth promoters such as granulocyte-colony stimulating factor (G-CSF), thus speeding up the time to neutrophil recovery.

Engraftment

Hematological engraftment is usually said to have occurred when neutrophils exceed 0.5×10^9/L and platelets 50×10^{11}/L. Hemoglobin is often not self-sustaining for 2–6 weeks after neutrophil and platelet engraftment and the patient may require one or two red cell transfusions as an outpatient. The appearance of neutrophils marks the end of a significant risk period for the transplant patient, who is now much more resistant to bacterial and fungal infection. Engraftment is faster and more reliable if larger stem cell doses are given and with sibling rather than unrelated donors; it also varies according to the source of stem cells used (Table 12.1). G-CSF decreases the length of hospital stay but does not reduce the early post-HSCT mortality. With some reduced-intensity conditioning regimes, there may be no period of neutropenia but simply a gradual shift from recipient to donor hematopoiesis. In these cases chimerism testing to demonstrate that the cells are of donor origin becomes even

Table 12.1 Speed and success rate of engraftment

Source	Neutrophils	Platelets	Success rate
Bone marrow	14–28 days	14–28 days	>97%
PBSC	10–21 days	14–28 days	>97%
Cord blood	21–56 days	28–100 days	90%

more important than after myeloablative conditioning. Patients therefore require hospitalization, usually in sterile isolation with protective measures to prevent infection during this period following bone marrow transplantation.

Immune reconstitution

Immune reconstitution is generally used to describe recovery of lymphocyte populations and immunoglobulin levels. These are usually studied 100 days and 1 year post-HSCT for malignancy, but more often after HSCT for primary immunodeficiency (PID). After fludarabine-containing regimes with alemtuzumab or with *in vitro* T-cell depletion, lymphopenia may persist for as long as 2 years, confirming the need for extended herpes virus and PCP prophylaxis in some patients, with aciclovir and co-trimoxazole, respectively. Persistent lymphopenia is associated with poor outcome in several studies, although this is closely linked to other adverse factors such as poor graft function, graft-vs.-host disease (GVHD) and its associated immunosuppression. More detailed tests of lymphocyte function and repertoire are useful after HSCT for PID but have limited use in predicting susceptibility to infection in adults. In pediatric patients, immunological reconstitution should be carefully monitored with the measurement of lymphocyte subsets. In particular, specific lymphocyte markers can be helpful, e.g. CD4+CD45RA+CD27+, which is a marker of recent thymic emigrants (lymphocytes that have emerged from the thymus having matured from lymphocyte precursors). Pediatric immunodeficiency patients and some pediatric hematology/oncology patients will require intravenous immunoglobulin (IVIG); most adults do not receive IVIG routinely, although they may be given it in the case of viral pneumonia or cytomegalovirus (CMV) reactivation. Initial indications of normal antibody production can be made by measurement of IgM and IgA, as well as isohemagglutinins, which are indicators of endogenous IgM production.

Chimerism testing and immune reconstitution

Chimerism tests on the patient's blood or bone marrow (BM) determine how much is derived from the donor and how much is residual recipient material. Most commonly chimerism results are expressed in terms of "percentage donor." Several misnomers abound: a patient is said to be a "complete" or "full" donor chimera when blood or BM are 100% donor derived and a "partial" or "incomplete" chimera when there are still recipient cells present.

Two methods are commonly used to monitor donor chimerism:
• XX/XY FISH after HSCT where donor and recipients are of different sex;
• polymerase chain reaction (PCR) to detect variable "DNA fingerprint" sequences between donor and recipient.

More detailed information can be gathered by examining T and B lymphocytes and neutrophils separately.

Some centers use PCR for all transplants in the interests of uniformity, but X/Y chromosome analysis remains a cheaper, quicker, and more sensitive test. It is also more accurate than PCR, which tends to have a slight bias towards either the donor or the recipient.

In HLA mismatch HSCT, chimerism can be measured by monitoring the appearance of donor HLA type by flow cytometry, although this is more generally used as a research tool. In congenital disorders it may be possible to test for the appearance of normal cells, e.g. the neutrophil respiratory burst will be corrected in a successful transplantation of chronic granulomatous disease and platelets of normal size will be formed in Wiskott–Aldrich syndrome. The simplest chimerism test on whole blood reflects myeloid and lymphoid compartments. Lineage-specific chimerism is achieved by isolating CD15-positive myeloid cells and CD3-positive T cells with immunomagnetic techniques, prior to analysis.

Chimerism testing is especially important after reduced-intensity conditioning, although the development of mixed chimerism varies enormously with different reduced-intensity regimens. In some circumstances a reduction in immunosuppression may allow a failing graft to recover, especially following minimal-intensity non-myeloablative regimens.

The meaning of partial chimerism

Chimerism testing helps determine engraftment, immune reconstitution and early relapse. Partial donor chimerism may result from graft rejection, incomplete donor immune reconstitution, relapse of malignancy or a combination of these. It is commonly seen in patients who have undergone reduced-intensity conditioning; 100% donor chimerism is the goal as this ensures complete engraftment, full donor immune reconstitution and the least chance of relapse, or most chance of full immune reconstitution in PID. However, when transplanting pediatric immunodeficiency diseases, stable lymphoid donor chimerism without myeloid donor chimerism may result in full cure, although this may wane over time. In contrast, partial donor chimerism after transplantation for malignant disease may herald relapse, either directly because recipient leukemic cells are reappearing or because inadequate donor immune reconstitution leads to poor GVL activity, allowing leukemic cells to re-emerge. In cases of partial chimerism where relapse has not yet occurred, early intervention with DLI is known as "pre-emptive DLI".

Partial donor chimerism is more common after reduced-intensity transplantation (RIT) than myeloablative transplantation. Accordingly, chimerism should be monitored more frequently after RIT. There may be lineage-specific partial chimerism after RIT and separate evaluation of the CD15-positive myeloid fraction and CD3-positive lymphoid fraction in the blood is recommended. A suggested schedule is given in Table 12.2 for adult RIC transplantation for malignancy: different RIC regimens tend to produce different patterns of partial chimerism. For example, the Seattle regimen (Fludarabine, Cyclophosphamide, 2G, Total Body Irradiation) progresses from 100% recipient to 100% donor over several months whereas the UCH regimen (fludarabine, melphalan, alemtuzumab) tends to give high donor chimerism in all lineages initially but progressively more recipient lymphoid chimerism with time.

For patients who have evidence of falling donor chimerism it may be necessary to reduce or stop anti-GVHD prophylaxis and/or to give a "boost" with either donor lymphocyte infusions (DLI) or a further infusion of donor stem cells. Which cells are used depends partly on the degree of HLA mismatching between donor and recipient.

100% donor chimerism is more likely to occur in patients developing GVHD, probably because there is a stronger immune response against recipient cells including leukemic clones. It is useful to titrate DLI infusions as chimerism rises because, not infrequently, attainment of 100% donor chimerism is coincident with the onset of GVHD.

Table 12.2 Suggested schedule for chimerism measurements follow RIC transplantation for adult malignancy

Interval	Sample	Total	Myeloid	T cell
1 month	blood			
2 months	blood			
Day 100	blood			
Day 100	BM			
6 months	blood			
9 months*	blood			
12 months*	blood			
12 months	BM			

* Lineage test at 9 and 12 months only if <100% at 6 months.

Monitoring for infection

Patients presenting with symptoms of infection, such as fever, need to be examined carefully and appropriate treatment instituted. Treatment will be guided by previous organisms isolated, but should include broad-spectrum Gram-positive and -negative antibodies, an antifungal agent and, if indicated, specific antiviral therapy. For many patients, ongoing monitoring of viral infection is necessary by measurement of whole blood PCR, particularly for infections such as cytomegalovirus (CMV), Epstein–Barr virus (EBV) and adenovirus. Weekly measurements in the early stages post-HSCT enable early detection of low levels of viremia. Patients who have evidence of viremia will require treatment and monitoring can help guide duration of treatment. Pre-emptive treatment of adenovirus with cidofovir, or of CMV with foscarnet or ganciclovir, can prevent progression to symptomatic disease.

Assessment of remission status, DLI and boosts

Remission status for malignant disease is usually assessed 100 days and 1 year post-transplant. Additional assessments may be performed at 6 and 9 months depending on the disease and initial remission status (Table 12.3). Assessment of bone marrow aspirate morphology will define remission to 95% certainty; chimerism testing or cytogenetic analysis will increase this to within 1% (chimerism testing is more universally applicable than cytogenetic analysis), but ideally matched related donor (MRD) assessment by molecular analysis or multiparameter fluorescence activated cell sorter (FACS) should be sought. MRD-positive patients will almost always benefit from accelerated withdrawal of immunosuppression or early DLI to stimulate potential graft-vs.-leukemia (GVL) effects.

Patients with an incomplete response at 100 days, including MRD positivity, should be assessed again at 6 months and 9 months. This allows time for immunosuppression withdrawal or DLI to take effect. Some centers monitor patients in remission at 100 days and again at 6 and 9 months; this may

Table 12.3 Assessment of disease remission status

	Aspirate	Trephine	Chimerism	MRD
AML	+		+	(BCR-ABL)
ALL	+		+	Ig; TCR; (BCR-ABL)
CML	+		+	BCR-ABL
CLL	+	+	+	Ig; FACS
FL[1]	+	+	+	t(14; 18); FACS
MCL[1]	+	+	+	t(11;14); FACS
Hodgkin's[1,2]		+	+	
Myeloma[3]	+		+	FACS

[1] with CT scan.

[2] consider PET scan.

[3] consider MRI spine; free light chains.

be wise where relapse is more common, as in ALL or where BM sampling may be variable such as myeloma.

Donor lymphocyte infusions

This is the only successful immunotherapy, especially for those with ALL and myeloma patients. GVL or graft-vs.-tumor (GVT) effect is believed to be the main reason that stem cell transplantation leads to long-term disease-free survival. This effect occurs when immune cells of the donor, principally T lymphocytes and natural killer (NK) cells, recognize and kill the recipient's hematopoietic and lymphoid cells. In doing so, donor immune cells eradicate the malignant clone of leukemia, lymphoma or myeloma. As GVL is part of the immune response of the donor against the recipient, it is associated with the occurrence of GVHD. Patients who suffer GVHD are, on average, more likely to benefit from the GVL effect than patients who do not develop GVHD. Although GVHD can be prevented by strong prophylactic measures such as donor T-cell depletion, this may increase the risk of relapse owing to a lack of GVL. In general, it is desirable to achieve a mild to moderate level of GVHD after transplantation for malignancy to foster some degree of GVL. However, not every patient who suffers GVHD will have an effective GVL response and unfortunately some with GVHD will still relapse. The effect of GVL also varies from one disease to another, with CML stimulating the best GVL response and ALL probably the weakest.

Immunological reconstitution

In the majority of cases evidence of neutrophil reconstitution will be sufficient to consider discharge from the bone marrow transplantation unit. In rare cases of patients transplanted for T lymphocyte immune deficiency, discharge may be delayed until there is evidence of lymphocyte engraftment. In whole marrow transplant this is usually within 4–6 weeks following transplantation but, in patients who have undergone a T-cell-depleted procedure, evidence of lymphocyte engraftment may not be available until 120 days or more after bone marrow transplantation.

Boost infusion for PID

For patients with PID, boost infusions of stem cells (with whole marrow product, or TCD) can improve falling chimerism or poor T-cell function. The stem cells should be harvested from the original donor source, and can be given as a day case without further conditioning. Boost infusions are most likely to improve T-cell function, but may not alter poor B-cell function.

Discharge from hospital

Discharge from hospital is another milestone in post-transplant life. Successful discharge depends on good liaison with the post-transplant care team and attention to a number of details (Table 12.4).

Follow-up visits

First 100 days

Patients are usually followed up at the transplant center for the first 100 days post-transplant. Thereafter an arrangement of shared care is likely, unless there is significant GVHD or other complications. During the first 60 days it is not uncommon to see patients twice weekly for CMV monitoring. Subsequently this may be decreased to weekly visits. Hickman lines require weekly flushing but may be removed before 100 days, allowing greater intervals between follow-up visits. Close observation is

Table 12.4 Criteria to be met before discharge

Engraftment/FBC	Neutrophils > 0.5; platelet independent; Hb adequate
Electrolytes/biochemistry	Stable renal function and Magnesium
GVHD	Controlled or resolving; adequate enteric absorption
Immunosuppression	Stable blood levels on oral treatment
Infection	Apyrexial on oral antibiotics for >24 hours
Prophylaxis	Local regime instituted
Medications	Indications and dosing explained
Home circumstances	Relatives and carers informed; transport arranged
Emergency contact	Clear advice given
Clearance of pre-existing viral infection	
Weight gain without parenteral nutritional support	(pediatric transplants)

required during the first 100 days, looking carefully at:

- engraftment status and transfusion requirement;
- GVHD and adjustment of immunosuppression;
- CMV status and treatment of reactivation;
- signs of opportunistic infection and starting prompt treatment;
- monitoring of side effects, especially those related to ciclosporin and tacrolimus:
  - hypertension;
  - renal impairment;
  - magnesium depletion;
- chimerism testing;
- central line hygiene;
- psychosocial support;
- continuing education.

First year

After 100 days, follow up is largely dictated by the requirements of individual patients. In difficult cases, active GVHD, CMV reactivation and poor graft function may demand frequent visits to clinic. Patients who do not suffer GVHD or opportunistic infection may rapidly return to work, or school, and relatively normal life. In the absence of complications, 1–2 monthly clinic visits are appropriate for most patients during the first year.

Patients who reactivate CMV may require treatment with ganciclovir or foscarnet, particularly if CMV is detected in the blood or in two separate sites. For those patients with poor graft function

DLI or "boost" infusions of donor cells may be required – regular chimerism monitoring will help guide this decision.

While some treatment for skin GVHD may involve the use of topical steroids or calcineurin inhibitors, severe GVHD or GVHD involving liver and gut may require significant doses of immune suppression, and usually requires inpatient treatment.

Other aspects of care

Specific complications may require further care sometimes as an inpatient. These include oxygen for pneumonitis, total parenteral nutrition for severe mucocitis or nutritional deficiency secondary to infection or gut GVHD.

Follow-up reviews

Patients whose home is a long way from the hospital may require a temporary base closer to the transplantation unit. This is particularly true for patients who have been referred to supraregional national services, such as those for immunodeficiency. The nature and frequency of follow up will depend on unit guidelines but will be influenced by:

- type of HSCT;
- complications.

Reviews usually become less frequent as the patient moves further from HSCT. Depending on the services local to the patient's home, some follow up may be possible at a local hospital rather than at the transplantation unit (Table 12.5).

Issues to address at follow up immediately following bone marrow transplantation

These issues will be dominated by short-term considerations such as resolution of acute GVHD, continuing hematological and immune reconstitution, and ongoing infective episodes.

Graft-vs.-host disease

Ongoing GVHD must be monitored closely. Stool volume and liver function tests, especially bilirubin and ALT, will need to be measured regularly to assess the extent of gut or liver GVHD. Skin GVHD should be assessed by recording of the areas of skin involved. Skin biopsy is usually needed to confirm presence of GVHD. Likewise abnormal liver function tests that continue to deteriorate without any other explanation or ongoing diarrhea with no infective cause identified may require more extensive investigation with liver biopsy and gut biopsy. Careful monitoring of immune suppression is required and immune suppression should be titrated against response. In cases of severe acute GVHD or

ongoing GVHD, immune suppression will need to be tailored very slowly. Attention should be paid to side effects of the immunosuppressive drugs. In particular, patients on steroids will need to have the following in order to prevent osteoporosis secondary to steroid treatment:
- regular eye check-ups for cataracts;
- bone mineral density performed;
- calcium supplements;
- vitamin D supplements and biphosphonates

Steroid sparing drugs such as calcineurin inhibitors and anti-inflammatory biologics (e.g. anti-TNF antibody) may be useful.

At subsequent follow ups the issues alluded to above still need to be considered. Patients receiving anti-GVHD prophylaxis may be able to discontinue prophylaxis by about 6 months following stem cell transplantation providing there has been no evidence of GVHD. Patients receiving treatment for GVHD will need to be monitored carefully and treatment tailored to response. By 6–9 months following transplantation, if there is evidence of T and B cell immune reconstitution with immunoglobulin production, then intravenous immunoglobulin substitution may be discontinued. It is advisable to recommence the vaccination programme 3 months after discontinuing intravenous immunoglobulin (to allow donor immunoglobin to wash out). Prior

Table 12.5 Example of follow-up schedule from a pediatric immunology BMT unit

Follow-up reviews: frequency depending on progress	• 2–6 weekly depending on clinical progress • 6 weekly until 6 months post BMT • 3 monthly until 1 year post BMT • 6 monthly until 2 years post BMT • Annually thereafter
Immunosuppressive drugs	• Ciclosporin until 6 months (6 weeks for TCD marrow) – give for longer if indicated • Steroids when indicated

Substitution therapy	• IVIG 3 weekly until satisfactory evidence of IgM, IgA and isohemagglutinins
	• Blood and platelet therapy
	  a Hb<8
	  b platelets <10–20 depending on patient

Anti-infective prophylaxis	• Nystatin: stop on discharge • Itraconazole: discontinue at 6 weeks if neutrophils above 0.5–1 • Aciclovir: discontinue when PHA positive • Co-trimoxazole: once a day until 2 years post-BMT with specific antibody production • Isoniazid: discontinue when PHA positive • Azithromycin: discontinue at 6–8 weeks post-BMT

to vaccination it is helpful to measure specific antibody levels and repeat these following vaccination to demonstrate evidence of antibody response. For children with PID, the national primary immunization schedule should be followed, with antibody responses documented before proceeding to live vaccines, e.g. MMR.

Anti-infective prophylaxis

Patients will be discharged on anti-infective prophylaxis such as nystatin or other antifungals, as well as HSV and CMV prophylaxis, aciclovir and co-trimoxazole as PCP, and bacterial prophylaxis. Antifungal prophylaxis can normally be discontinued at 6 weeks after stem cell transplantation if the neutrophil count is above 500 cells/µL. Aciclovir is normally discontinued at 6 months providing there is no ongoing herpes virus infection and the patient is not on significant immunosuppression for GVHD. Co-trimoxazole is conventionally discontinued when there is evidence of specific polysaccharide antibody production, usually 2 years after transplantation. For patients who have undergone a splenectomy or who have evidence of splenic dysfunction, lifelong antibiotic prophylaxis with penicillin will be necessary.

Growth and development

For children it is important to measure growth and development. Plotting of height and weight against centiles provides a useful measurement of growth progress. Particular concerns need to be addressed for those who have received radiotherapy as well as chemotherapy. Measurement of sex hormones may be necessary when pre-pubertal patients approach puberty.

Thyroid function

It is important to measure thyroid function and thyroxine levels at each visit. Up to 40% of patients develop thyroid function following bone marrow transplantation – not only patients who have received radiotherapy but also those who have received only chemotherapy – and it may be necessary to initiate thyroxine replacement.

Further reading

Andre-Schmutz, I., Dal Cortivo, L., Fischer, A., Cavazzana-Calvo, M. (2005) Improving immune reconstitution while preventing GvHD in allogeneic stem cell transplantation. *Cytotherapy* **7**: 102–108.

Moss, P. (2001) Developments in the treatment of post-transplant viral disease. *Best Pract Res Clin Haematol* **14**: 777–792.

Peggs, K.S., Thomson, K., Hart, D.P. *et al.* (2004) .Dose-escalated donor lymphocyte infusions following reduced intensity transplantation: toxicity, chimerism, and disease responses. *Blood* **103**: 1548–1556.

Ranke, M.B., Schwarze, C.P., Dopfer, R. *et al.* (2005) PDWP of the BMT. Late effects after stem cell transplantation (SCT) in children – growth and hormones. *Bone Marrow Transplant* **35**(Suppl. 1): S77–81.

Skinner, R., Cant, A.J., Davies, E.G., Foot, A., Finn, A. (2002) Immunisation of the immunocompromised child. Best Practice Statement. London: Royal College of Paediatrics and Child Health.

Chapter 13

Immune recovery following hematopoietic stem cell transplantation and vaccination

A.R. Gennery, D. Barge and G. Spickett

Immune reconstitution

Hematopoietic stem cell transplantation (HSCT) aims to replace defective or malignant recipient cells with normal donor cells or, in autologous transplantation, to rescue bone marrow following lethal chemotherapy/radiotherapy or, in autoimmune disease, to "wipe the slate clean" by removing aberrant dysregulated T cells and replacing them with normal T cells. The timing and speed at which different cell lineages return depends on factors including the underlying condition, HSC source, conditioning therapies, and presence or absence of graft-vs.-host disease (GVHD). It is important to be clear what is meant by hematological and immune reconstitution. In simple terms hematological engraftment is the appearance of donor cells in peripheral blood, beginning with short-lived cells, such as platelets and neutrophils, which should be found within a few weeks of HSCT; their presence implies that donor HSC have repopulated the recipient bone marrow and are differentiating into mature cells. The presence of longer-lived donor cell lineages, such as lymphocytes (immune reconstitution), may simply represent "peripheral engraftment" of pre-existing mature lymphocytes present in the donor stem cell source, without engraftment of pluripotent stem cells. Alternatively, pre-existing T-lymphoid precursors derived from the donor stem cells may have migrated to the recipient thymus, completed maturation and been released into recipient's peripheral blood. Engraftment of donor HSC within the bone marrow should lead to the continuous production of immature lymphocytes, which develop into mature lymphocytes in the recipient's bone marrow or thymus. It is not clear whether all patients develop a diverse range of mature lymphocytes capable of responding to all antigens or whether "holes" in the T- and B-cell receptor repertoire may leave the patient susceptible to particular infections such as pneumococcus. When assessing immune recovery following HSCT it is important to be clear precisely which aspect of immune recovery is being measured. Increasingly sophisticated laboratory investigations give a more detailed picture of immune function and perhaps better predict long-term protection from infection.

Measuring immune reconstitution after HSCT

After HSCT the prolonged period of profound multifaceted immunodeficiency explains the high risk of opportunistic infection. A number of factors determine the speed and completeness of immune reconstitution. Counting the numbers of platelets, red cells, neutrophils, and the different types of lymphocytes gives a rough guide to immune reconstitution, but says little about function. However, in specific conditions such as congenital neutropenia, bone marrow failure or severe combined immune deficiency (SCID), where very low numbers of specific cell lineages or lymphocyte subsets are a feature of the disease for which HSCT has been performed, the appearance of such cells is usually a good marker of "cure."

Myeloid function

More sophisticated neutrophil investigations, including the assessment of the intracellular killing apparatus, the neutrophil oxidative burst, by nitroblue tetrazolium reduction test (NBT) or a flow cytometric assay using dihydrorhodamine are really only of use after HSCT for a neutrophil disorder such as chronic granulomatous disease (Fig. 13.1).

When considering platelet reconstitution, analysis of platelet number is usually all that is needed. In conditions where small or large platelet size is a feature of the disease, e.g. Wiskott–Aldrich syndrome, determination of platelet size will confirm whether emerging platelets are of normal size, and thus of donor origin. To date, more complex tests such as HLA typing of platelets have not been universally successful.

T-lymphocyte reconstitution

Development of T-lymphocyte function depends on two separate mechanisms, peripheral expansion of mature T cells and naive T-cell production by the thymus. If the donor stem cell source has been depleted of T cells (as after a mismatched HSCT), then T cells seen will usually be derived from stem cells that develop into lymphocyte precursors, which are then "educated" in the thymus.

An initial indication of T-cell reconstitution will be found by looking at absolute CD3 numbers in the peripheral blood. A number of factors influence the timing of this, including:
- conditioning;
- use of anti-T cell serotherapy (e.g. ATG, alemtuzumab) pre-HSCT;
- HSC source – whole or TCD marrow, UCSC;
- GVHD;
- immunosuppressive treatment (e.g. ciclosporin A, steroids).

In general, T cells >200 cells/µL are seen by about 6 weeks post-HSCT if whole marrow is

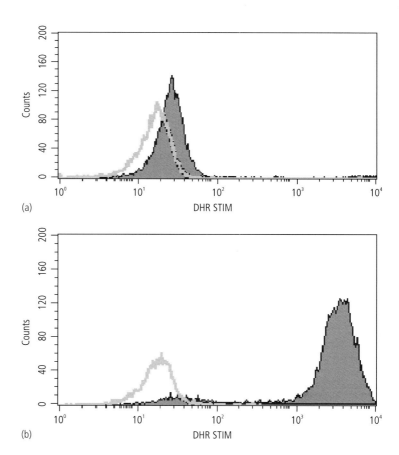

Fig. 13.1 Histograms showing (a) severely reduced oxidative burst prior to BMT and (b) normal oxidative burst post BMT. x-axis = fluorescence of dihydrorhodamine; y-axis = number of events. Data shown are gated on neutrophil population: pale grey = unstimulated; dark grey = stimulated with PMA.

given. However, this is due to repopulation of the peripheral circulation by mature T lymphocytes present in the donor marrow.

T-cell thymogenesis takes approximately 4 months (120 days) from HSCT, as donor stem cells have to engraft in the bone marrow, T-cell precursors must migrate to the thymus and T-cell maturation then occurs within the thymus, before mature, naive T cells emerge. These newly emerged thymic emigrants can be identified by the presence of T-cell receptor excision circles (TRECS), measured by PCR. A surrogate marker of newly emerged thymic emigrants is the CD45RA+/CD27+ marker, which can be measured by flow cytometry (Fig. 13.2).

Proliferative responses to mitogens such as phytohemagglutinin (PHA) can be a helpful, although very crude, test of T-cell function. Absence indicates severely deficient T-cell immunity and is seen soon after HSCT and in patients immunosuppressed for ongoing GVHD. Detailed examination of the diversity of T-cell receptors by spectrotyping will give some indication as to the breadth of the T-cell receptor repertoire.

B-cell function

Full B-cell reconstitution is reflected in the generation of specific antibody in response to antigen challenge, either following vaccination, or after natural exposure to the infectious agent.

B-cell reconstitution after bone marrow transplantation (BMT) recapitulates normal B-cell development. In patients without chronic GVHD there are 3 phases to B-cell reconstitution: in phase 1 there is a gradual increase in B-cell number; phase 2 is characterized by B-cell proliferation with supranormal B-cell counts; and finally phase 3 is characterized by normalized B-cell numbers. Phase 1 may be short (1–3 months) in autologous transplant recipients, and longer (3–4 months) in allograft recipients without chronic GVHD. Phase 2–3 B cells resemble neonatal cells with features of immature B cells.

The first useful investigation of B-cell reconstitution is B-cell enumeration. Examination of B-cell subsets can also be useful. The use of the CD27 marker as an indicator of a memory B-cell sub-

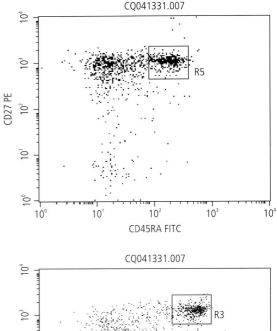

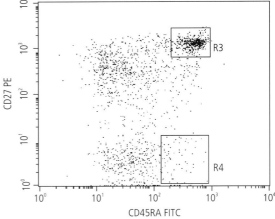

Fig. 13.2 Dot plots show naive T-cell populations. Top plot is gated on CD3+CD4+ T cells, bottom plot on CD3+CD4– T cells. R5 is naive CD4+ T cells (CD4+ CD45RA+ CD27+) and R3 naive CD8+ T cells (CD4– CD45RA+ CD27+). R4 is effector CD8 T cells (CD4– CD45RA+ CD27–).

set may be helpful in determining whether class-switched memory cells have been formed. Looking at surface immunoglobulin at the same time will determine whether Ig class switching from IgM to IgG and IgA has occurred. Other useful tests of B-cell function include measurement of serum IgM, IgA, IgG and IgG subclasses. Isohemagglutinin titers are a useful measure of endogenous IgM response; this is especially helpful in patients receiving IVIG or SCIG where IgG levels simply refer to those in the IgG product, not the patient's endogenous IgG production, whereas IgM responses must be made by the patient as IVIG does not contain IgM. The measurement of specific responses to vaccine antigens, such as tetanus, *Haemophilus influenzae* type B (HiB) and *Pneumococcus* or infective antigens known to have been encountered by the patient is helpful but should only be assessed at least 3 months after IVIG has been discontinued. Care should be taken to relate measurements to age-related normal values.

Factors influencing immune reconstitution

Conditioning

For children with SCID, an infusion of whole marrow or of TCD stem cells will allow T-cell engraftment, but for all other conditions rejection is very likely if no pre-BMT conditioning is given. Immune reconstitution differs after full myeloablation or reduced-intensity conditioning. Following reduced-intensity conditioning there is a greater risk of graft rejection or "slipping" donor chimerism, and regular chimerism assessment needs to be made to monitor this. Infusion of donor stem cells can consolidate poor or falling donor chimerism and improve immunological reconstitution. The combination of fludarabine with Campath-1H in reduced-intensity conditioning regimens leads to a longer period of lymphopenia, with concomitant risk of viral reactivation, particularly with cytomegalovirus (CMV), Epstein–Barr virus (EBV) and adenovirus.

Stem cell source

The quality of stem cells is the same whether taken from bone marrow (BM) or peripherally mobilized blood stem cell pools (PBSC). However, BM and PBSC grafts give different patterns of immune reconstitution depending on the proportion of early pluripotent and self-renewing stem cells to lineage-committed late progenitor cells and on number of accompanying accessory cells, particularly T-cell subsets, contained in the stem cell allografts.

For example, allografts of recombinant human GCSF-treated PBSCs contain 2–4 times more CD34-positive cells than those from untreated BM. The total number of T cells, monocytes, and natural killer cells in a PBSC allograft is almost 10 times higher than those in a BM allograft and this is reflected in the faster time to engraftment seen in patients who receive PBSC. However, PBSC are associated with a greater risk of GVHD. A CD34-positive stem cell count of $>3 \times 10^6$/kg is associated with more rapid neutrophil, monocyte and lymphocyte engraftment and a decreased risk of invasive fungal infection.

Engraftment after cord blood stem cell transplantation is slower than for PBSC or marrow transplants, and is related to the stem cell dose and perhaps the smaller number of lineage committed late progenitor cells.

Graft-vs.-host disease (GVHD)

Complete immune reconstitution depends on the generation of new T cells from hematopoietic stem cells. While the transfer of mature donor T cells (as in whole marrow HLA sibling HSCT) improves short-term immune function, immune function at 1 year or more correlates with the number of CD45RA+CD27+ naive T cells, suggesting that later immune function depends on how well the thymus generates new T cells from stem cell-derived T-cell precursors. Thymic function is modified and impaired by GVHD and direct thymic damage from chemo/radiotherapy. Active chronic GVHD inhibits thymopoiesis and, even after GVHD has resolved, the number of thymic derived mature T cells is still lower than in patients who have not had GVHD.

Adults given T cell-depleted grafts can generate new T cells (as shown by increasing TREC levels) but chronic GVHD severely depresses this, a finding consistent with a GVHD-mediated destruction of lymphoid niches for the regeneration of T-cell immunity. Recipients of T-cell-depleted grafts have lower TRECs than unmodified allograft recipients in the first 9 months following transplantation, reflecting the delay in production of new T cells. Lower TREC values correlate strongly with an increased risk of severity of opportunistic infections.

Table 13.1 Differences in T-cell responses from newly emerged thymic T cells and peripherally expanded mature T cells

Thymopoiesis	Peripheral T-cell expansion
Better in children	More in older patients
Responses to new antigens	Poor responses to new antigens
Full polyclonal TCR repertoire	Frequent oligoclonal TCR repertoire
Normal T-cell pool	Only starting population of peripheral T cells, so incomplete T-cell pool levels
New T cells with CD45RA+CD62L+ phenotype	Peripheral T cells of CD45RO+ phenotype
Expansion driven by MHC peptide signals as positive selection	Expansion driven by peripheral MHC peptide stimulation of dividing memory T cells

Age

In younger patients T-cell (CD3) regeneration is faster and involves expansion of CD45RA+CD27+ naive cells derived from thymopoiesis, probably because the thymus is much more active in young children, whereas in older patients (greater than 18 years of age) CD3-positive T-cell levels rise more slowly and do so more because of peripheral expansion of T cells, rather than generation of new T cells (Table 13.1).

In adults, T-cell-depleted HSCT using an unrelated adult donor is associated with prolonged T-cell lymphopenia compared with adults who received TCD BMT from a related donor. In children normal T-cell populations are seen just as soon after related or unrelated BMT. Factors that may account for the more profound lymphopenia in adults include involution of the thymus, which may lead to prolonged immunodeficiency after unrelated donor transplantation (Table 13.2).

Vaccination schedules

Timing of vaccination depends on the progress following HSCT. If the patient is receiving immunoglobulin replacement this should be continued until increasing levels of IgA and IgM suggest that there is endogenous immunoglobulin production. For patients with ongoing immune suppression or poor immune function due to GVHD, vaccination should be delayed. All children who have received an allogeneic HSCT should be considered for re-immunization, according to agreed unit guidelines. Usually re-immunization commences 12 months after an HLA-identical sibling donor HSCT or 18

Table 13.2 Clinical events and diseases that decrease thymic function and prevent T-cell reconstitution

Thymic atrophy due to aging
Cancer chemotherapy
Thymus irradiation
GVHD
Ciclosporin therapy
Serious systemic illness or stress responses

months after any other allogeneic HSCT. If re-immunization is to be undertaken, the full primary immunization schedule should be followed (Table 13.3).

Re-immunization of allogeneic or autologous HSCT recipients should commence 12 months after an HLA-identical sibling donor, and 18 months after allogeneic or syngeneic HSCT, providing that:

• there is no evidence of active chronic GVHD;
• the child has been off all immunosuppressive treatment for at least 6 months;
• the child has been off IVIG for at least 3 months.

Care should be taken in assessing polysaccharide antibody responses to pneumococcus. Some patients following HSCT make inadequate polysaccharide responses, probably explaining the increased late susceptibility to pneumococcal infection seen after HSCT. In part this is due to poor splenic function, which may be secondary to disease or radiotherapy. The pneumococcal response should be assessed by measuring pneumococcal-specific antibody response to pneumococcal vaccination. This may help determine whether long-term antibiotic prophylaxis is necessary. Patients who are unable to make polysaccharide responses

Table 13.3 Re-immunization schedule following HSCT with HLA-identical sibling, allogeneic or syngeneic donor

At 12 months post-HSCT
   (or 3 months after discontinuing IVIG)
	Diphtheria, tetanus, acellular pertussis, inactivated polio, conjugated HiB and conjugated 7 valent
	   pneumococcal vaccine (for immunodeficient patients serological responses should be measured)

At 13 months post-HSCT	Diphtheria, tetanus, acellular pertussis, inactivated polio, conjugated HiB and conjugated meningococcal C
At 14 months post-HSCT	Diphtheria, tetanus, acellular pertussis, inactivated polio, conjugated HiB and conjugated 7 valent pneumococcal vaccine, and conjugated meningococcal C
At 18 months post-HSCT	MMR
At 24 months post-HSCT	HiB/meningococcal C conjugated vaccine
At 25 months post-HSCT	MMR and conjugated 7 valent pneumococcal vaccine
At 30 months post-HSCT	Polysaccharide pneumococcal vaccine

Any other allogenic HSCT: re-immunization schedule as above but commencing at 18 months post-HSCT.
Autologous HSCT: re-immunization schedule as above.

should remain on long-term antibiotic prophylaxis as there is a danger of invasive pneumococcal disease. This is particularly important for patients who have had irradiation involving the spleen. An adequate response to polysaccharide antigen is generally defined as a fourfold rise, or greater, antibody level from baseline (pre-vaccination) provided that the final antibody value is within the protective range given by the laboratory.

Measles and *Varicella zoster*

Significant contact with measles or chicken pox/shingles requires treatment until patients are at least 1 year post-HSCT and at least 12 months off all immunosuppressive treatment. Significant contact is defined as play or direct contact for more than 15 minutes, on the ward, at school or in the household. If the contact with a confirmed measles case is less than 14 days the patient should receive intramuscular human normal immunoglobulin or intravenous immunoglobulin, which will give protection for approximately 4 weeks unless the patient is still on immunoglobulin replacement. The patient who has significant contact with an individual with chicken pox requires either high-dose oral aciclovir from 7 to 21 days following the initial contact or, if less than 72 hours from the contact, should receive intramuscular zoster immunoglobulin or IVIG if not already receiving replacement. The protection lasts approximately 4 weeks. Whichever method of prophylaxis is used,

the patient and family should be informed to contact the specialist unit should any suspicious skin lesions develop in order that early treatment with intravenous aciclovir may be considered.

Long-term changes in immune function

Patients with full donor chimerism, good levels of neutrophils and continued emergence of naive T cells from the recipient thymus should have broad-spectrum, long-term immunity. Patients whose T-cell immunity is due to peripheral expansion of T cells given with the graft may develop "immune exhaustion" after 15 or more years post-HSCT. Immunization of the recipient and the donor before transplantation may be more effective in improving antibody immunity after transplantation irrespective of patient or donor age, total body irradiation and GVHD. Antibody levels in the first year after transplantation are affected primarily by donor and recipient antibody levels pre-HSCT (this clearly does not apply to immunodeficient patients).

Further reading

Fallen, P.R., McGreavey, L., Madrigal, J.A. *et al.* (2003) Factors affecting reconstitution of the T cell compartment in allogeneic haematopoietic cell transplant recipients. *Bone Marrow Transplant* **32**: 1001–1014.

Haynes, B.F., Markert, M.L., Sempowski, G.D., Patel, D.D., Hale, L.P. (2000) The role of the thymus in immune reconstitution in aging, bone marrow transplantation, and HIV-1 infection. *Annu Rev Immunol* **18**:529–560.

Skinner, R., Cant, A.J., Davies, E.G., Foot, A., Finn, A. (2002) Immunisation of the immunocompromised child. Best Practice Statement. London: Royal College of Paediatrics and Child Health.

Slatter, M.A., Bhattacharya, A., Abinun, M., Flood, T.J., Cant, A.J., Gennery, A.R. (2005) Outcome of boost hemopoietic stem cell transplant for decrease in donor chimerism or graft dysfunction in primary immunodeficiency. *Bone Marrow Transplant* **35**: 683–689.

Slatter, M.A., Bhattacharya, A., Flood, T.J. *et al.* (2003) Polysaccharide antibody responses are impaired post bone marrow transplantation for severe combined immunodeficiency, but not other primary immunodeficiencies. *Bone Marrow Transplant* **32**: 225–230.

Chapter 14

Prevention of infection following discharge after hematopoietic stem cell transplant

H. Harvey and A. Reed

Introduction

Returning home following hematopoietic stem cell transplant (HSCT) provokes a range of emotions in the transplanted individual and their carers. They are frequently elated yet anxious about returning home; these feelings are regularly replaced by frustration at the restrictions imposed upon them at home. Increasingly patients are discharged to their own home or to a home environment outside the hospital (half-way house) much earlier than previously. After an allogeneic HSCT, especially from a matched unrelated donor, patients receive greater immunosuppressive treatment, are slower to engraft and so are more susceptible to infection than autologous transplant patients. Graft-vs.-host disease (GVHD) will increase the degree of immunosuppression, as will its treatment. This chapter will explore prevention of infection in the home environment and why this is necessary. Much of this information is based on adopting a sensible, cautious approach to the immunocompromised individual, as little evidence-based research is available. While the transplant unit will have no control of their patients following discharge, there is practical advice that can be given to reduce the risk of infection immediately following transplant. Any restrictions that are recommended depend on the patient's immune system and should be reviewed at each outpatient visit at the specialist center.

Laboratory tests for immunity

Tests that may indicate a satisfactory degree of immunity include:
- blood neutrophil count >1.5 × 10^9/L;
- CD3 (T-lymphocyte) count >200/µL;
- phytohemagglutinin (PHA) response – positive.

Once satisfactory immunity has been demonstrated then the restrictions given below may be relaxed. This will occur much earlier for patients receiving autologous transplants than for allogeneic transplants, especially if the latter suffer from complications of transplant, e.g. GVHD.

Medications

Antimicrobial agents

Following HSCT the patient will be given prophylactic medications in order to prevent infection. They usually include the following.
- Co-trimoxazole to prevent opportunistic infections such as *Pneumocystis* and infections due to encapsulated bacteria (e.g. *Haemophilus influenzae*, *Streptococcus pneumoniae*, meningococci). The patient may need to continue on this until they have demonstrated a specific antibody response to pneumococcus.
- Aciclovir or another antiviral agents to prevent *Herpes simplex* and cytomegalovirus (CMV) infection, usually given for six months providing the patient has >200/µL T cells and is no longer on significant immunosuppressive treatment.
- An antifungal agent such as itraconazole, usually until the patient has had a neutrophil count of 1.5 × 10^9/L or above (approximately six weeks following HSCT), although this may need to be continued in patients with GVHD.

Immunoglobulin replacement

If this has been started during transplant the patient will be required to continue treatment until they have adequate B-cell function. (Chapter 5 gives the indications for use of intravenous immunoglobulin.) Once the patient has evidence of producing IgA and IgM they can discontinue treatment. Three months following discontinuation of this therapy they should be vaccinated with inactivated vaccines. (See Chapter 13 for the vaccination protocol.)

Home environment

Patients will be returning to a wide range of accommodation but this should be clean, warm, and have running water and electricity. If their accommodation is deemed to be highly unsuitable for a safe transfer home then alternative arrangements should be discussed with the social worker. While ideal conditions will not be available for all patients, attempts should be made to make the home environment as safe and hygienic as possible.

Fresh flowers and plants, although the traditional gift for ill patients, are not recommended in the home as they will be heavily contaminated with *Aspergillus* and other fungal spores. Silk flowers and artificial plants provide a suitable alternative. Providing the HSCT patient is not receiving immunosuppressive treatment and has a CD3 count $\geq 200/\mu L$ then these restrictions can be relaxed.

Cleaning

Microorganisms, e.g. staphylococci from skin scales, and *Aspergillus* and other fungal spores that can cause serious infection, are found in dust, so the home environment needs to be dust free. Daily dusting with a damp, clean cloth is recommended to remove dust from horizontal surfaces until the patient's neutrophil count is constantly greater than $1.5 \times 10^9/L$. Following this the family can be encouraged to return to their normal cleaning regime using their regular cleaning products. The rooms that the patient is likely to use should be vacuumed by a carer on alternate days. HEPA-filtered vacuum cleaners are available, which prevent dust being dispersed back into the environment.

Vacuuming should be done when the patient is not in the room. Cleaning of the home should not be done by the HSCT patient until satisfactory immunity has been established.

Toys

Toys should be cleaned on a regular basis. Hard toys should be cleaned with a detergent solution on a weekly basis, soft toys cleaned weekly in a washing machine.

Professionals such as play workers should not bring external toys and equipment into the home.

Home improvements

As dust from building work is likely to be heavily contaminated with *Aspergillus* and other fungal spores that can cause serious invasive infection in HSCT patients, home improvements that create dust should not be carried out either immediately before or after the transplant; work should probably be postponed until the patient is off immunosuppressive treatment and has a T-cell count greater than $200/\mu L$. Patients receiving allogeneic HSCT usually remain on antifungal prophylaxis until approximately 6 weeks post-transplant, which provides some protection from fungal infections, but unnecessary exposure to fungal spores is still not recommended. It is advised that no bare plaster is left on walls as this will create dust; therefore all walls must be painted or papered.

Personal hygiene

Hand washing

Good hand hygiene is well recognized as being vital in reducing the spread of infection in hospital and in the general population. Microorganisms on the hands may be resident or transient organisms. Resident organisms are part of the normal skin flora, and usually include coagulase-negative staphylococci and *Corynebacteria* (diphtheroids). These are not easily removed and are located deep in the epidermis. They do not usually cause infection in immunocompetent individuals, but can cause infection associated with implanted and intravascular devices. In immunocompromised patients skin organisms can also cause local infection, e.g. at intravenous line sites. Transient organisms are those that are acquired through contamination. Examples of transient organisms are Gram-negative bacilli (*Escherichia coli*, *Klebsiella*, *Pseudomonas*, *Salmonella*) and gastrointestinal viruses, e.g. rotavirus. These are easily removed by washing the hands with soap and water. Liquid soap is preferred to bar soap as microorganisms can survive well on the surface of bar soap. Liquid soap should not be topped up in its container, rather a new container used each time. The nozzle should be kept clean to prevent colonization with bacteria.

The patient should ensure that they wash their hands regularly, using liquid soap, especially:
- following toileting;
- prior to and following food preparation;
- after gardening or touching plants or soil;
- after touching pets or animals;
- after changing nappies;
- after touching other secretions or excretions or items that might have had contact with human or animal feces, such as clothing or bedding.

It is important that young children are supervised when washing hands and taught how to do so properly prior to discharge. Hands need to be washed correctly to remove microorganisms. Each area of the hand needs to be covered including the commonly missed areas (thumbs, finger tips and inter-digital spaces). Drying of the hands is also important as the majority of microorganisms (90–95%) will be removed during the washing process and the remainder on drying. Towels should not be shared with family, household members or pets. Skin integrity is important because if the patient has dry skin or sore hands they may not wash them as often as is necessary. If the hands do become cracked it could lead to an increase in bacterial colonization and therefore infection. Individuals washing their hands frequently should use an emollient.

Hand-washing technique

- Wet hands, apply soap.
- Rub palm to palm.

- Rub back of both hands.
- Rub palm to palm with fingers interlaced.
- Rub backs of fingers (interlocked).
- Rub all parts of both thumbs.
- Rub both palms with fingertips.
- Rinse hands under running water and dry thoroughly on a clean towel.

Teeth and mouth care

Teeth should be brushed after eating using a soft toothbrush in order to reduce the build-up of bacteria. A soft brush will reduce the risk of bleeding if the patient has a low platelet count. Dentures should be cleaned daily using a conventional cleaning product in accordance with the manufacturer's instructions.

Hair and shaving

An electric shaver or clippers, rather than a razor blade, should be used until the patient has a neutrophil count of 1.5×10^9/L or above and a platelet count of 50×10^9/L or above.

Bathing and showering

A bath or shower should be taken daily to reduce bacterial colonization and for comfort. Soap or shower gel should be mild to help maintain the integrity of the skin. The shower head should be cleaned weekly using chlorine-based disinfecting solution such as 1% hypochlorite and the shower should be run for 5–10 minutes prior to use to ensure that any microorganisms in the shower head (e.g. *Legionella*) are flushed through the system. Ideally this should be done by someone other than the patient and while the patient is not in the room. Baths should be taken alone and not with other siblings or partners in order to minimize contact with organisms from their skin and perineum. Bath toys or equipment (e.g. loafers) that retain bath water should not be used as they will be heavily colonized with microorganisms. Patients should also avoid bathing in spa baths, jacuzzis or hot tubs as they are frequently contaminated with *Pseudomonas*. Baths and showers should be kept clean and bidets are not recommended as they are very difficult to clean thoroughly.

Care of the central venous lines (CVL)

Many patients return home with a CVL *in situ*; before doing so the transplant center needs to consider the following.
• Why does the CVL needs to be left in?
• Is the patient and/or carer able to cope with a CVL?
• Is the home environment suitable?
• Can hospital care be easily accessed if the patient has a temperature or shows signs or symptoms of infection?

If it is decided to leave the CVL in it is essential that the patient and/or their carer is confident and competent in caring for this device. They should be aware of the following.
• How and when to change the exit site dressing. This should be done in a clean environment at least twice a week. If the dressing becomes wet or soiled it should be changed immediately. The dressing applied should be waterproof.
• How to flush the CVL if they are expected to do this. All transplant centers should have protocols and a training package for flushing CVLs at home.
• Keeping the lumens clean and dry, taking particular care when in the bath (showering is preferable). The patient should be told not to go swimming or use a hot tub or jacuzzi with the CVL *in situ*.
• Keeping the CVL secure to avoid it becoming dislodged if accidentally pulled.
• Knowing what to do if the CVL is damaged/punctured. The patient should carry clamps with them at all times in case this occurs.
• Action to be taken if the HSCT patient is pyrexial.

Diet and food preparation

Healthy eating should be encouraged following discharge, remembering that patients will be keen to eat their favorite foods and snacks that may not have been available to them in hospital. It may be necessary to encourage increased calorie intake in some patients and expert advice from dieticians may be required.

Following discharge from the HSCT unit patients remain at risk from complications associated with gastrointestinal infections, either from organisms that they are currently colonized with or from food-borne sources. In order to reduce the likelihood of gastrointestinal illness due to food-borne infection the following precautions should be taken until the patient has a stable neutrophil count of 1.5×10^9/L or above.

Food hygiene in the kitchen

Good standard hygienic practices should be performed in the home. These include:
• washing hands prior to and after handling food, especially raw meat, poultry and fish;
• thoroughly washing all utensils and surfaces with hot soapy water after contact with raw meat, poultry and fish, and following each episode of food preparation;
• ensuring all foods are stored correctly according to their packaging and are consumed within their "best by" date;
• if food is to be frozen it should be cooled quickly, then immediately placed in the freezer in order to reduce the opportunity for bacteria to grow;
• keeping cooked and uncooked meats separately in a refrigerator (uncooked below cooked), as uncooked meat can contaminate other foods that are eaten without further cooking.

Food preparation and cooking

Care needs to be taken with food preparation and cooking. The following advice should be given to patients and their carers.
• Ensure all meat, poultry, eggs and fish are cooked thoroughly, e.g. meat and poultry are no longer pink in the middle and eggs do not have "runny" yolks.
• Foods containing uncooked eggs should not be consumed, e.g. homemade mayonnaise, hollandaise sauce, tiramisu.
• Ensure milk and dairy products are made from pasteurized milk only.

- Avoid soft cheeses and live (bio) yoghurts.
- Ensure fresh vegetables are peeled and cooked thoroughly.
- Fresh fruit should be washed and peeled. Avoid fruit that is bruised or mouldy.
- Avoid unpackaged food from a delicatessen counter or takeaway foods from other outlets, especially street vendors, as food hygiene cannot be guaranteed.
- Pepper and other spices should be added at the beginning of the cooking process rather than at the end. *Aspergillus* spores may contaminate pepper and other spices.
- Any food that smells or looks "off" should not be consumed.

Drinking water

If the patient is lymphopenic (<200 lymphocytes/µL) fresh tap water should be avoided due to potential contamination with *Cryptosporidium* and *Legionella*. To make tap water safe it should be boiled for 1 minute then, when cool, kept refrigerated in a covered container. Ice should be avoided if made from tap water. Bottled water may be of poorer quality than mains water. Water that comes from wells or a bore hole in an area that has a small population should not be drunk as microbiological quality cannot be guaranteed.

Bottle feeds

All bottles and feeding equipment should be cleaned and disinfected prior to use, using a steam or microwave sterilizer and stored dry. The feed should be made up following the manufacturer's instructions unless advised otherwise by the dietician. Feed can be prepared up to 12 hours in advance. We recommend that the milk is cooled rapidly, then refrigerated. Teats should be replaced monthly or sooner if they become damaged.

Dummies and teething rings

These should be disinfected (e.g. using 1% hypochlorite solution) prior to giving to the child. If a dummy or teething ring becomes contaminated a clean one should be given. Dummies and teething rings should be replaced monthly or sooner if they become damaged.

Social contacts and leaving the home

Visitors

Following discharge from the HSCT unit the patient remains immunocompromised and so the number of visitors should be restricted. All visitors to the patient's home should be encouraged to remove their outdoor shoes, then wash their hands using liquid soap. Visitors who may be suffering from a communicable infection, e.g. respiratory illness, diarrhea or cold sores (*Herpes simplex*) should not visit. Although healthy adult visitors to the patient should not pose a problem, it is advisable that children, especially infants, should not visit in the early stages following discharge because they are more likely to be excreting or carrying viruses, or incubating infectious diseases such as chicken pox (*Varicella zoster*). There are some obvious exceptions to this rule. Patients who have young siblings or children of their own are encouraged to mix with their own young family; however, sensible precautions should be taken if a family member is unwell, e.g. the patient should not kiss any individual with a respiratory illness or herpetic lesion. They should, where possible, avoid changing the nappy of an infant with diarrhea or an infant who has recently received live polio vaccine, as the virus will be excreted in the feces for several weeks.

Socializing

It is important that the patient does not become a prisoner in their own home; however, care must be taken when going out. Crowded places, such as shopping centers, football matches, nightclubs, swimming pools, and places with lots of young children such as soft play facilities, should be avoided. It is advisable to go to the park, go for walks or go to the local shops during off-peak times. This should be encouraged, as after a long time in a protective environment the patient will need to be re-established in their home surroundings. Their energy levels will be low due to illness and inactivity, therefore it is vital that they regain their strength and energy during their period of semi-isolation at home.

Children of school age are usually not encouraged to return to school for 3–6 months following HSCT, depending on immune reconstitution. However, during this time the child's education must not be forgotten. The transplant center, usually through the hospital teaching service, should ask the child's local education authority to arrange home tuition. Most children are keen for home tuition as they don't want to fall behind their peer group; having been away from school for a long time, they want to "fit in" without further differences between themselves and their peer group. The home tutor also provides some interest and distraction during a time when their activities are restricted.

As children are unable to have face-to-face contact with their friends it is especially important that they are encouraged to maintain friendships. Children can write and draw pictures to their friends, have telephone conversations and contact via e-mail, texting, photographs and videos. Prior to transplant the HSCT co-ordinator may encourage the child's parents to tell the class teacher about the transplant process and ask the teacher to allow the class to send pictures, etc., so that the child receiving the transplant continues to feel involved with their peer group and is not forgotten by their classmates.

The restriction with regard to socializing and other contacts should be in place until the patient has a CD3 count of 200/μL; however, the transplant team may allow small deviations (such as a child having 1 or 2 friends over to play) before this target is reached. Table 14.1 indicates the contacts to be avoided.

Contact with animals

Pets

Animals are a part of normal everyday life for many individuals; however, patients are at increased risk of infection acquired from their pets. It seems sensible to advise against getting any new pets during the initial recovery phase following HSCT; however, it is probably reasonable to have contact with pets already owned providing sensible precautions are taken (e.g. hand washing after contact and no contact with feces or cat litter). A pet's health is important for all pet owners; the health of pets in contact with an HSCT patient is even more important; pets should be up-to-date with immunizations, kept clean, and veterinary advice should be sought quickly if the pet is unwell in order to prevent transmission of potential infection to the immunocompromised individual.

Commercially produced pet foods are usually of high quality in order to minimize contamination. Any fresh products, meat or poultry fed to pets should be well cooked in order to reduce the risk of gastrointestinal illness. Pets should be fed regularly

Table 14.1 Contacts and activities to avoid until satisfactory immunity

Adults	If the adult is unwell
Children and babies	With the exception of siblings
Changing nappies	
School, nurseries, playgroups	Soft play areas for children
Crowded places	Bars, clubs, sports stadiums, shopping malls
Pets	
Animal litter	
Home improvements and other dusty environments	
Unboiled tap water	
Takeaway foods and food from street vendors	Any food or drink that may not have been hygienically prepared
Swimming and water sports	Crowded areas
Farms and zoos	
Travel to foreign countries	

to minimize the risk of them scavenging or hunting for food. Restrictions apply until the patient has a satisfactory immunity.

Pets that may pose particular health risks to HSCT patients
Cats

Individuals who are immunocompromised are at increased risk of contracting toxoplasmosis from cat feces (or from undercooked meat). Toxoplasmosis is a parasitic infection caused by *Toxoplasma gondii* and is found in the tissues of the majority of warm-blooded animals. However, the only hosts for its definitive life cycle are the cat family. In the immunocompetent individual exposed to *Toxoplasma* the illness is usually self-limiting, with duration of 2–5 weeks characterized by lymphadenopathy. Asymptomatic infection also frequently occurs. However, toxoplasmosis in the immunosuppressed individual, which may be due to reactivation of infection acquired previously or a primary infection, may result in severe central nervous system or pulmonary disease. To prevent primary infection in HSCT patients litter trays should be placed away from areas where food preparation and consumption occur and should be cleaned daily. Ideally the cleaning of litter trays should not be the responsibility of the HSCT patient. If this is unavoidable the individual should wear disposable gloves and wash their hands thoroughly immediately after cleaning the litter tray.

Dogs

Puppies in particular are likely to be infected with *Campylobacter*. The mouths of dogs will also harbor a number of organisms that may be pathogenic in humans, including *Pasteurella multocida* and *Capnocytophaga*; both these organisms can causing overwhelming infection in immunocompromised patients. Dogs should therefore not be encouraged to lick patients, especially if there are any breaks in the skin or wounds.

Birds

Bird droppings can be a source of yeasts such as *Candida* spp., *Cryptococcus neoformans* and other organisms such as *Mycobacterium avium* or *Histoplasma* (not endemic in UK). Bird cages should therefore be cleaned daily, preferably not by the HSCT patient. If this is unavoidable, the individual should wear disposable gloves and wash their hands thoroughly afterwards.

Fish

Mycobacterium marinum is found in fish tanks; therefore, immunocompromised individuals should avoid cleaning fish tanks. Where this is not possible disposable gloves should be worn and hands should be washed thoroughly immediately afterwards.

Animals that should be avoided by HSCT patients

These include:
- reptiles – snakes, lizards;
- ducklings and chicks;
- exotic pets – monkeys;
- rodents – mice, rats, guinea pigs.

Table 14.2 indicates the specific infective risk from these animals. In addition, many of these animals are likely to cause scratches or bite and the risk of infection is therefore increased. Handling these animals or their fomites should therefore be avoided. If contact does occur the individual must wash their hands thoroughly immediately

Table 14.2 Infection associated with animals

Animal	Risk
Cats	*Toxoplasma*
Dogs	*Campylobacter, Pasteurella, Capnocytophagia*
Birds	*Cryptococcus neoformans, Mycobacterium avium, Histoplasma*
Fish	*Mycobacterium marinum*
Reptiles	*Salmonella*
Ducklings and chicks	*Salmonella, Campylobacter*
Lambs	*Chlamydia*
Exotic pets	*Salmonella*, shigellosis
Rodents	*Leptospira interrogans, Pasteurella multocida, Staphylococcus, Streptobacillus moniliformis*

afterwards. Bites from any animal should receive immediate medical attention as antibiotic prophylaxis may be warranted.

Farm and zoo visits

These should be avoided in the early period following transplant and direct contact, e.g. with lambs, is particularly hazardous. Visits to enclosed aquaria may provide a good alternative.

Gardening

Gardening is enjoyed by many adults; however, the HSCT patient should take extra caution when gardening. There is a risk of contracting *Cryptosporidium* or toxoplasmosis from animal or human feces that may be found in the soil or fungal infection that may be associated with rotting vegetation. In the immunocompromised host this can disseminate and become life threatening. Therefore the HSCT patient should:
• wear protective gardening gloves to protect hands from feces, scratches, and splinters;
• remove gardening gloves after use and put in a safe place such as the garden shed – the individual should be reminded not to place the gloves on kitchen worktops or eat or drink with gloves on;
• wear long-sleeved and long-legged clothes in order to protect against scratches, splinters and bites;
• wash hands thoroughly after gardening.

Return to work, school or college

Most HSCT patients are able to return to their work or school environment 3–6 months following their transplant. The time scale is dependent upon their immune reconstitution, working environment and feeling of wellbeing.

Work

The level of immune reconstitution necessary for returning to work depends upon the type of job in which the patient is employed. Individuals who have sedentary employment will probably find it easier to return to work than those who have more physically demanding jobs. Those who work in dirty conditions, such as plumbers and builders, or those occupations associated with a high risk of exposure to infection, such as farm or abattoir workers, may be advised not to return to work until their immune reconstitution is more advanced than those working in clean environments, due to the risk of acquiring diseases. The patient should be encouraged to talk to their employer prior to returning to work in order for the employer to understand their needs and for them mutually to decide on the most appropriate way of returning to work (e.g. part time, flexitime) and what duties they will be able to undertake.

This is often a major turning point for the transplanted individual as it is often viewed as returning to normality, but may also result in the patient feeling less special. All individuals will feel differently in this situation; therefore their care needs to be appropriate for them.

School or college

For a child returning to school it may be appropriate for a specialist nurse to visit the school prior to the child's return in order to talk to the child's teacher and perhaps the pupils about the transplanted child's experience and what the class can expect from them. Contact with a college tutor may also be appropriate to allay any fears about the pupil's return. Teenagers and young adults may face special problems as they may be very self-conscious of their appearance and unwilling to discuss their illness with their peers.

Information for the teacher or tutor

For the younger child the teacher will need to know to what level the child can join in with their peer group. They will usually be told that the child should be encouraged to join in with all activities (with the exception of contact sports if the child has a low platelet count) but that it may take time to build up their confidence and energy levels. Often, the teacher and parents will decide to allow the child to return to school initially on a part-time basis, gradually building up the time spent at school. It is usually best to try not to make the child "special" within the group.

The class teacher or tutor should also be aware of any medications that the HSCT patient may require during school time and their usual policies should be followed regarding their administration.

The school or college should be aware of the risk that infectious diseases pose to the patient. Generally, coughs and colds should be well tolerated by the patient at this stage; however, if there is an outbreak of a more serious infection, e.g. chickenpox, influenza, this should be reported to the individual or child's carers as soon as possible as prophylactic treatment may be available – zoster immunoglobulin for chickenpox and antiviral agents, e.g. oseltamivir, for influenza A or B. The school may wish to inform the parents of the other children in the class of the situation so that they can contact the school on the first day of their child's absence. The parents will be aware that they need to contact the child's transplant center if this situation arises. Usually if the patient is receiving immunoglobulin and an antiviral medication (e.g. aciclovir) they are unlikely to contract chickenpox; however, if they are not receiving these medications they may need prophylactic treatment. This is often decided by the length of time following the transplant and the degree of immune reconstitution. If the individual is immunized and has made good specific antibody responses then the transplant center may decide not to recommend prophylactic treatment.

Information for the other pupils

This will be varied depending on the age group of the children involved. Children are naturally curious and can cope with complex information when required. It is usually advisable to inform the class if the child has any obviously different features, such as alopecia, so that the children can be prepared. They should also know why the HSCT patient has been absent for such a long period. However, this information should be brief so that the child returning to school does not become the focal point of interest to the class group, as this may be intimidating for the transplanted child.

Swimming and water sports

Swimming is a very popular pastime enjoyed by children and adults alike, and is recommended as an effective and enjoyable form of exercise and relaxation. Diarrheal illnesses can be transmitted by swimming/bathing in contaminated water, such as in swimming pools, lakes, rivers, and the sea. It has been reported that *Cryptosporidium* and *Giardia* have varying degrees of chlorine resistance; they have low infectious doses and high excretion concentrations, so swimming pools, etc., become contaminated quickly and swallowing a few mouthfuls of contaminated water is sufficient for disease transmission. In the immunocompetent host *Cryptosporidium* infection causes diarrhea, abdominal cramps, anorexia, pyrexia, nausea and vomiting; it is self-limiting, lasting for 4–7 days. Importantly, the individual could remain infectious for up to 8 days after the illness has resolved. In the immunocompromised host *Cryptosporidium* can be fatal as there is no absolute curative therapy available. Therefore HSCT patients are strongly advised against swimming until their immune system is fully reconstituted. For children, swimming is not usually recommended until they have demonstrated good specific antibody responses (as children are more likely to swallow the water).

Travel abroad/holidays

Travel abroad is not usually recommended for patients during the first 6 months following HSCT, both because they are immunocompromised and because if they become unwell abroad it may be difficult to return to the transplant center for assessment and treatment. Once the individual is able to return to school/work it is usually acceptable for them to travel to developed countries. They should adopt the same restrictions as they are required to do at home with regard to eating/drinking and swimming. Camping outdoors when normal facilities are not available is not recommended. A transplanted individual wishing to travel to a developing country should ideally wait until they can demonstrate good specific antibody responses. Even with good specific antibody

responses the individual, like any other traveller, should always avoid the following in developing countries in order to minimize the risk of acquiring water-borne or food-borne infections:
• raw fruit and vegetables (including fresh fruit juices);
• tap water, including ice made from tap water;
• unpasteurized dairy products;
• food and drinks from street vendors;
• raw or undercooked eggs.

Travel to developing countries should be discussed with the transplant center well in advance of the proposed trip. The HSCT patient may require additional prophylactic medications or some vaccinations, depending on where they are proposing to travel. This will be decided by the transplant center using advice from national guidelines. This advice is updated regularly, taking into consideration diseases prevalent in specific areas at the time of travel. Generally, inactivated vaccinations pose no significant threat to transplanted individuals but live vaccinations, such as BCG, should be avoided unless the individual is travelling to a region where the disease being vaccinated against is prevalent. Importantly, vaccination of family members is recommended in order to reduce the exposure of preventable diseases to the transplanted individual.

Patients should also be advised:
• to keep out of the sun, as the skin will be very sensitive due to chemotherapy and total body irradiation;
• if in the sun to wear total sun block, long sleeves and a hat – sun block for the lip area is particularly useful for patients prone to oral *Herpes simplex*;
• patients who had antibodies to positive *Herpes zoster* pre-transplant (i.e. evidence of previous infection) may develop shingles;
• if body temperature is above 37.5°C, patients should seek advice.

Hobbies and sports

Most hobbies and sports are safe to pursue once restrictions are lifted with regard to mixing. Water sports, for reasons discussed earlier, should be avoided until the patient has good specific antibody responses. Contact sports such as rugby, or sports that carry increased risk of injury such as abseiling, should be avoided if the patient has a low platelet count.

Religion

Patients who previously frequented places of worship may be keen to re-establish their routine; crowded places should be avoided but there may be an opportunity to attend their places of worship during quieter periods or for the cleric to visit the patient for prayer. A common sense approach should be adopted to avoid unnecessary exposure to infection in the early days following discharge.
• It is advisable for the patient not to drink from the communal communion cup as the cup is not cleaned between individuals.
• Careful consideration is required when using holy water as it is a potential source of contamination. The individual should not be immersed in this water.
• Circumcision should not be performed for religious reasons until the individual has a fully functional immune system and then should only be performed in an operating theatre environment within a hospital setting. The transplant center may recommend prophylactic antibiotics.

Sex

The HSCT patient can rekindle sexual relationships on their return home following transplantation. However, they should be advised to avoid sexual practices that could result in oral exposure to feces. The patient needs to be cautious about sexually transmitted diseases (STDs) and therefore they should be encouraged to have a monogamous partner and to use a condom to prevent STDs. Low sexual desire is not uncommon following HSCT, which can be attributed to depression, altered hormone levels, medications, or concerns about body image. Difficulty with arousal may occur in both males and females; this is often psychological in origin. Females may initially find that their vaginal mucosa is dry; therefore a lubricating product should be recommended.

Substance abuse

After HSCT there are particular reasons for extra caution regarding substance abuse.

Alcohol

Alcohol should be avoided for approximately 3 months following transplant, as the patient may have altered liver function due to the conditioning regimen. Following this period of time it should be discussed at each outpatient visit. Some medications may alter the individual's tolerance to alcohol and this should be discussed with the transplant team. Beers containing live yeasts (e.g. homebrew and "white" beers) should be avoided until satisfactory immunity has been demonstrated.

Smoking and tobacco

The HSCT patient may have had repeated chest infections resulting in chronic lung damage, which may only be evident on lung function or chest CT scans. Chemotherapy and radiotherapy may also cause pulmonary changes; cigarette smoking may exacerbate this damage. Where possible, the patient should avoid smoke-filled rooms.

Cannabis

Cannabis may contain high counts of *Aspergillus*, which can convey a risk of life-threatening infection to the immunocompromised individual; the HSCT patient should avoid this drug.

Users of intravenous substances

As with the normal population, advice needs to be given regarding single use and sharing of needles. If the patient is known to be an intravenous (IV) drug user it is very important for the transplant team to acknowledge this. As with all IV drug users advice

and support should be given regarding the health risks associated with this type of abuse and how to stop. However, time should be taken to explain to the patient the particular risks to them and the importance of good hygiene practices.

Conclusion

Returning to a "normal" lifestyle may be difficult for the HSCT patient, especially if they have suffered years of ill health and have been hospitalized for a significant period of time. Restriction of activity and diet can be reduced in line with immune reconstitution that may vary from individual to individual. If the patient does not develop serious complications, such as disease relapse or GVHD, then it can be expected that immune function will be completely restored after 2 years post-transplant. The transplant coordinator will be able to advise patients on reducing restrictions following transplant so that they can live life to the full.

Further reading

Ayliffe, G.A.J., Fraise, A.P., Geddes, A.M., Mitchell, K. (eds) (2000) *Control of Hospital Infection*. London: Arnold.

Bannister, B.A., Begg, N.T., Gillespie, S.H. (2000) Infections in immunocompromised patients. In: *Infectious Disease*, 2nd edn. Oxford: Blackwell Science, pp. 404–415.

Castor, M.L., Beach, M.J. (2004) Reducing illness transmission from disinfected recreational water venues: swimming, diarrhea and the emergence of new public health concern. *Pediatr Infect Dis J* **23**: 866–870.

Centers for Disease Control and Prevention. (2000) Guidelines for preventing opportunistic infections among hematopoietic stem cell transplant patients. *MMWR* **49** (RR10): 1–120.

Mooney, B.R., Reeves, S.A., Larson, E. (1993) Infection control in bone marrow transplantation. *Am J Infect Control*, **21**: 131–138.

Schlossberg, D. (ed.) (2004) *Infections of Leisure*, 3rd edn. Washington DC: ASM Press.

Chapter 15
Social and psychological aspects of care

M. Allan and D. Holder

Introduction

This chapter describes the social, practical, emotional and psychological issues that affect patients, their families and carers. There are limited studies directly related to the social aspects of hematopoietic stem cell transplantation (HSCT) and the policy frameworks and procedures referred to relate to the UK.

Social workers are most likely to be the professionals dealing with social aspects of HSCT. The social workers' professional skills, values, and practice will be influenced by the values, goals and organizational structures of the settings in which they work. Practice will also be influenced by local and national economies and policy frameworks.

Working together – social worker and the clinical team

The modern social worker works as part of a multidisciplinary team, in partnership with the medical team and in coordination with the nursing liaison staff, to provide the necessary support to the HSCT patient and their families. The acknowledgement that social issues can have an impact on the patient's ability to deal with their treatment successfully has been recognized in England since the 1890s when the first trained social workers, known as almoners, were appointed to hospitals. Figure 15.1 shows Lady Almoner receiving an award (MBE) for her services and the modern-day multidisciplinary team at work.

The social worker is hospital based within the vicinity of the transplant ward and has easy accessibility to the families, medical and nursing staff involved in the care of the HSCT patient. Therefore, the response to urgent and serious issues can be addressed with minimum delay. Communication is very important, so fixed regular meetings should be set in place to exchange information and keep all members of the team informed about the patient's progress.

This chapter has been written by different contributors with different patient groups and therefore, for clarity, has been divided into three sections looking at aspects of social and psychological care covering the different age groups:
- Section I – adults;
- Section II – children;
- Section III – teenagers.

Section I: working with adults as patients

Putting the patient at the center of the care process, considering all aspects of their life and that of their carers and families has been central to the recent policy frameworks for cancer care. The Calman Hine report (A Policy Framework for Commissioning Cancer Services, 1995), The Cancer Plan (2000) and, more recently, the National Institute for Clinical Excellence (NICE) publication, Improving Supportive and Palliative Care for Adults with Cancer (2004), all include references to the social and emotional needs of patients and their carers. Social workers have responsibilities under the Community Care Act (1990). This act requires social services departments to assess for, and provide services to adults with a wide variety of social needs, including those with cancer. All of this pro-

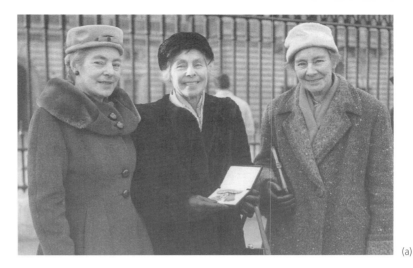

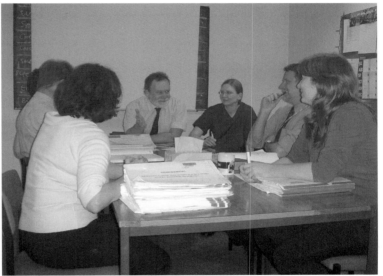

Fig. 15.1 (a) Grace Nicholson, Lady Almoner from Royal Victoria Infirmary, Newcastle upon Tyne, receiving an MBE at Buckingham Palace (1955). (b) The modern-day multidisciplinary team in action.

vides social workers with a legal and policy framework for working with patients, their families and carers.

Although the focus of this chapter is HSCT, it is necessary, in looking at the social aspects for patients, to start at the point of diagnosis, when most patients and their carers will encounter some social consequences of their illness. In identifying these consequences it is then possible to go on to describe the challenges the patients face during and following recovery from transplant.

Following the confirmation of a serious illness such as leukemia there is an initial shock. This is followed by a feeling of being ill-equipped to deal with what lies ahead, facing the possibility of death, and then somehow finding an inner strength or a strategy to get through the difficulties and to gain a heightened appreciation of life. Achieving this degree of acceptance and apparent success does not come easily. Many patients describe their initial reaction to diagnosis as a death sentence. Once they realize that death is not imminent, they worry about how they are going to live. Concerns about employment and finance are usually high on the list. They worry also about the effects on their partners, families, and carers. Those with children are concerned about them and how to explain what is happening. They are devastated by the thought that they may not see them grow up. Others may have caring responsibilities to older or other dependent relatives. Some patients have other disabilities or health problems. They may have existing housing problems or serious financial difficulties. Helping patients to identify and tackle these issues will hopefully provide them with a basic survival kit to get through their treatment and recover from their transplant.

Identifying social aspects of care

The NICE document, Improving Cancer and Palliative Care for Adults with Cancer (2004), includes a chapter on social support services, which has been written in consultation with the Social Care Institute for Excellence (SCIE).

Drawing on a study conducted for Cancer Relief Macmillan Fund, it points out that "The social impact of cancer is considerable." The document sets out the range of needs for social care and support that people affected by cancer can experience at different stages of the patient pathway (Table 15.1). It also acknowledges that "The social implications of cancer may extend beyond the patient's immediate family and carers to relatives, friends, employers and work colleagues," and identifies the areas that social care encompasses (Table 15.2).

Table 15.1 Patient's social needs

Emotional support, engaging in social activities, companionship or befriending; making contact with health and social care professionals
Help with personal care, e.g. bathing and dressing
Advice on work and employment issues and assistance to secure financial support, e.g. help in making a benefit claim
Help inside and outside the home, e.g. cleaning and shopping
Practical aids, including wheelchairs and other equipment
Help to care for children and other dependents

Table 15.2 Available help

Practical help
Personal care for patients
Preservation or enhancement of social networks
Emotional support
Income maintenance
Provision of information on local and national resources
Access to safe living environments which comply (at least) with minimum standards
Provision of respite care

Supporting the patient – what can help?

Having accepted the importance of the social implications and consequences of cancer diagnosis and treatment, and having identified what these needs might be, it is now possible to relate these directly to patients with a malignancy receiving chemotherapy treatment and a HSCT.

In order for any social issues to be identified and addressed, a relationship between the patient and the social worker must be established that allows honest and straightforward communication to take place. Social work has, at times, been on the receiving end of negative publicity in the press and media. Under-resourcing and shortages of staff have not always helped to promote a positive image of the social worker. This may lead to difficulties in assessment of need because some patients and their carers may be reluctant to ask for help or reject it if it is offered. Patients may feel it is an intrusion of their privacy, an attack on their independence or an inference that they are not coping. It is important, therefore, to reassure patients and their carers that professional interventions are intended to be helpful and not intrusive, threatening, or judgmental. Social workers who are well integrated into the multidisciplinary team are likely to have less of a problem in being accepted. They can be introduced as just another member of the team in a non-threatening way. It is also useful if patients can be helped to accept that it is "normal" to be experiencing difficulties and to feel frightened or vulnerable at such a time in their lives, and that social workers are there to help them deal with very difficult circumstances.

Assuming the patient and their carers accept the offer of an assessment of their social needs, it is then possible to support the patient through their treatment, transplant and recovery. Tables 15.1 and 15.2 identify a range of social care needs and issues for patients and their carers. Looking at these in greater depth will provide some information on what can be done to meet these needs.

Emotional support

Once a patient has received a diagnosis of a hematological malignancy, they will know that they have many months of aggressive chemotherapy ahead of them. This may be followed by a stem cell transplant and then many more months of recovery. Throughout this period, emotional support may come from a variety of sources. It may come from the health and social care professionals or from friends and family. Some patients seek out support from complementary therapists or voluntary organizations set up to offer services to cancer patients. They can only do this, however, if they are aware of the existence of such services. It is the responsibility of health and social care professionals to ensure that information is available for patients and their carers.

Others may feel they are supported and encouraged by fellow patients. Relationships with other patients can have negative as well as positive implications. Things work well when both patients are going through similar problems and can relate to each other's needs. Black humour is often a feature of these positive relationships. Patient relationships, however, can be terribly upsetting if things go wrong for one of the patients, leaving the others feeling threatened, vulnerable, and sometimes guilty. It is at these times that professionals need to be aware of the patient's concerns, to be able to offer a listening ear, and to understand the distress that is being experienced. Emotional support, in whatever guise, is extremely important throughout the patient's treatment and recovery. Recognition of the needs of carers, partners, families, and friends is already well documented. The strain of caring for a loved one with a life-threatening condition can be immense and the emotional needs of the carer may be as great as or greater than that of the patient. There may be sexual problems or concerns about infertility. It is important that carers and partners have their concerns acknowledged and are offered support to deal with them.

Help with personal care

Patients undergoing months of chemotherapy and a HSCT will at times have their ability to self care compromised by fatigue and the side effects of treatment. Those without a carer within their family or close circle of friends may need help from community social or nursing services. Assessing for and accessing such services can be done by a social worker. As most of the patients will be in the younger age groups, i.e. under 50 years, this support from social services is provided by the younger persons' disability teams. Where the social worker covers a regional unit, liaison with other local authorities outside of the immediate catchment area is necessary to ensure that the patient can have a safe discharge. Provision of services will, of course, always be subject to local resources and availability. However, planning ahead and giving information about the patient's illness to the local authority providing the service in good time should ensure that an appropriate assessment of need is made, and that these needs are met whenever possible.

Work, employment, education and finance

Concerns about work, future employment, and finances are usually high on the agenda for adult patients and their families. Most patients will have been unable to work during the months of chemotherapy leading up to their transplant. Even those lucky enough to have full pay for six months followed by a further six months of half pay will be unlikely to have completed their treatment before payment from their employer ceases. Some, especially those in physically demanding jobs or without secure contracts of employment, may lose their jobs completely. Work and financial worries can be particularly problematic for the self employed, especially those in very small or one-man businesses.

For many patients the diagnosis of a hematological malignancy will lead to a reduction of income at some stage during treatment and recovery. It is very important, therefore, that patients have access to appropriate advice. The benefits system is complex and having the services of a benefits adviser is invaluable in helping patients understand and claim their entitlements. Most local authorities provide benefits advice, as do the Citizens Advice Bureau. The Macmillan Fund also has a benefits advice line. Completing unfamiliar benefit forms can be daunting and confusing for some patients who may be dealing with a number of other worries or concerns. Offering help with the completion of forms is often greeted with gratitude and relief.

Having treatment that extends over many months or even years can be an expensive business. All patients, but especially those on low incomes or welfare benefits, feel this financial strain. Table 15.3 indicates additional cost pressures.

Patients on certain benefits are entitled to help with outpatient treatment visits and in some circumstances with help for close relatives to visit them in hospital. They may also be entitled to other help from the Social Fund. Appropriate benefits advice should ensure that patients and their families are able to obtain their entitlements from the benefits system. For those not on benefits, but whose income falls below a certain level, the Macmillan Fund can help with grants to cover a wide range of needs. Applications to this fund can be made by Macmillan nurses or social workers.

Another major expense for patients is prescription costs. It is helpful, therefore, for patients to be given information about who is exempt from charges and how to get help or obtain a prepayment certificate if they are not exempt. Some pa-

tients are still at school or attending institutions of higher education when they are diagnosed. Their treatment will mean an interruption of their studies and this can be a source of worry to the individual. However, once the school, college, or university is aware of the situation they are usually extremely supportive and accommodating to the student, and offer as much practical and emotional support as possible to enable them to take time out or to continue with their studies at a less demanding rate.

Help inside and outside the home

Throughout chemotherapy treatment and recovery from transplant, patients will experience extreme fatigue and immunosuppression. Those who do not have a partner or carers may need a carer to be provided by the local authority to do their shopping and keep their home clean. Fresh food, the safe storage of it, and a clean environment are important in minimizing the risk of infection. Some local authorities may not provide a domestic service, or perhaps only a limited service. In this instance the patient may have to employ private help. Where this causes financial hardship the social worker needs to explore sources of financial support.

Practical aids and equipment

Some patients are badly affected by their treatment, or have other health problems or disabilities. This means that they may need assessment for aids and/or adaptations to their home to maximize their independence. The most expedient way to obtain an assessment is for the patient to be assessed by the occupational therapist or physiotherapist while they are an inpatient. In certain circumstances it may be necessary for a home assessment visit to be done prior to discharge. This is normally arranged by the occupational therapist but may also involve social workers, other members of the multidisciplinary team, and community-based workers. This can enable a whole package of care to be put together and important links to be made between hospital- and community-based services prior to discharge.

Table 15.3 Additional cost pressures for patients with prolonged illness

Frequent outpatient visits, parking fees
Family visiting hospital during inpatient care
Prescription costs
Increased child care costs
Need for clothing to keep pace with weight changes
Replacing bedding affected by night sweats

Where the patient has already been discharged, the local social services department becomes responsible for assessing and providing aids and equipment. Providing as much information as possible to that local authority will be helpful in assessing and meeting the patient's needs.

Care for children and other dependents

For patients who have caring responsibilities for children, older relatives or relatives with physical or learning disabilities, there is an added dimension to their areas of concern. It is imperative that these concerns are alleviated as soon as possible so that the patient does not feel pressurized into returning to these responsibilities before they are physically and emotionally fit enough.

Where children are involved, a partner, extended family, and friends are often able to rally round and arrange care for the children, thus preventing, as far as possible, major disruption to their daily routine. This maintenance of routine can be a great reassurance to children who are confused by the sudden departure of one of their parents or carers into hospital. It is especially helpful if care can be given by adults known to and close to the child or children. If patients lack close family or friends able to care for their children, the social worker can assist with more formal arrangements. Wherever possible this should allow the child or children involved to remain in their own community or school and to maintain links with friends. Children having to be looked after by the local authority in these circumstances are very rare.

Once patients have acceptable child care arrangements in place, they will be concerned about what they should tell their child or children about their illness. Some parents may disagree on whether the children should be told anything. Some may feel that by not saying anything they are protecting the child. Others want to talk to their children but do not know how to begin or what to say. Talking through these concerns with a social worker or other healthcare professional can help to sort out these concerns. Booklets, specially written for children, may help in this situation. Our local unit has a booklet for parents to use to explain a blood disorder to children. The booklet, called "What's

the matter with Mum?", is based on the life of a family whose mother was a patient on our unit and the family wanted their experience to be used to help other families tackle this often difficult area. Another useful booklet, "Talking to children when an adult has cancer" (published by Macmillan), gives invaluable advice to healthcare workers and parents or carers. It explains why it is helpful to talk to children about cancer affecting a significant adult in their life. It suggests when, how, and what children should be told, and describes the kinds of reactions children are likely to display and the questions they are likely to ask. It gives reassuring advice on how to deal with emotional or behavioral changes in the child, and how to deal with the child's own social network in school and with friends.

Patients who care for older relatives or relatives with physical or learning disabilities can be equally concerned about what will happen to those for whom they have responsibility during their illness. Social workers can assist in accessing alternative care, and as far as is practicable, keeping the patient in touch with their relatives. These patients also need to explain to their relatives what has happened. They are, however, often reluctant to do so because the physical health of the person they are caring for is so fragile or they may also have concerns about their mental health or their ability to understand what is happening. Patients with these additional worries will need time and support to talk through concerns. This will hopefully bring some peace of mind and acceptance of their situation and allow them to proceed with their treatment.

Support for carers

The importance of family members and carers in supporting the transplant patient has recently been acknowledged by the National Institute of Clinical Excellence (2004). The physical toll of additional responsibility and the emotional stress experienced by carers needs to be recognized and appropriate support given. A carer's involvement in the transplant journey, with the patient, can help them feel part of the whole process and have equal access to all members of the multidisciplinary team.

Enabling carers to identify their own needs early on in the process may head off problems at a later stage. In order to meet such needs, staff should be aware of local resources. There may, for instance, be organizations that provide complementary therapies for cancer patients and their families and carers. There may be support groups or counseling services within or outside the hospital unit.

It may be that carers have practical needs. Obtaining financial support to fund a convalescent break with the patient or to enable a carer travelling from a long distance to spend valuable time with the patient may be the priority. It is also possible that the local social services department may provide relevant practical support.

Assessing social issues and quality of life pre-transplant

Patients who have had their initial chemotherapy in units associated with their transplant center will already have had the opportunity to discuss the social consequences of their diagnosis and their concerns about transplant during their admissions for treatment and frequent outpatient visits. For those who are referred from other hospitals, the assessment of social issues can be done by means of a simple letter given to the patient by a transplant nurse specialist. This can be done at one of the early meetings during the transplant work up by asking the patient to complete a single-sheet tickbox questionnaire. This allows the patient to express concerns about particular social issues and request help with them. In some units personal interviews with all patients are possible and this is obviously preferable. It is helpful for the patient to use a personally held record which allows easy access to information.

By the time they are admitted for transplant the patient and their families and carers should have already dealt with a number of social consequences of their diagnosis. The transplant, however, confronts them with another life-threatening situation, further treatment, and a prolonged period of recovery. There is limited literature dealing exclusively with social issues for patients with hematological malignancies. There is, however, more extensive literature on quality of life (QoL) issues for HSCT survivors and it is this literature that is useful in understanding what is important for patients and how to support them through recovery. QoL is associated with a positive attitude to life, which is dependent on interpersonal relationships and autonomy by individuals with leukemia (Bertero and Ek, 1993). Related to this is the need for security, support, respect, information and conversation. A study by Ferrell *et al.* (1992) discusses the particular significance of QoL for HSCT survivors who are faced with the demands of acute transplant symptoms as well as chronic illness demands following transplant. The study developed a model illustrating the impact of HSCT on QoL. The model identifies four domains (Table 15.4).

Within the domain of social wellbeing, patients identified the following factors as being significant:

- appearance;
- financial burden;
- roles and relationships;
- affection/social relationships;
- care giver burden;
- leisure activities;
- return to work.

Most patients will identify to a greater or lesser extent with the significance of these issues in relation to their social readjustment following transplant. For many, they represent a loss of control over important areas of their lives. Such loss of control is often frightening, and challenges even the most able in coping with the impact and recovery from transplant. For some patients it may be some time after transplant before the full impact is felt. This can be illustrated by Case Study 1.

Table 15.4 Factors affecting quality of life for HSCT patients

Physical wellbeing and symptoms
Psychological wellbeing
Social wellbeing
Spiritual wellbeing

Case Study 1

Two years after a sibling donor allogeneic HSCT for acute my-eloid leukemia, a 45-year-old man contacted the social worker. Throughout treatment and transplant he had always been cheer-ful, positive and, apart from some assistance with benefit ap-plications, had not acknowledged any other social or emotional difficulties. Following transplant he developed graft-vs.-host dis-ease (GVHD) and lost 25.4 kg (56 lb) in weight. This prolonged his recovery period. His employer was taken over by another company and he lost his job. He was now physically well enough to return to work but had lost all his confidence.

His weight loss had made him very conscious of his changed appearance. He was now living completely on benefits, some-thing he had never done before. Managing on much-reduced income had become a huge practical problem as well as lowering his self-esteem.

His marriage had broken down prior to his diagnosis and he had no children. He lacked a special relationship in his life and now felt he would never find one. He also felt he had exhausted the goodwill of his few close friends. He had stopped going out or involving himself in activities he had previously enjoyed. He had applied for several jobs but had been unsuccessful.

In subsequent discussions with the social worker, he revealed that he had always been a very private man. Despite many other previous problems, e.g. an unhappy childhood, divorce, and other health problems, he had always coped. The impact of the trans-plant, however, had made it impossible for him to employ his pre-vious coping strategies. The use of a cognitive-therapy approach enabled this patient to gain a better understanding of himself.

Practical advice enabled him to seek out appropriate support from the employment services and with this, together with input from the post-transplant clinical team, he began to establish con-trol over the social aspects of his life, regain some self-esteem and move on.

He was also able to acknowledge and allow his close friends (who were his carers) to express their concerns and access sup-port.

Section II: working with children and families

Working with children as patients raises a number of different issues that need to be addressed prior to and following transplant. A Framework for the Assessment of Children in Need and their Families was originally produced in 2000, with a fourth impression in 2005. The framework has been de-vised to provide a systematic way of analyzing, understanding and recording what is happening to children within their families and community, with the aim of gaining a clear professional judgment. It acts as a key element of the Department of Health's work to support local authorities in implementing Quality Protects, the Government's program for transforming the management and delivery of chil-dren's social services.

One of the aims of the framework is to encour-age the working together of health services, Social Services, and agencies in assessing children in need and their families. This is to be achieved by provid-ing a common language in which to understand the needs of children, resulting in shared values about what is in children's best interests. This framework is in conjunction with the Working Together to Safeguard Children document produced in 1999 and the Children Acts of 1989 and 2004.

The framework clearly sets out to provide for the more complex needs of some children. The document highlights the responsibility of Social Services and hence the social worker has the lead responsibility for assessing the needs of children. It is within this context that the social aspects of HSCT within a pediatric setting will be explored.

Communicating with children and their families

When working with children and their families there are several aspects of communication that need to be considered, as follows.
• Is the child old enough to understand the use of language?
• Does the child understand the native language?
• Is the child mature enough to understand the significance of what is being said?

The importance of communicating with a child itself should not be overlooked. Each child needs to be assessed individually regarding their ability to understand their situation and to understand the use of language.

In addition, in some units a number of children admitted may be of a different nationality and language problems may occur, not only with the child but also with their family. It is usually recom-mended that family members do not act as inter-preters for the parents or carers, as only selected information may be passed on. The use of a professional interpreter ensures that the parents gain a full understanding of the child's treatment program throughout the transplant episode. In providing support for these families it is also very important to be sympathetic towards their cultural needs.

Preparation for admission

For some children a transplant can be planned in advance. Therefore, the parents will have some time at home with their child to organize and plan for their child's future admission. Preparation for admission may be carried out in the home or hospital setting. A visit to the family home, arranged in coordination with the social worker and hospital liaison sister, allows a joint discussion on the impending admission of the child and the implications for the family arising from this. The liaison sister can discuss the medical aspects with the parents, and the social worker can discuss any social problems the parents may envisage as a result of the child coming into hospital.

The visit to the home provides a more comfortable setting, and parents feel more in control and less inhibited than in a hospital environment. The relaxed atmosphere of their home is also more conducive and it has been noted that parents are more able to discuss topics around the transplant, without feeling inhibited as they may do in a clinical setting. They are also more able to absorb and retain information, which might otherwise have been forgotten or misunderstood had the meeting taken place in a hospital room.

The typical social questions that arise are usually around siblings, relatives, work, accommodation, and money. For example, they may have other children to take into consideration, and discussions with the social worker can help to identify and develop a clearer understanding with regard to the care needs. The social worker can be supportive by helping the family to organize a routine at home that will create as little upheaval as possible for the family when the child is admitted into hospital. Parents will very often express their uncertainties around the medical aspects of the transplant, and the liaison sister will respond to these questions

The information gathered from a pre-transplant meeting can also provide many positive aspects

that will aid the social worker in making preparations with the medical and nursing teams in planning for the child's future admission. A named nurse and nursery nurse will be appointed to work with the family. They will be briefed by the social worker and liaison nurse to enable them to gain an understanding of the family. The nursery nurse is then able to buy special appropriate toys for the child and prepare the room for the child's admission. Extra personal touches will be added to the room to try to make the room special for the child. The visit also allows the social worker to make preparations in advance of the parents arriving on the ward by:

- giving an insight into the positive and negative feelings the parents and the child may have towards the transplant;
- enabling the sharing of information with the medical and nursing team to give them an understanding of the family and their needs;
- presenting an analytical and philosophical approach to the family situation;
- planning and organizing admissions, which allows for each part of the pre-transplant procedure to be timed – this can be effective in the planning of bed space and help maintain the efficient running of the unit.

A minority of parents from planned admissions can become anxious and stressed during the build-up to their child coming into hospital and telephone regularly for reassurance. However, generally parents of planned admissions appear to be more positive and remain so throughout the HSCT procedure. During the child's admission into hospital, they form a consistent routine with the child, which can lead to a more positive outcome. It has been observed that parents who remain optimistic throughout the transplant tend to be more understanding of their child's needs. Therefore, the transplant can be a positive experience for the child and, in view of this, the time spent in hospital can be shorter than anticipated.

Emergency admissions

Unfortunately, planned admissions cannot always be possible and a number of babies or children with congenital disorders, such as immune deficiencies, are referred urgently by other hospitals and admitted onto the transplant unit as an emergency. In this situation the parents can present quite differently from the parents of children from a planned admission. They arrive on the unit totally unprepared mentally or physically, with no prior understanding of a transplant or what this entails. Parents will have been informed by the consultant that their baby or child has a life-threatening illness. They can find it difficult to grasp and understand the concept of the illness, especially as the child may look healthy, although they may have had previous hospital admissions with infections. The thought of a transplant is very frightening for them. They are in shock and disbelief, and may show fear, anxiety, and depression. Parents may develop symptoms of post-traumatic stress disorder (PTSD), which invariably stays with them throughout the transplant.

Psychological distress

Physical evidence suggests a large number of parents experience some kind of psychological distress during their child's transplant, which can have adverse effects on their understanding and reasoning process. A study by Manne *et al.* (2004) of 111 mothers of children who survived HSCT examined the prevalence and predictors of anxiety, depression, and PTSD. The results showed that approximately 20% of mothers had clinically significant distress reactions. When sub-threshold post-traumatic stress disorder was included, nearly one-third of mothers met the criterion for persistent distress. The report also claimed that watching one's child undergo transplantation can potentially lead to the development of long-term psychological distress responses. This study heightens awareness for social workers to possible post-traumatic stress disorder and psychological distress among parents of children undergoing HSCT.

Symptoms of PTSD include:
- intrusive worries of re-experiencing aspects of the traumatic event;
- avoidance of reminders of the traumatic event;
- numbing of emotions;
- hypervigilance.

Discussions with parents in this situation can be very daunting for the social worker, as the parents are so stressed and anxious that quite often they do not absorb information given to them, and discussions may need to be repeated several times before they are fully able to understand. Patience and understanding on the part of the medical and nursing team is very important, as the parents need to be able to process the information and thus gain an understanding of the treatment process for their child. It has been noted that most parents, including the parents of planned admissions, remain in an anxious frame of mind throughout the transplant. However, those parents fortunate enough to have had a home visit prior to admission appear to handle the anxiety much better.

Parents staying with the child

The expectation by medical and nursing staff is for the parents or carers to stay with the child during the transplant to provide nurturing and care. Basic living accommodation is normally provided by the hospital to enable them to do so. In the case of children or babies requiring a highly specialized transplant, e.g. for severe combined immunodeficiency (SCID) for which there are only two such units in the United Kingdom (Newcastle and London), parents may need to travel long distances from different parts of the country to stay with their child. This may be for the duration of the transplant, which is usually several weeks or months. They may feel pressured into giving up their jobs, or in some circumstances are granted leave without pay by their employer. In the case of the main earner this can have a drastic effect on their self esteem and on their ability to provide for their family. Parents may also be compelled to leave other children at home to be looked after by relatives. This, together with the physical effects on their child of the treatment program throughout the transplant, can take its toll and adds to a continually stressful situation for the parents.

How the social worker can help

The social worker's prime aim is to keep the parents in a positive, proactive frame of mind, to enable them to provide the bonding, nurturing, and loving care the child requires during the long stay in hospital. This ensures a more loving environment, which will keep the child happy and contented, allow the patient to develop naturally, and aid the transplant recovery process. Procedures that reduce fear and anxiety help heighten the sense of self efficacy (Egan, 2001). The time leading up to the transplant and after the transplant can be a roller-coaster of personal experiences. The experiences of parents are unique in that they have many extraordinary situations to contend with; their needs may vary from help with financial issues, housing problems, work issues, and family problems to emotional support. The trust and understanding of the social worker, nursing and medical staff is imperative to guide them through the many emotional phases they may experience. The provision of positive support throughout the transplant, the use of alternative therapy, together with actively working in partnership with the transplant team can be instrumental in achieving a positive end result for the patient.

The support a social worker needs to provide to each individual family can vary and will depend on their individual needs. Case Study 2 below is an example of the support delivered by the HSCT social worker.

Case Study 2

A five-month-old baby (X) with a SCID urgently required a transplant. The family consisted of mother, father and an older child (Y), aged 3 years, who was found to be a donor match.

The family, of Asian background, lived 100 miles from the transplant unit. The mother was born and brought up in the UK, but the father was born and raised in Pakistan and spoke little English. It was an arranged marriage. They settled well in England and lived in a two-bedroom rented property. The father had not been able to obtain full-time work, but found employment as a casual labourer working 3–4 days per week. Their income was topped up with Tax Credits.

The parents and siblings had uprooted themselves from their home town to come to Newcastle to stay temporarily in a one-bedroom apartment at the transplant center. The accommodation was extremely basic.

The agreement was that the mother would stay permanently on site to care for her sick child but the father would only stay from Tuesday to Friday. Y would attend nursery on Wednesday

and Thursday, which would allow the father to spend time with X. The father would return home on Fridays to continue to work three days per week. Y would accompany the father and be cared for by the mother's sister while the father was at work.

The mother married soon after leaving school, quickly becoming pregnant with her first child. She developed limited parenting and daily living skills, and regretted not having been involved in the nurturing of her first child. She believed this had affected their mother–child relationship. The father has lived in the UK for just over three years. He was very involved and relaxed in the caring of their first child. He did most of the cooking and household tasks.

Y spoke Punjabi most of the time with occasional English words. She had no set boundaries and quickly became disruptive when she believed her needs were not being addressed. She tended to bite and spit to draw attention to herself. She had a poor appetite and her parents allowed her a diet of milk rather than persevere with set eating habits.

This assessment was centered on addressing the needs of X in hospital and a family-centered approach was necessary to meet the needs of the family (as outlined in the Framework for Assessment of Children in Need, 2005). For some families the process of assessment is in itself a therapeutic intervention. Being able to look at problems in a constructive manner, with a professional who is willing to listen and who helps family members to reflect on what is happening, is often enough to help them find solutions. The services of an interpreter were used to gain a full understanding of the needs of both parents. A health visitor and social worker from their home town were contacted. The views of nursing and medical staff were gained. Through the process the following were identified.

The mother had limited parenting and daily living skills. Hence the mother had little concept of her commitment to the care of X both during the life-threatening illness and afterwards. The mother displayed very little confidence and self esteem. Y received a poor diet, and no boundaries or routines had been established for her daily life. Mother and father did not communicate in a meaningful way with each other, nor with close family. They had limited income and did not discuss financial matters. Their family home had limited space and would be inappropriate when they returned.

It was necessary to apply to charity organizations for financial support to aid the family with travelling costs and the additional income they would need during the transplant process. Intervention included a task-centered approach and a cognitive behavioral method.

The mother was keen to develop a close parental bond with X and gain confidence in her parental skills. Liaising with medical and nursing staff, a task-centered approach was developed that involved the mother spending time with X. In return she received positive loving responses from X, raising her confidence and self esteem.

A cognitive behavior approach was used working with the parents to help them gain an understanding of each other's needs. They did not communicate in a meaningful way, and each blamed the other for problems that arose. A cognitive behavior therapy approach allowed them to identify the repetitive negative behavior patterns they had both established. This allowed them to understand their lack of consideration for each other's needs and thus be more sympathetic and understanding towards each other. Interactions of distressed couples are often characterized by reciprocated negative behavior: if one spouse behaves negatively, the partner is likely to respond in kind, and thus starts a chain of escalating negative interactions (Hawton, 1996).

To deal with the inappropriate housing situation a letter was sent to the local housing office to support the parents' application for more appropriate housing to address the health needs of X. To provide for the assessed needs of Y the social worker liaised with a private nursery. It was agreed that Y would attend the private nursery 2 days per week to establish her into daily routines and learn the value of playing and sharing with other children. It was hoped that this would improve her behavior. The nursery staff would also help to toilet train her and reduce the need for nappies. She would be encouraged to establish good eating habits and set her into eating routines. Her use of English would be encouraged. The social worker negotiated with a charity to fund her nursery fees.

Following the interventions used the parents reported that Y was eating well and at appropriate times. She used the toilet and no longer needed to wear nappies. Her use and understanding of the English language was more frequent. She was a happier and more affectionate child, displaying less antisocial behavior. She no longer spat or bit. The intervention techniques appeared to have had a positive effect on both parents and child. The parents interacted in a much more understanding way with Y and also as a family with each other. Improving the parents' ability to address the needs of their children in a proactive way created a better quality of life.

Discharge and multidisciplinary working

When the time draws near for discharge the baby or child may first go to a halfway house. The halfway house is, as the name suggests, halfway to being discharged home. The period spent by the parents in the halfway house allows time to adjust in the caring for their child without nursing involvement. Many parents initially feel very insecure and fearful of caring and administering medication. They are reluctant to take over the responsibility of their child. However, their confidence returns in time and they are soon keen to return home. For patients living nearer the transplant unit the child may be discharged home and have frequent follow-up visits as an outpatient.

Before the child returns to their own home the social worker will prepare for the family's return home. Contact will be made with the various agencies and statutory authority able to provide the anticipated ongoing support the family are expected to need. A multidisciplinary meeting is often set up with the appropriate people to discuss the needs of the family. This is essential to provide support to enable them to resume their daily living routine. The needs of the family vary according to the needs of the child and the family circumstances.

Problems that need to be addressed following discharge include the following:
- The child will not be able to:
  - mix with other children;
  - travel on public transport;
  - frequent public places.
- The parent will need extra support and time for:
  - caring for a recovering child;
  - administering medication;
  - attending hospital outpatient appointments;
  - ensuring other siblings/dependents are cared for (taking them to school, babysitting);
  - housework, shopping.

Children who are defined as in need under the Children Act 1989 are those whose vulnerability is such that they are unlikely to reach or maintain a satisfactory level of health and development, or their health and development will be significantly impaired without the provision of services. Social Services alone cannot promote the social inclusion and development of these children and families. However, in partnership with others Social Services can play a vital role.

Section III: working with teenagers as patients

As a natural part of adolescent development, a young person begins to form their own values, ideas and opinions. They begin to confide more in their peers, rather less in their parents, whose opinions they are often rejecting. Peers can provide an opportunity for debate and can act as a sounding board when decisions have to be made. The physical segregation necessary as part of the HSCT process denies the young person this crucial support, thus adding to their sense of emotional isolation.

Consent to treatment

An issue for consideration when working with teenagers is that of consent to examination and/or treatment. Before a teenager can be examined and treated a health professional must obtain their consent. Teenagers aged between 16 and 17 years are presumed to have the competence to give consent themselves. The case of Gillick[1] laid down the principle that a child under the age of 16 years can be allowed to give consent rather than their parents, if the child has demonstrated that they have the mental and emotional maturity, intelligence, and comprehension to understand the procedures involved. A teenager's capacity to consent to examination is a matter of clinical judgement. Each transplant unit needs to determine the approach that will be taken with regard to this. In our transplant unit both the parent and the teenager are encouraged to sign the consent form for HSCT. It is seen as best practice that parents and the teenager are involved in all of the discussions from diagnosis through the trajectory of treatment. This can cause conflict in some situations: for example, the teenager may not want their parent(s) involved and may wish to refuse any further treatment, whereas the parent or parents may be adamant that they want the treatment to continue.

Where both the teenager and the parent refuse to give consent, treatment can be given if it is deemed to be in the best interests of the child. Legal advice would need to be sought and action may be taken through the courts, if appropriate.

Dependence/independence

A life-threatening illness raises independence-vs.-dependence issues for any teenager as their situation dictates that they become more reliant on their carers at a time when they are establishing their own way of doing things and experiencing an increased level of freedom they did not have when they were younger. This potential for conflict is particularly prevalent in the HSCT situation, because the procedure can make many patients very sick indeed, thus increasing their dependence. In addition, the patient and the carer have far less opportunity to have a break from one another, the isolating environment provides no distractions whatsoever, and their environment is extremely physically restrictive. Teenagers naturally spend little time with parent(s). Even in the home, they tend to retreat to their own space. The teenager's space on the transplant unit is consequently "invaded" by the carer and medical staff, impacting on privacy at a stage of personal development that makes self-consciousness a huge issue and privacy more important than at any other stage of life. The teenager can regress emotionally, and accept care or want to be "cared for," with the parent becoming even more protective and providing less opportunity for the patient to have control.

Education and work

The transplant procedure interferes with social life, school, college, and work. Students have their academic life disrupted at a stage when it is vitally important and at a time when there is less opportunity to catch up on missed studies. Examinations may be missed or may have to be taken in a hospital setting. Some teenagers are employed, and have to rely on the co-operation and understanding of employers. As the absence from work can be protracted and employers have commitments to meet, this support can wane. Employed patients can incur significant financial costs, which cannot be compensated for by the state benefit system. For

---

[1] Gillick v. West Norfolk and Wisbech Area Health Authority (1985). 3 ALL ER 402 (HL). This was a test case in English Law regarding the competence of a child under the age of 16 to give consent or agree to a treatment.

teenagers who are aged 16 and over, because benefits such as Disability Living Allowance, Income Support, and Incapacity Benefit cannot be paid when the person is in hospital for more than 28 days – supposing that benefits have been awarded in the first place – financial hardship is significant. In addition, there is a huge financial cost to the family, as carers are not able to follow their own employment, and if the young person officially qualifies for a benefit in their own right (but is not actually receiving anything) parents cannot claim for them as dependents.

Emotional issues

On an emotional level, the teenage HSCT patient fluctuates constantly between not wanting anything to do with their friends – because they feel that their emotions are not understood – and wanting friends to support and sympathize. One hindrance to maintaining friendships is related to poor body image. Teenagers are extremely self-conscious, as they associate how they are judged and how they judge others by physical appearance. They can therefore become ashamed of how they look and cannot be reassured about their appearance as long as they are not happy with their own view of themselves. This sometimes results in them metaphorically and actually keeping friends at arm's length.

Prior to and during the transplant procedure, the teenager is obviously very concerned as to whether the process will be a success. They are old enough to realize that they need the transplant in order to survive, but there is a part of them afraid that they may be hastening death because the procedure is risky. Being at an age when they challenge the opinions and views of adults, they wonder whether the doctors could be wrong. This is in contrast to the younger age group, who are much more accepting of the medical explanations given. This older group are much more aware, and therefore worry much more, about the acute and chronic side effects of the treatment, i.e. GVHD, infertility (with its associated implications for future personal relationships), and psychological impact. Within the isolation context they also have to deal with feelings of loss (freedom, normal life, etc.), fears, sadness, and anger.

At the end of the procedure teenagers/young adult patients can experience different psychological outcomes and have an altered view on life in general. Many have lost confidence in everything and are less trusting because of what has happened to them and the speed with which it happened. There are others who consider themselves invincible and follow a path of increased risk taking. Almost all struggle with the period of readjustment. Having been forced to mature more quickly than normally, they often find themselves marginalized by their peers and/or isolate themselves, because they no longer have the same things in common and have missed out on the community of relationships because of their absence from the "scene."

Although never free from the fear of relapse, many young people are grateful to have had the opportunity of a healthy future. Now aware of mortality, they are determined to achieve their potential and appreciate life that much more than they did previously, when they took their life for granted.

Support for donors

Donors will either be recruited from one of the volunteer donor panels or be a sibling of the patient or, rarely, a parent. Donor panels will provide some counseling to their volunteers at the time of their registration, whereas sibling donors are more likely to have direct contact with the transplant team. Support for related donors is an area often neglected due to time and staffing constraints. It is important, therefore, that someone within the transplant team is identified as being available to offer support. It will help if sibling donors are informed and educated from the beginning of the process, and that they are supported and offered counseling after the transplant. The teenager/young adult patient may be much more aware of the psychological impact on a family if a sibling is their donor. They have to cope with feelings of guilt and relief in equal measure at the implicit/explicit pressure placed on the family member who is a match.

There may be special circumstances where additional support may be needed, if, for instance, there has been a difficult or estranged relationship between the donor and the patient, or if the transplant fails or the patient has an early relapse. Full information from the start of the process can prevent problems developing later.

Death and bereavement

All patients and their families and carers should have been informed of the potential risks involved in transplant prior to the procedure. They should know that there are chances of dying during the transplant, or of relapsing afterwards. Some relapsing patients will respond to further treatment and achieve a second remission; some will not and will need to face death. Reactions to relapse and impending death will vary from person to person, and it is important that each person's individual needs are acknowledged and their wishes met if at all possible. It is also important to respect the spiritual and cultural needs of the patient and involve the relevant spiritual leaders. Many patients may have already made wills but others may need the opportunity to do so.

This may involve patients and their carers being offered choices about where they would like to be cared for in the terminal stages of their illness. Meeting such wishes will often help those left with the grieving process. Early contacts with community nursing teams and hospices can make it possible to transfer a patient to their preferred place of care even when death is very near. Some patients will opt to remain in the hospital, where they know the staff and feel secure. It is important that, if appropriate, such discussions take place at a time when the patient feels able to make these important decisions.

The Department of Health's (DoH) document "When a Patient Dies. Advice on Developing a Bereavement Service in the NHS" (2005) offers comprehensive guidance on relevant issues relating to death and bereavement, and encourages hospitals to develop clear policies.

Families or those taking responsibilities for the funeral of their loved one need to know the basic sequence of events following the death in terms of registering the death and arranging the funeral. Each unit needs to be clear about who provides this information. Families may also need to know that, for those on certain benefits, financial help for the cost of the funeral may be available.

The DoH document states that "The vast majority of people who have been bereaved neither seek nor need focused professional help or counseling in connection with their bereavement. Their families and social networks within the community often offer all the informal help they need."

This may be true for some, but it is important to recognize the special circumstances related to transplant. Even though patients and their families have been aware of the risks, transplant will have offered hope and the chance of a cure, making the loss more difficult to accept. The patient may be very young or leaving very young children. Sibling donors may have particular needs or feel guilt. Other life events or previous losses may complicate grief.

Some bereaved relatives and carers gain comfort and reassurance by returning to the hospital and talking to the consultant and members of the multidisciplinary team. The consultant may be able to make a home visit; this can provide some answers, or a deeper understanding of the causes of the death. It will also provide the professionals involved with clues as to whether further or more formal bereavement support is needed. Discussions can then take place with the bereaved as to whether this would be helpful and what local resources there are to provide it.

Conclusion

Social need within cancer care is acknowledged and defined within existing policy frameworks and can be linked to QoL issues for survivors of HSCT. The identification of social need early on in the treatment process gives the patient and carers the best possible opportunity to resolve problems prior to transplant and to feel more comfortable about acknowledging other needs if they arise. Having someone integrated into the multidisciplinary team who is able to assess for and support patients with the social issues arising out of their diagnosis is extremely important. Such interventions can enhance a patient's QoL and contribute to a successful re-adjustment to life post-transplant.

Acknowledgements

We would like to thank Jan McBride and Anne Wilson for their contribution, especially on the section dealing with teenagers as patients. Their help has been invaluable.

Further reading

Expert Advisory Group on Cancer (1995) A Policy Framework for Commissioning Cancer Services (Calman Hine report): A report by the Expert Advisory Group on Cancer to the Chief Medical Officers of England and Wales. Available from www.dh.gov.uk

Bertero, C., Ek, A.C. (1993) Quality of life of adults with acute leukaemia. *J Adv Nurs* **18**: 1346–1353.

Children Act, 1989 (2004) The Stationery Office. Also available from www.ops.gov.uk

Department of Health (2001) The NHS Cancer Plan.

Department of Health (2005) When a Patient Dies. Advice on Developing a Bereavement Service in the NHS. Available from www.dh.gov.uk

Egan, G. (2001) *The Skilled Helper: A Problem Management and Opportunity Development Approach to Helping*, 7th edn. California: Wadsworth Publishing, Brooks/Cole Publishing Co.

Hawton, K., Salkovskis, P.M., Kirk, J., Clark, D.M. (eds) (1996) *Cognitive Behaviour Therapy for Psychiatric Problems*. Oxford: Oxford University Press, Chapter 10, p. 340.

Ferrell, B., Schmidt, G.M., Rhiner, M., Whitehead, C., Fonbuena, P., Forman, S. (1992) The meaning of quality of life for HSCT survivors, Part 1. *Cancer Nurs* **15**(3): 153–160.

Ferrell, B., Schmidt, G.M., Rhiner, M., Whitehead, C., Fonbuena, P., Forman, S. (1992) The meaning of quality of life for HSCT survivors, Part 2. *Cancer Nurs* **15**(4): 247–253.

The Stationery Office (2005) Framework for the Assessment of Children in Need. Available from www.dh.gov.uk

National Institute for Clinical Excellence (2004) Improving Supportive and Palliative Care for Adults with Cancer. Available from ww.nice.org.uk

Macmillan Cancer Relief (2002) Talking to Children when an Adult has Cancer. Available from www.macmillan.org.uk

Manne, S., DuHamel, K., Ostroff, J. *et al.* (2004). Anxiety, depressive and post traumatic stress disorders among mothers of paediatric survivors of haemopoietic stem cell transplantations. *Pediatr* **113**(6): 1700–1705.

Molassiotis, A. (2000) Social issues. In: Grundy, M. (Ed), *Nursing in Haematological Oncology*. London: Balliere Tindall, pp. 258–267.

The NHS and Community Care Act 1990, HMSO. Available from www.opsi.gove.uk/acts/

Useful contacts

Leukaemia Care. www.leukaemiacare.org.uk 24/7 Care line 0800 1696680.

Macmillan cancer relief. Cancer line 0808 8082020. www.macmillan .org.uk

Working Together to Safeguard Children 1999. Department of Health, Home Office and Department for Education and Employment. The Stationery Office, London.

Chapter 16
Long-term follow up of transplant recipients

R. Skinner and G. Jackson

Introduction

International Bone Marrow Transplant Registry (IBMTR) data record approximately 45,000 hematopoietic stem cell transplants (HSCTs) (30,000 autologous, 15,000 allogeneic) performed annually (2003 IBMTR/ABMTR Summary Slides, Current Use And Outcome Of Blood And Marrow Transplantation 2003, available at http://www.ibmtr.org/SERVICES/summary_slides.html). Ultimately, the steady reductions in transplant-related mortality (TRM) should be reflected in improving long-term survival, which is already at least 50% for most common indications for HSCT, and substantially better for certain conditions.

However, long-term follow-up is essential as survivors of HSCT are at high risk of developing late adverse effects of treatment due to a number of factors:
- previous treatment – many HSCTs are performed for patients with poor prognosis disease who have received a great deal of prior treatment involving several cytotoxic drugs and frequently radiotherapy (RT);
- conditioning treatment – which usually involves intensive and high-dose chemotherapy and often RT;
- graft-vs.-host disease (GVHD) and other specific complications of allogeneic HSCT.

The wide variety of chemotherapy agents used (nearly all of which have well-described late toxicity profiles), and the use of total body irradiation (TBI), mean that potentially any tissue or organ system may be affected by late adverse effects of HSCT. In recipients of HSCT, most of the adverse effects that are attributed to RT incorporating particular fields (involving specific organs or tissues) are due to TBI rather than local RT.

Although HSCT is felt to offer the best chance of cure in many of these patients, considerable late toxicity may be inevitable in a significant proportion of patients. There is preliminary evidence that over 90% of survivors of HSCT performed in childhood for hematological malignancy experience at least one late adverse effect of treatment, and over 70% suffer three or more. Chronic toxicity may become more apparent with time and increasing age, and patients may develop increasing impairment of vital organ systems (e.g. cardiac, pulmonary, renal). This may lead to an increased risk of premature major illness or early death, which is most devastating in survivors who undergo HSCT in childhood or early adulthood. Moreover, in addition to the impact on individual patients, late adverse effects of HSCT impose a significant burden on the healthcare system.

Most pediatric, and many adult, hematology/oncology centers undertake long-term follow up of survivors of HSCT, although many different models and settings are used. Usually this follow up has been performed in the same unit that performed the HSCT, most often by the same clinicians, with the additional involvement of other specialists as appropriate. However, the rapidly growing number of adult survivors of HSCT, whether performed in childhood or adulthood, has led to the emergence of a unique group of patients with complex needs. Many transplant teams have responded to these pressures by developing dedicated long-term follow-up clinics with multidisciplinary teams including:

- medical staff (age specific), with close liaison with other specialists (e.g. endocrinologists, ophthalmologists, dermatologists);
- specialist nurses;
- psychologists;
- social workers.

Most transplant units perform lifelong follow up of survivors of HSCT in view of the continued uncertainty about the future prognosis of many late adverse effects.

Although nearly all of the published literature about the occurrence of late adverse effects after HSCT describes patients who have received bone marrow as a source of stem cells rather than peripheral blood or umbilical cord blood, the profile of late adverse effects is probably broadly similar after these newer techniques due to chemotherapy and RT received prior to and during conditioning.

Most of the adverse effects of chemotherapy and RT in pediatric and adult HSCT recipients are the same as those seen in patients receiving the same treatment in the non-HSCT setting. In particular, the great majority of late toxicity seen in recipients of autologous HSCTs is readily explicable on this basis, although high treatment doses and/or additive effects may lead to unusual or accentuated toxicity in a significant minority. However, survivors of allogeneic HSCT are at additional risk of a range of severe and potentially life-threatening manifestations of chronic graft-vs.-host disease (cGVHD), other immune-mediated disturbances (e.g. hematological cytopenias), and delayed immune reconstitution.

Most conditioning regimens for HSCT have been based on TBI (of which cyclophosphamide and TBI [CyTBI] has been the commonest) or on chemotherapy alone (of which busulfan and cyclophosphamide [BuCy] has been the prototype). In general, TBI-based regimens are more likely to lead to serious late adverse effects, particularly in children, including:
- endocrine toxicity:
  - primary hypothyroidism;
  - impaired growth;
  - delayed or arrested puberty;
  - infertility;
- neurocognitive and educational toxicity;

- cataracts;
- secondary malignancies.

However, although it is often stated that the long-term toxicity of BuCy is less than that of CyTBI, it is important to recognize that there is less long-term experience with BuCy and that it is not devoid of late toxicity (e.g. infertility is very common).

A high index of suspicion is needed for early detection and optimal management of these complications, so survivors of HSCT should undergo long-term follow up in a setting that allows adequate opportunity for careful review of their physical, mental, and psychological health. Active surveillance should allow early detection and appropriate management of incipient or established late adverse effects and so reduce the frequency of severe complications, and morbidity and mortality, as well as the impact on health services.

However, clinical investigation is complicated by the knowledge that there is a very wide range of severity of clinical abnormalities seen after HSCT. Furthermore, it may be unclear whether early diagnosis and perhaps treatment of subclinical toxicity improves the outcome. Unfortunately, the detailed prospective and longitudinal research necessary to understand the true significance of subclinical abnormalities is seldom available.

Table 16.1 summarizes the most frequent and important late adverse effects of HSCT. Most of these can be monitored at patient annual reviews. Table 16.2 provides a suggested checklist for clinical assessment and surveillance investigations to be performed or considered at regular intervals during long-term follow up. The exact checklist will vary according to local protocols and the nature of the long-term follow-up clinic's workload (e.g. age of patients, indications for HSCT, etc.). Some units may wish to perform additional investigations in patients receiving HSCT for specific or rarer indications. It is important that the follow-up team and the patient (and family where appropriate) appreciate the rationale and benefits to be gained.

Although yearly review is often adequate, more frequent assessment is appropriate in circumstances such as adolescence, when growth and pubertal development should be monitored; also, patients with significant complications, e.g. active cGVHD,

Table 16.1 Summary of potential late adverse effects of HSCT

Impaired quality of life

Secondary malignancy
- Solid tumors
- Hematological (predominantly myelodysplastic syndrome [MDS]/ acute myeloid leukemia [AML])

Hematological
- Immune-mediated cytopenias

Immunological
- Delayed immune reconstitution
- Immune dysregulation
- Autoimmunity

cGVHD and its sequelae

Visual
- Cataract
- Keratoconjunctivitis sicca
- Chorioretinitis

Auditory
- Sensorineural deafness
- Impaired speech development*

Craniofacial/dental
- Impaired craniofacial skeletal growth*
- Dental

Oral
- Xerostomia
- Lichenoid lesions/leukoplakia
- Oral/salivary gland tumors

Endocrine
- Thyroid dysfunction
- Pituitary dysfunction
- Growth impairment*
- Pancreatic/metabolic dysfunction

Gonadal/reproductive
- Female – ovarian failure, adverse pregnancy outcome, early menopause
- Male – Sertoli cell failure, Leydig cell failure
- Both sexes – delayed/arrested puberty,* sexual dysfunction, sub/infertility

Neurological
- Leukoencephalopathy
- Vasculopathy
- Central nervous system infection
- Central nervous system tumors
- Peripheral neuropathy

Neuropsychological
- Functional impairment*
- Cognitive impairment*

Cardiovascular
- Myocardial
- Pericardial
- Coronary artery disease

Respiratory
- Obstructive disease
- Restrictive disease
- Late-onset pulmonary syndrome

Renal
- Radiation nephritis
- Glomerular impairment
- Proximal tubular impairment
- Isolated hypertension
- Proteinuria/nephrotic syndrome
- Cancer-associated hemolytic–uremic syndrome

Lower urinary tract
- Hemorrhagic cystitis
- Bladder tumors

Musculoskeletal
- Joints – sclerodermatous contractures, arthropathies
- Muscular – polymyositis, weakness
- Skeletal – osteoporosis, avascular necrosis, slipped epiphysis,* scoliosis,* osteochondroma

Skin
- Manifestations of cGVHD
- Alopecia
- Benign pigmented nevi
- Skin tumors

* Specific to children and adolescents.

and patients still within 5 years of transplant should be monitored every 3–6 months.

Although the risk of developing a new onset of some late adverse effects decreases with very long-term follow up (e.g. in TBI recipients, the chance of developing primary hypothyroidism for the first time diminishes after 10 years post-transplant), this is not true for some other complications (e.g. secondary malignancies, where the risk continues

to increase with time). Nevertheless, once a patient is 10 years post-HSCT and has reached final height (for those transplanted in childhood), it may be possible to reduce the frequency of follow up to every two years. However, there is very little clear published evidence concerning the best follow-up schedule.

This chapter will discuss the major long-term complications of HSCT with the exception of the

Table 16.2 Checklist for post-HSCT long-term follow-up clinic

Consider the following at least yearly (unless otherwise indicated) in clinic. Additional investigations may be appropriate in presence of abnormal symptoms/signs, or may be indicated in particular groups of patients.

History
Employment/school*
Quality of life (including sexual function)
Growth – height,* weight
Nutrition
Pubertal development*
Fertility issues ⎫ At appropriate age/time
Joint pain (especially hip, knee)
Vision
Dental health
Compliance with medications, e.g. anti-infective prophylaxis
Immunization up to date (as appropriate)
Health education as appropriate, including healthy eating, smoking, sunlight, breast examination

Examination
NB Wide variety of symptoms/signs of cGVHD
Skin (cGVHD, nevi, suspicious lesions) – consider clinical photography
Thyroid palpation
Central nervous system examination
Ophthalmoscopy (cataracts)
Blood pressure
Height (including sitting height if possible),* calculate height velocity,* weight ⎫ 3–6 monthly until puberty and growth completed
Pubertal assessment (Tanner stage)*

Investigations
Full blood count
Biochemical profile (incl U+Es, LFTs, albumin, protein, calcium, phosphate, magnesium)
Ferritin
Thyroid function tests (T_4, TSH)
LH, FSH, estradiol[†]/testosterone ⎫ After 10 years age
Inhibin B (if available)
IGF-1* ⎫ In TBI recipients if concern about growth
Bone age*
Fasting glucose and lipids
Hemoglobin A_{1c}
Immunoglobulins, lymphocyte subsets (if concern about delayed/poor immune reconstitution)
Urinalysis (hematuria, proteinuria, glycosuria)
Urine cytology (if previous severe hemorrhagic cystitis)
Echocardiogram ⎫ Yearly if previously abnormal or if new symptoms,
Pulmonary function tests ⎭ 3–5 yearly if previously normal and no symptoms
Chest X-ray (if symptomatic or PFTs severely abnormal)
Consider BMD scan (especially in patients treated for GH deficiency or hypogonadism)

* Appropriate for children and adolescents.
† Not helpful if on hormone replacement treatment.
Adapted with permission from Table II, Skinner, R., Leiper, A.D. (2005) Appendix B, Survivors of allogeneic bone marrow transplantation. In: Skinner R, Wallace WHB, Levitt GA, on behalf of Late Effects Group (eds), *Therapy based long term follow up. Practice Statement*. United Kingdom Children's Cancer Study Group.

more common manifestations of cGVHD (which are covered in Chapter 10).

Quality of life/psychological issues

It is not surprising that some patients with life-threatening illnesses who have undergone potentially lethal intensive therapy, and who face the prospect of potential ill health and long-term follow up for the rest of their lives, may face psychological problems in coping with everything they have endured previously and in coming to terms with their uncertain future. It is more remarkable that most long-term survivors of HSCT do adjust well to all that they have to deal with. However, patients' personal, medical, and employment circumstances, relationships, and support mechanisms change with time, and as a consequence they may need support from social workers and/or psychologists even long after HSCT. Therefore, a clinical psychologist is an important member of the follow-up team.

Sexual difficulties can arise after HSCT. Psychological problems, relationship difficulties, vaginal dryness, male sexual dysfunction due to hypogonadism with low testosterone concentrations (see "Gonadal/reproductive" below), difficulties with conception, and other health concerns may all contribute to reduced libido and sexual difficulties. Although these problems are often concealed from healthcare professionals, sexual function can be restored if individual problems are addressed.

Children and adolescents also face considerable disruption of school and college education, with potentially major adverse effects on their future plans. Despite the practical and emotional difficulties of reintegration, for both the patient and their family, it is important to encourage consistent attendance at school as soon as the child's isolation restrictions permit and they are well enough, both to avoid further compromise of their education and to encourage the beneficial effects of re-establishing normal peer contact and support.

Secondary malignancy

Over the first 2 years after HSCT for malignant disease, relapse of the original malignancy is one of the commonest reasons (indeed the commonest in children) for HSCT failure. However, survivors of HSCT also have a greater lifelong risk of developing another (secondary) malignancy (Table 16.3). The increased risk is highest in older patients and is related to:
- chemotherapy;
- RT;
- prolonged immunosuppression usually in the context of cGVHD;
- other risk factors for developing malignancy (e.g. smoking).

Chemotherapy, especially with alkylating agents and topoisomerase II inhibitors such as epipodophyllotoxins, is associated with myelodysplasia or acute myeloid leukemia typically in the first few years following an autologous HSCT, whilst RT (including TBI) is linked with the later (typically 5 years or more post-HSCT) onset of solid tumors, especially brain, thyroid, oral, salivary gland and skin malignancies.

Prevention and early detection are very important. Patients should be aware of the increased risk of malignancy, and advised to avoid additional cancer risks such as cigarette smoking and prolonged sun exposure.

Table 16.3 Secondary malignancy following HSCT

Type	Examples	Notes
Hematological	Myelodysplasia/acute myeloid leukemia	Usually after autologous HSCT
	Non-Hodgkin's lymphoma	Often occur early post-HSCT driven by Epstein–Barr virus infection in profoundly immunosuppressed patients
Solid tumors	Brain	Especially in patients who received TBI during conditioning
	Thyroid	

Hematological

Immune-mediated cytopenias may occur individually (e.g. isolated neutropenia) or in combination (e.g. concurrent or sequential anemia and thrombocytopenia) in recipients of allogeneic HSCT, often in the context of cGVHD. Further immunosuppressive (e.g. steroids) or immunomodulatory (e.g. intravenous immunoglobulin) treatment may be required.

Immune reconstitution

The immune system recovers slowly in patients who have had an allogeneic HSCT. Recovery is slower in older patients, recipients of mismatched, unrelated cord or haploidentical transplants, and patients with cGVHD, particularly those on immunosuppressive therapy. Both humoral and cell-mediated immune reconstitution may be delayed, leading to a wide range of infective risks.

Autoimmune disorders

Immunological recovery can be associated with the development of immune dysregulation, leading to autoimmune disorders including:
- hypo- or hyperthyroidism;
- myasthenia gravis;
- diabetes;
- hepatitis;
- allergies and atopy (may be transferred from the donor's immune system).

Infections

Patients who have undergone HSCT have a greater risk of infections, particularly within the first 12 months after an allogeneic transplant. See Chapters 6, 7 and 8 for infections in the HSCT patient. After 12 months the risk of life-threatening infection falls but still remains above normal, particularly in alternative donor HSCTs, where immune reconstitution can be slow, and in patients with cGVHD receiving prolonged immunosuppressive treatment. A high index of suspicion for opportunistic infections is important in such patients, since they are at much higher risk of developing potentially lethal viral or fungal infections at a later stage post-HSCT than was previously observed when most HSCT were performed using donor HLA-identical sibling donors.

Patients and their carers should be given appropriate anti-infective prophylaxis and advice about recognition of symptoms suggestive of infection, as well as a clear indication of how to seek prompt and appropriate medical advice (see Chapter 14) and specific advice about reimmunization (see Chapter 13). It is important to liaise with the patient's primary care physicians to provide advice about ongoing strategies for prevention and treatment of infection.

Specific infections that may present relatively late post-HSCT include the following.

Pneumocystis jirovecii

HSCT recipients are most at risk of this infection during the first 12–18 months post-HSCT, the duration of susceptibility depending on the type of transplant and the length of immunosuppressive treatment. Patients should receive specific prophylaxis against *Pneumocystis* until it is considered that they have achieved satisfactory immune reconstitution, and they are no longer on immunosuppressive therapy. Oral co-trimoxazole is the most commonly used prophylactic agent, but alternatives (e.g. intravenous or nebulized pentamidine) may be used in patients intolerant of co-trimoxazole.

Varicella zoster virus (VZV)/*Herpes simplex* virus (HSV)

All VZV-seropositive patients and those with a history of VZV infection after HSCT should continue to receive prophylaxis with aciclovir or valaciclovir throughout the time they remain on immunosuppressive therapy, to prevent reactivation of both VZV and HSV infections. All patients who develop reactivation of these viral infections should be treated promptly with aciclovir, which may initially need to be given intravenously.

Bacteria

Patients who have undergone allogeneic HSCT, particularly recipients of unrelated donor HSCTs or patients with cGVHD, are highly susceptible to recurrent bacterial infections, especially with encapsulated bacteria such as *Streptococcus pneumoniae* (pneumococcus), *Haemophilus influenzae* (Hib) and *Neisseria meningitidis*. Susceptibility to these organisms may be due to a number of factors including:

• persistently low levels of opsonizing antibodies;
• low CD4 counts;
• poor reticuloendothelial function (particularly in the context of hyposplenism after TBI);
• long-term use of immunosuppressive therapy (especially corticosteroids).

Long-term antibiotic prophylaxis is recommended in addition to immunization specifically with pneumococcus (both polysaccharide and conjugated vaccine preparations), Hib and meningococcal C vaccines, starting approximately 12–18 months post-HSCT (i.e. when satisfactory immune recovery is expected). Chapter 13 gives further details on post-HSCT reimmunization. Traditionally penicillin-based prophylaxis (predominantly phenoxymethylpenicillin, with amoxicillin as an alternative) is used in all patients and compliance should be encouraged. Penicillin resistance should be monitored and, if appropriate, alternatives should be considered. Alternative prophylaxis (e.g. erythromycin) should also be considered in those who are allergic to penicillin.

Hepatitis C and other blood-borne viruses

Infection with hepatitis and other blood-borne viruses is much less common following the introduction of universal blood and donor screening in the UK. Both donor and recipient should be screened appropriately for infection before transplant. Some longer-term follow-up patients may, however, have developed hepatitis C before the universal screening of blood products and should be managed jointly with infectious disease physicians or hepatologists.

Visual

Ocular complications of transplantation are common, particularly after TBI, and close liaison is required between the transplant team and ophthalmology services.

Cataract formation, usually bilateral, is an important, relatively common complication, usually occurring after three years or more. It is usually seen in patients who have received TBI. High-dose single-fraction TBI is associated with a higher risk of cataracts (up to 100% in some pediatric reports) than low-dose single-fraction TBI or fractionated TBI (about 35%). Cataracts may also occur in patients who have received high-dose or prolonged steroids for severe GVHD. If vision is significantly impaired, surgical removal of the cataract(s) may be indicated, with good functional results.

Dry eyes may result from damage to the lachrymal glands either due to "keratoconjunctivitis sicca" associated with cGVHD, or from the effects of TBI, or both. Artificial tears, careful eye toilet, prompt treatment of infectious complications, and careful ophthalmological follow up are important.

Although uncommon after HSCT, cytomegalovirus (CMV) chorioretinitis may occur in isolation without evidence of systemic reactivation. It should be considered in patients presenting with visual disturbance and treated both systemically and topically.

Auditory

Sensorineural deafness is mainly seen in autologous HSCT patients who have received platinum chemotherapy (especially cisplatin or high-dose carboplatin) either before HSCT or during the conditioning regimen. Previous RT to a field including the ears may exacerbate hearing damage, as may treatment with aminoglycosides, e.g. gentamicin, amikacin, or other ototoxic drugs. This complication is serious in a young child, as it may have severe adverse consequences on their speech development and hence educational attainment.

Craniofacial/dental

Children receiving RT to a field incorporating the face (including cranial RT) may suffer impairment of craniofacial skeletal development, occasionally leading to considerable disfigurement (usually with higher RT doses), while RT including the jaw may result in later dental abnormalities affecting the teeth themselves (e.g. dental aplasia, enamel hypoplasia) or their roots (e.g. hypoplasia) in 50–90% of survivors.

Oral

Long-term oral toxicity, usually occurring in patients treated with TBI or those with cGVHD, may manifest as:
• xerostomia with difficulty in chewing and swallowing (present in up to 40% of TBI recipients);
• lichenoid lesions;
• leukoplakia;
• oral or salivary gland tumors (benign or malignant).

Regular oral examination and dental assessment are important components of long-term follow up.

Endocrine

Endocrine complications are relatively common after HSCT, especially in children, and it is important that there is close cooperation between the transplant and endocrine teams. The range of problems seen includes thyroid, pituitary, and pancreatic dysfunction. Occasionally, prolonged steroid treatment (usually of cGVHD) leads to adrenal suppression, which is usually reversible.

Thyroid

Thyroid complications of HSCT include overt and subclinical (compensated) hypothyroidism and thyroid neoplasms, and are predominantly due to RT given to a field incorporating the neck, most frequently administered as TBI. Autoimmune thyroid disease may also lead to hypo- or hyperthyroidism.

The incidence of compensated primary hypothyroidism (normal free thyroxine but high TSH) after fractionated TBI ranges between 15 and 25%, while overt primary hypothyroidism is seen in around 5% of patients. Unfractionated (i.e. single dose) TBI (which is no longer used in most centers) is associated with a higher incidence of compensated (60%) and overt hypothyroidism (15%). Patients should undergo annual thyroid palpation (for nodules and tumors) and thyroid function tests, bearing in mind that these complications typically occur 3–5 years post-HSCT (hypothyroidism) or later still (tumors). Both the patient and their primary care physician should be aware of the risk of hypothyroidism. Thyroid tumors are 125 times more common post-HSCT than in a healthy, age-matched population. Both adenomas and carcinomas may occur.

Pituitary/growth impairment

Pituitary complications of HSCT result primarily from RT (including previous cranial RT). They are of most importance in the pediatric age range, where growth hormone (GH) deficiency may lead to impaired growth resulting in short stature, skeletal disproportion (due to loss of spinal growth) and reduced bone mineral density (BMD). GH deficiency is more likely in children who have previously received both cranial RT and TBI. Dynamic GH testing is indicated in children with a slow height velocity. Initial limited data led to concerns regarding a possible increased risk of relapse in leukemia survivors treated with GH, but extensive surveillance has provided no evidence to support this and most pediatric endocrinologists offer GH treatment for documented GH deficiency in a child with slow growth velocity post-HSCT. Adults may develop the adult GH deficiency syndrome with adverse effects on cardiovascular lipid profile, body composition, BMD, and quality of life.

Pancreatic/metabolic

The metabolic syndrome is an important and

increasingly recognized complication of HSCT, manifesting with:

- diabetes mellitus or impaired glucose tolerance despite hyperinsulinemia (denoting insulin resistance);
- hyperlipidemia;
- hypertension (in some patients);
- abdominal obesity (in some patients).

The true prevalence of this syndrome remains unclear, but was reported as 39% in one small cross-sectional study of patients 3–18 years after HSCT performed in childhood. The pathogenesis of the metabolic syndrome is unclear but is likely to be mutifactorial with contributions from both RT and chemotherapy.

Factors contributing to the development of post-transplant lipid abnormalities include treatment with corticosteroids, ciclosporin and sirolimus. Serum lipid profiles should be checked regularly during follow up. Prevention and management of hyperlipidemia include maintaining a stable body weight, regular exercise, a low-fat diet and treatment with a statin. All therapies including statins should be introduced with care, particularly for post-transplant patients who are still on multiple drug therapies.

Diabetes mellitus (either type 1 or type 2) may also occur occasionally in the absence of other metabolic abnormalities.

Gonadal/reproductive

Gonadal toxicity of HSCT is due to either RT, chemotherapy (especially high-dose alkylating agents), or both.

Most patients undergoing TBI develop permanent germ cell failure (Sertoli cell failure in males, ovarian failure in females), leading to infertility. The effects of chemotherapy-only conditioning are more variable – many children receiving high-dose busulfan suffer severe germ cell failure, while many receiving cyclophosphamide alone (e.g. for aplastic anemia) do not. Although subsequent recovery of germ cell function is reported in some patients after chemotherapy conditioning, and occasionally after TBI, successful conceptions are relatively rare (especially after TBI) and females remain at risk

of premature menopause. When pregnancy does occur in a female survivor of HSCT, miscarriage, twin pregnancies or premature delivery of a low-birthweight infant are more common (especially due to uterine vascular damage when TBI is given to pre-pubertal girls), and expert antenatal and obstetric care is required. However, the majority of pregnancies appear to go to term and result in the birth of normal infants. Many adult patients, especially women, require long-term sex hormone replacement treatment to reduce the adverse effects of hypogonadism on cardiovascular and bone health.

Children may experience delayed or arrested pubertal development. This is more common in girls, up to half of whom need hormone replacement treatment for delayed menarche after TBI. More rarely, boys who receive higher doses of testicular RT, principally those with previous testicular relapse of acute leukemia who are given testicular boost RT as well as TBI, may suffer Leydig cell failure of testosterone production, necessitating testosterone treatment to restore pubertal progression.

Neurological

Leukoencephalopathy is a potentially devastating complication of HSCT, predominantly associated with cranial RT and TBI, and may present with a variety of symptoms and signs. The long-term outcome is variable, with some patients deteriorating inexorably and others changing little with time. Vascular events, including cerebrovascular accidents (CVAs) or transient ischemic attacks (TIAs), and less well-defined but often recurrent migrainous episodes, are well described, probably related to RT and potentially neurotoxic chemotherapy such as methotrexate.

Patients with cGVHD may suffer "vasculitic" syndromes. Furthermore, patients with GVHD requiring prolonged immunosuppression are more vulnerable to central nervous system infections, manifesting as meningitis or discrete localized infections, often with opportunistic organisms, while those treated with thalidomide for cGVHD may develop a predominantly sensory peripheral neuropathy.

Patients treated with TBI or cranial RT have an approximately 50 times increased risk (rising with increasing duration of follow up post-HSCT) of brain tumors, especially gliomas, meningiomas and lymphomas.

Neuropsychological

Children who have received cranial RT (and, to a lesser extent, TBI) may develop a range of adverse neuropsychological outcomes, including functional deficits (e.g. impaired fine motor or visual–spatial skills) and/or cognitive dysfunction (e.g. in memory, attention skills, intelligence), with potentially major effects on psychosocial function and educational performance. Neuropsychological toxicity, which is aggravated by neurotoxic chemotherapy (e.g. busulfan, intrathecal or high-dose intravenous methotrexate), is greater in children who are younger at treatment (especially less than 3 years old) and those who have received higher RT doses (typically as separate treatment episodes of cranial RT and TBI). In some patients, cognitive impairment may only become evident after very long-term follow up.

Cardiovascular

Late cardiac complications are usually seen in patients of any age who have received large doses of anthracyclines as part of their chemotherapy prior to HSCT, with the degree of toxicity varying from subclinical left-ventricular impairment in up to 25% of children to cardiomyopathy or overt cardiac failure in about 3–7%. Pericardial disease, most commonly manifested by an effusion, may be a rare presentation of cGVHD, sometimes as part of "polyserositis" also including pleural effusions or ascites.

In addition, RT to a field including the heart increases the risk of early-onset coronary artery disease. Some of the other late adverse effects of HSCT, notably the occurrence of sex hormone and/or GH deficiencies (again usually related to RT), may exacerbate this increased risk of atherosclerosis. Furthermore, patients with the metabolic syndrome (see "Pancreatic/metabolic" above) are at increased risk of atherosclerotic cardiovascular disease. Careful attention to a healthy lifestyle, including smoking-related issues, is important.

Respiratory

Respiratory complications represent major late adverse effects of HSCT. Up to 20% of HSCT recipients develop symptomatic chronic pulmonary damage, while abnormal pulmonary function tests (PFTs) may be seen in up to 50% of long-term survivors. Many patients, particularly children, may have very mild or even no symptoms, despite markedly abnormal PFTs. Patients with other risk factors for respiratory disease are more likely to develop chronic pulmonary damage after HSCT. Respiratory late effects may be broadly categorized as:
- obstructive;
- restrictive;
- elements of both.

Fewer children than adults appear to develop clinically overt, especially obstructive, disease. Patients who are transplanted from donors with asthma may themselves develop asthma.

Obstructive disease is predominantly associated with allogeneic HSCT, especially in the context of cGVHD following mismatched transplants, and may range in severity from mild abnormalities in spirometry to a clinical picture of progressive airways obstruction refractory to bronchodilator or even immunosuppressive treatment. Restrictive disease, which is usually attributed to prior or conditioning chemotherapy (especially bleomycin, busulfan or methotrexate) or RT, may include isolated abnormalities in gas transfer (manifest by reduced diffusion capacity [transfer factor]), or a classical restrictive defect with reduced lung volumes.

The clinical spectrum of chronic obstructive and restrictive non-infective pulmonary disease is best described as late-onset pulmonary syndrome (LOPS). The predominant symptoms are:
- breathlessness;
- cough;
- wheeze (sometimes);
- fever (occasionally).

Clinical examination, which often reveals crackles and wheezes, and chest radiography are usually non-discriminatory, but high-resolution CT scanning may reveal the extent and severity of disease. Histological entities underlying LOPS include:

- bronchiolitis obliterans (BO);
- bronchiolitis obliterans with organizing pneumonia (BOOP);
- interstitial pneumonia (lymphocytic or non-classifiable);
- diffuse alveolar damage (DAD).

Although it is often difficult to relate specific histological diagnoses to clinical outcome, BO is often associated with remorseless obstructive disease, while both BO and BOOP appear to be associated with cGVHD.

Pulmonary toxicity (both clinical features and abnormalities in PFTs) will be exaggerated in patients who smoke after transplant and is also more likely to occur in patients who have suffered pulmonary damage due to infection before, during or after transplant. PFTs with measurement of spirometry, lung volumes and transfer factor should be evaluated at least annually in symptomatic patients or those already known to have abnormal PFTs, and every 3–5 years in other patients.

Patients who continue to smoke will also be at greatly increased risk of lung cancer. This is difficult to quantify, but the effects of smoking and previous therapies seem to be synergistic in increasing the risk.

Gastrointestinal

Chronic gastrointestinal complications of HSCT occur mainly in the context of cGVHD, which may lead to:

- esophageal strictures (presenting as dysphagia);
- malabsorption (pancreatic or intestinal);
- or non-specific symptoms including:
  - nausea;
  - vomiting;
  - diarrhea;
  - abdominal pain;
  - weight loss.

Previous gastrointestinal surgery or RT and chronic intestinal infection may also cause long-term symptoms.

Hepatic

Chronic hepatic complications of HSCT may result from cGVHD (see Chapter 10), drug toxicity, hepatitis C (see "Infections" above) and iron overload.

Although hepatic veno-occlusive disease is a fairly common early complication of HSCT, there is very little published information about its long-term outcome, but chronic sequelae appear to be rare. Other drugs received before (e.g. 6-thioguanine) or during HSCT (e.g. methotrexate) may contribute to hepatic dysfunction, but long-term toxicity is uncommon.

Iron overload

Iron overload occurs frequently after HSCT (Table 16.4). Relatively little is known about the long-term effects of iron overload in HSCT patients, although it has been associated with extensive organ toxicity in survivors of HSCT performed for thalassemia, including cardiac failure, cirrhosis, insulin-dependent diabetes mellitus, and other endocrinopathies. In patients with chronic hepatitis C, iron overload may accelerate the development of cirrhosis. Excessive iron stores decline slowly over several years but removal of iron by venesection in heavily overloaded patients improves cardiac and hepatic function (and may normalize previously elevated serum transaminase levels). Hemochromatosis is relatively common among Caucasians and the possibility of genetic hemochromatosis con-

Table 16.4 Causes of iron overload in survivors of HSCT

Multiple red blood cell transfusions
Ineffective erythropoiesis
Excessive intestinal iron absorption
Genetic hemochromatosis (rarely)

tributing to post-transplant iron overload should be considered. In such patients, it is appropriate to have a lower threshold for commencing a venesection program.

Renal

Late renal complications are relatively rare, but hypertension is described in some survivors (up to 16% after childhood HSCT), sometimes in isolation, or alternatively as a component of radiation nephritis (usually following TBI), which may present with:

- chronic glomerular impairment;
- hematuria;
- anemia (sometimes);
- in addition to hypertension.

Glomerular toxicity may be due to previous or current drug toxicity, especially long-term ciclosporin or tacrolimus in patients with cGVHD, or persist occasionally as a result of incomplete recovery from acute renal failure during the early post-HSCT period. Renal tubular (especially proximal tubular) toxicity may be due to previous chemotherapy prior to HSCT (especially in patients with solid tumors undergoing autologous HSCT, who have often received prior ifosfamide or platinum therapy).

Rarely, cGVHD may present with proteinuria or the nephrotic syndrome. Occasionally, recipients of autologous HSCTs may develop cancer-associated hemolytic uremic syndrome, usually presenting within weeks but sometimes later after mitomycin C, and occasionally other cytotoxic drugs.

Lower urinary tract

Oxazaphosphorine cytotoxic drugs (cyclophosphamide or ifosfamide) or RT to a field including the bladder (including TBI), or both, may cause hemorrhagic cystitis, presenting with:

- hematuria;
- dysuria;
- frequency;
- urgency.

Although this is principally an early complication of HSCT, it may recur occasionally during later follow up, especially in the context of cGVHD or viral infection (e.g. BK virus, adenovirus, CMV). Patients who have suffered from severe hemorrhagic cystitis have an increased risk of subsequent bladder malignancy, and should be investigated if they develop new or increased lower urinary tract symptoms (e.g. hematuria).

Musculoskeletal

Common skeletal complications of HSCT include:

- osteoporosis;
- avascular necrosis (AVN).

Other complications that may be seen after HSCT performed in childhood include:

- slipped epiphyses (especially upper femoral);
- scoliosis.

Osteochondroma may follow RT (including TBI) at any age.

Long-term treatment with corticosteroids is the primary risk factor for osteoporosis, while GH deficiency, gonadal failure, and lack of exercise may all contribute. Patients ≥ 40 years of age should have a baseline BMD assessment (DEXA scan) and by the osteoporosis team. Selected younger patients considered to be at higher risk (e.g. due to long-term steroid treatment) may also benefit from BMD measurement and appropriate lifestyle advice (see below). Bone loss can be reduced by:

- minimizing glucocorticoid dose and duration;
- optimizing dietary calcium and vitamin D intake and supplementation;
- undertaking adequate amounts of weight-bearing exercise;
- commencing hormone replacement therapy (where appropriate).

Steroid treatment and RT are the main risk factors for AVN, which is more common in males, but rare in younger children (under 10 years old). This diagnosis should be considered in any patient developing hip or knee problems (particularly joint pain), especially those who have received previous long-term or high-dose steroids. MRI imaging should be performed and the orthopedic team consulted.

Patients with extensive cGVHD may develop sclerodermatous joint contractures (see Chapter 10), whilst auto-immune arthropathies may be a manifestation of immune dysregulation post-HSCT (see "Immune reconstitution" above). Polymyositis and generalized muscle weakness may also occur in patients with cGVHD.

Skin

In addition to the cutaneous features of cGVHD (see Chapter 10) and secondary malignancies (see above) of the skin, benign pigmented nevi occur more commonly and numerously in survivors of HSCT. Alopecia may be seen, sometimes related to cGVHD but also occasionally due to previous RT (especially in patients who have received both cranial RT and TBI on separate occasions).

Conclusion

Despite the long list of many different complications above, it cannot be stressed too strongly that most long-term survivors of HSCT return to a relatively normal and full life. Careful attention to lifestyle and regular detailed follow up, together with close links with and easy access to other medical teams, will allow emerging complications to be treated promptly and effectively, thereby minimizing the risks of chronic morbidity.

Further reading

Afessa, B., Litzow, M.R., Tefferi, A. (2001). *Bronchiolitis obliterans* and other late onset non-infectious pulmonary complications in hematopoietic stem cell transplantation. *Bone Marrow Transplant* 28: 425–434.

Bhatia, S., Bhatia, R. (2004) Secondary malignancies after hematopoietic cell transplantation. In: Blume, K.G., Forman, S.J., Appelbaum, F.R. (eds), *Thomas' Hematopoietic Cell Transplantation*, 3rd edn. Oxford: Blackwell Publishing, pp. 962–977.

Boulad, F., Sands, S., Sklar, C. (1998) Late complications after bone marrow transplantation in children and adolescents. *Curr Probl Pediatr* 28: 277–297.

Brennan, B.M.D., Shalet, S.M. (2002) Endocrine late effects after bone marrow transplant. *Br J Haematol* 118: 58–66.

Cohen, A., Rovelli, A., Bakker, B. *et al.* (1999) Final height of patients who underwent bone marrow transplantation for hematological disorders during childhood: A study by the Working Party for Late Effects – EBMT. *Blood* 93: 4109–4115.

De-Marco, R., Dassio, D.A., Vittone, P. (1996) A retrospective study of ocular side effects in children undergoing bone marrow transplantation. *Eur J Ophthalmol* 6: 436–439.

Deeg, H.J., Socie, G. (1998) Malignancies after hematopoietic stem cell transplantation: many questions, some answers. *Blood* 91: 1833–1844.

Duell, T., van-Lint, M.T., Ljungman, P. *et al.* (1997) Health and functional status of long-term survivors of bone marrow transplantation. *Ann Intern Med* 126: 184–192.

Flowers, M.E.D, Deeg, H.J. (2004) Delayed complications after hematopoietic cell transplantation. In: Blume, K.G., Forman, S.J., Appelbaum, F.R. (eds), *Thomas' Hematopoietic Cell Transplantation*, 3rd edn. Oxford: Blackwell Publishing, pp. 944–961.

Leiper, A.D. (2002) Non-endocrine late complications of bone marrow transplantation in childhood: Part I. *Br J Haematol* 118: 3–22.

Leiper, A.D. (2002) Non-endocrine late complications of bone marrow transplantation in childhood: Part II. *Br J Haematol* 118: 23–43.

Nysom, K., Holm, K., Michaelsen, K.F. *et al.*(2000) Bone mass after allogeneic BMT for childhood leukemia or lymphoma. *Bone Marrow Transplant* 25: 191–196.

Sanders, J.E. (2004) Growth and development after hematopoietic cell transplantation. In: Blume, K.G., Forman, S.J., Appelbaum, F.R. (eds), *Thomas' Hematopoietic Cell Transplantation*, 3rd edn. Oxford: Blackwell Publishing, pp. 929–943.

Sanders, J.E., Hawley, J., Levy, W. *et al.* (1996) Pregnancies following high-dose cyclophosphamide with or without high-dose busulfan or total-body irradiation and bone marrow transplantation. *Blood* 87: 3045–3052.

Skinner, R., Leiper, A. (2004) Bone marrow transplantation. In: Wallace, W.H.B., Green, D.M. (eds), *Late Effects of Childhood Cancer*. London: Arnold, pp. 304–320.

Skinner, R., Leiper, A.D. (2005) Appendix B, Survivors of allogeneic bone marrow transplantation. In: Skinner, R., Wallace, W.H.B., Levitt, G.A., on behalf of Late Effects Group (eds), *Therapy based long term follow up. Practice Statement*. United Kingdom Children's Cancer Study Group.

Socie, G., Cahn, J.Y., Carmelo, J. *et al.* (1997) Avascular necrosis of bone after allogeneic bone marrow transplantation: Analysis of risk factors for 4388 patients by the Societé Française de Greffe de Moelle (SFGM). *Br J Haematol* **97**: 865–870.

Socie, G., Salooja, N., Cohen, A. *et al.* (2003) Nonmalignant late effects after allogeneic stem cell transplantation. *Blood* **101**: 3373–3385.

Thomas, B.C., Stanhope, R., Plowman, P.N., Leiper, A.D. (1993) Endocrine function following single fraction and fractionated total body irradiation for bone marrow transplantation in childhood. *Acta Endocrinol* **128**: 508–512.

Chapter 17
Hematopoietic stem cell transplantation – the future

A.J. Cant and G. Jackson

Introduction

Stem cell transplantation has evolved dramatically over the last two decades. The development of stem cell harvesting, DNA-based tissue typing, better supportive care, and lower-intensity conditioning have helped to increase the safety and effectiveness of transplantation beyond recognition. Previously hematopoietic stem cell transplantation (HSCT) was viewed with great trepidation by the patient, nurse and doctor alike; now it has become a much more routine procedure with a justifiably much higher expectation of a favorable outcome. There is little doubt that more progress will be made over the next decade. In this chapter we review areas where progress is being, and will be made. Table 17.1 highlights the areas where research is ongoing.

Umbilical cord stem cell transplantation (USCT)

Transplantation of umbilical cord-derived stem cells from related and unrelated donors has become a routine technique on pediatric transplant

Table 17.1 Ongoing research

Umbilical cord stem cell transplantation
Haplo-identical stem cell transplantation
Graft engineering
Genetic engineering and gene therapy
Mesenchymal stem cells
HSCT for auto-immune disease

units and in this setting the promise of cord blood stem cells has been largely fulfilled. Initial successful studies with related cord blood transplants in children were rapidly followed by similar success in the unrelated setting. A recent single-center series reporting USCT for primary immunodeficiency (Bhattacharya *et al.*, 2005) showed 86% cure rate with full immune reconstitution in all cases. Cord blood has many advantages:

- easy to collect;
- causes no harm to the donor;
- easy to store;
- easy to maintain in a frozen state.

In the unrelated setting the product is immediately available for recipients who are found to match cord bloods in the various banks around the world. Worldwide approximately 150,000 cord blood units are stored in 35 cord blood banks in 21 countries. Several thousand cord transplants have now been performed. While engraftment and immune recovery are slower after cord transplantation than after transplantation of cells harvested from siblings or unrelated donors, it is durable and there appears to be a lower incidence of graft-vs.-host disease (GVHD).

The investment required to maintain cord blood banks demands that this product should also be useful for adults who require an allograft. Single cord transplants in adults have been performed but often the cell dose/kg body weight is low, and engraftment may be slow and incomplete. The early transplant mortality has been high and infectious complications remain a major concern. Three main strategies are emerging to improve the results of cord blood transplantation in adults and older children, as follows

• Cord blood units are pooled or given in a sequence to increase the cell count and engraftment. Crossed immunological rejection does not seem to occur, and engraftment rate and quality seem to be improved using a pooled or sequential approach.

• Methods to expand cord blood stem cells are being explored. This more complicated, difficult and labour-intensive approach has not yet developed fully, but a greater understanding of stem cell biology may allow sufficient improvement to allow successful adult transplants using umbilical cord blood.

• Combining a cord graft with a haplo-identical CD34-positive graft from a family donor. Successful engraftment has been seen with this technique but experience is limited and this approach needs to be further explored.

Cord blood stem cell transplantation in adults is becoming a reality, opening up the possibility of every patient who requires an allograft having a suitable donor. In the past potential non-Caucasian allograft recipients could not always receive HSCT because, as fewer people from ethnic minorities offer to be volunteer donors, suitable donors are harder to find. Cord blood banks that have a more comprehensive ethnic profile may help all ethnic groups to benefit from the advances seen in stem cell transplantation.

Haplo-identical stem cell transplantation

HLA-matched hematopoietic stem cells may be obtained from siblings, unrelated donors and umbilical cord blood. Unfortunately, a substantial minority of patients do not have a suitable matched stem cell donor, particularly if they have rare HLA haplotypes. In the UK the majority of potential donors on the registries are Caucasian and so non-Caucasians may have few or no potential donors. Parents give half their tissue types to each child, and so parents and some siblings can be used, as so-called haplo-identical or half-identical donors. Over the years investigators have explored the possibility of using haplo-identical donors. This type of transplant has been used in infants with severe combined immunodeficiency (SCID) for many years, but it has been felt that the risk of GVHD and graft rejection was too high to contemplate this type of transplant for older children and adults with other conditions. However, improved supportive care and GVHD prophylaxis means that this technique is being re-evaluated. (See Fig. 17.1.)

Graft engineering

Graft engineering is not new. Red cell depletion for

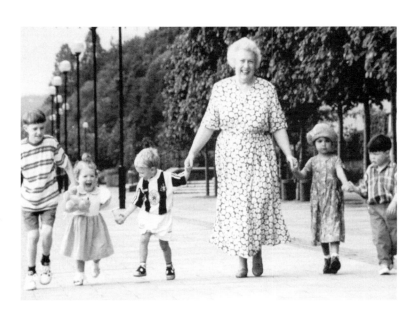

Fig. 17.1 Children who had successful transplants with the President of the "Bubble Foundation UK," Newcastle upon Tyne. Image © the Bubble Foundation UK, Newcastle General Hospital, Newcastle upon Tyne, UK; used with permission.

ABO incompatibility, T-cell depletion to prevent GVHD and CD34-positive cell selection have all been introduced to improve the safety and efficacy of stem cell transplantation. These relatively crude attempts at graft engineering have brought significant but not complete success. It is likely the science of graft engineering will advance rapidly over the next decade, particularly in the following areas.

• Prevention of cytomegalovirus (CMV) infection. T-cell engraftment is vital to prevent potentially fatal CMV infection but is also associated with GVHD. Selection of specific anti-CMV T cells pre-transplant and the development of anti-CMV T-cell clones may allow selective add-back of those T cells to become the mainstay of CMV prevention.

• Removal of allo-reactive T cells is another important area of research. Identifying and removing allo-reactive T-cell clones may allow researchers to produce grafts that are not associated with GVHD but result in rapid recovery of the immune system, better graft-vs.-tumor (GVT) effects, but with a reduced risk of CMV and other opportunistic infections.

• Enhancement of GVT effect is another area of interest and research. A better understanding of and exploitation of minor histocompatibility differences between donor and recipient may allow a GVT effect without GVHD. Other factors that enhance the GVT effect may come to light, including potential exploitation of antigenic differences between tumor and the patient's normal tissue.

• It is likely that the interaction between the incoming T cells and other components of the immune system with host tissue will be better understood. Polymorphisms in inflammatory cytokine genes may help to identify patients at particularly high or low risk of GVHD, enabling GVHD prophylaxis to be adjusted accordingly.

• Chronic GVHD remains poorly understood and, although the autoimmune features are better recognized, the key interactions that produce this disorder, which is difficult to manage, remain to be elucidated. Only by understanding the immunological basis of this disease can we develop effective long-term solutions to both localized and generalized chronic GVHD.

Genetic engineering and gene therapy

Hematopoietic stem cells have been the first target for genetic engineering. Inserting sequences of DNA containing normal genes into the patient's own hematopoietic stem cells has been performed in an attempt to cure a number of genetic disorders including immunodeficiencies and hemophilia. A carefully conducted trial of gene therapy in 12 infants with X-linked SCID was initially very successful, with correction of the defect and immune reconstitution in 10 patients. However, 3 patients developed T-cell leukemia caused by the switching on of an oncogene adjacent to the DNA cassette inserted by gene therapy. As long as DNA cassettes can only be inserted at random, the risk of switching on a malignant process will remain a concern. Once the techniques are refined, transplantation of genetically engineered autologous stem cells is likely to become more routine and more effective.

Mesenchymal stem cells

The discovery that the marrow contains non-hematopoietic mesenchymal stem cells that can differentiate to form cells of different sorts of connective tissue has led to interest in exploiting these non-hematopoietic stem cells to repair other organs. Enormous interest in replacing damaged myocardial tissue has been fueled by the successful repair of cardiac damage in mice and rats. Significant progress has yet to be made in humans but the principles of non-hematopoietic stem cells being used to repair damaged tissues are being established. Stem cell therapy for acute myocardial damage may switch over the next few years from interesting animal experiments to mainstream cardiac care.

In the allograft setting, mesenchymal stem cells with hematopoietic stem cells may help regenerate bone marrow stromal cells, so improving the microenvironment in which HSCTs differentiate, thus speeding up immune reconstitution and lessening the risk of infection and GVHD.

HSCT for auto-immune disease

Over the past 20 years case reports have suggested that auto-immune disease could be cured by HSCT. More recently a larger series has been published, auditing around 700 patients who have received HSCT for severe auto-immune disease that has been unresponsive to conventional immunosuppressive treatment (Tyndall and Saccardi, 2005). About one-third of patients remain disease free after HSCT, although this varies according to the exact auto-immune disease being treated. HSCT for auto-immune disease is believed to work because autoreactive T cells are removed by pre-HSCT chemotherapy and then replaced by non-autoreactive T cells. For most conditions T-cell-depleted autologous marrow has been given and, for conditions such as juvenile idiopathic arthritis (JIA), about two-thirds of patients benefited. More recently allogeneic HSCT has been attempted in these conditions and, while long-term remissions are seen, the risk of GVHD is not insignificant. With decreasing transplant-related mortality and more sophisticated ways of preventing GVHD, it is likely that allogeneic HSCT will be used more often in auto-immune disease.

Conclusion

Stem cell transplantation has been an exciting area of medical breakthroughs over the last 30 years, with thousands of lives saved through the application of this technique to an enormously varied population of patients. We have developed a much greater knowledge of the HLA system, how stem cells work, and how to look after our patients after the procedure. We have learned to follow patients long-term, to understand the potential for long-term complications and how to prevent these problems. We have learned that stem cell grafts have longevity and that many patients can live full lives of normal span after stem cell transplantation. The future looks just as promising and if we make the same progress in the next 30 years then we can look forward to curing many more patients and returning them to complete and fulfilling lives. In short, stem cell transplantation is likely to be a continued success story. We look forward to continuing to update this book so that the potential of the techniques discussed in this final chapter become the standard techniques of the future.

Further reading

Bhattacharya, A., Slatter, M.A., Chapman, C.E. *et al.* (2005) Single centre experience of umbilical cord stem cell transplantation for primary immunodeficiency. *Bone Marrow Transplant* **36**: 295–299.

Tyndall, A., Saccardi, R. (2005) Haematopoietic stem cell transplantation in the treatment of severe autoimmune disease; results from phase 1/11 studies, prospective randomised trial and future direction. *Clin Exp Immunol* **141**: 1–9.

Index